AF668553

Second Edition

Medicinal Chemistry I

Course Code **BP 402T**

for **Fourth Semester Bachelor in Pharmacy**

As per the latest syllabus prescribed by Pharmacy Council of India

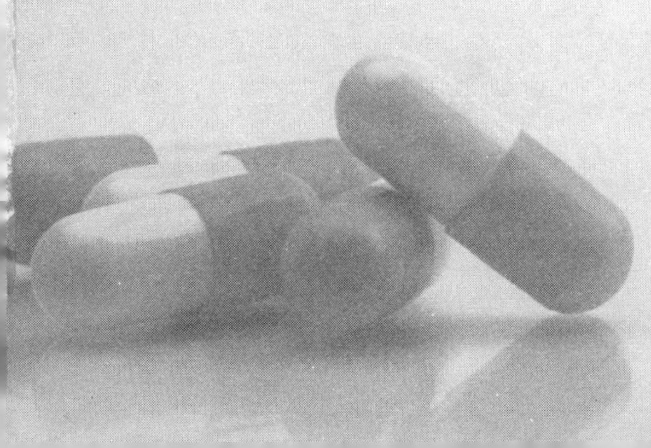

Second Edition

Medicinal Chemistry I

Course Code **BP 402T**

for **Fourth Semester Bachelor in Pharmacy**

As per the latest syllabus prescribed by Pharmacy Council of India

K Ilango MPharm PhD FIC
Professor and Principal
Tagore College of Pharmacy
Chennai – 600 127

P Valentina MPharm PhD
Professor and Principal
PERI College of Pharmacy
Chennai – 600 048

CBSPD

CBS Publishers & Distributors Pvt Ltd

New Delhi • Bengaluru • Chennai • Kochi • Kolkata • Lucknow • Mumbai
Hyderabad • Jharkhand • Nagpur • Patna • Pune • Uttarakhand

Disclaimer
Science and technology are constantly changing fields. New research and experience broaden the scope of information and knowledge. The authors have tried their best in giving information available to them while preparing the material for this book. Although all efforts has been made to ensure optimum accuracy of the material, yet it is quite possible some errors might have been left uncorrected. The publisher, the printer and the authors will not be held responsible for any inadvertent errors or inaccuracies.

Second Edition

Medicinal Chemistry I

Course Code **BP 402T**

for **Fourth Semester Bachelor in Pharmacy**

As per the latest syllabus prescribed by Pharmacy Council of India

ISBN: 978-93-49057-11-1

Copyright © Authors and Publisher

Second Edition: 2025
Reprint: **2026**
First Edition: 2019

All rights reserved. No part of this book may be reproduced or transmitted in any form or by any means, electronic or mechanical, including photocopying, recording, or any information storage and retrieval system without permission, in writing, from the authors and the publisher.

Published by Satish Kumar Jain and produced by Varun Jain for
CBS Publishers and Distributors Pvt Ltd
4819/XI Prahlad Street, 24 Ansari Road, Daryaganj, New Delhi 110 002, India.
Ph: 011-23289259, 23266838
Website: www.cbspd.com
e-mail: delhi@cbspd.com

Corporate Office: 204 FIE, Industrial Area, Patparganj, Delhi 110 092, India
Ph: 011-49344934 Fax: 011-49344935 e-mail: publishing@cbspd.com; publicity@cbspd.com

Branches

- **Bengaluru:** Seema House 2975, 17th Cross, K.R. Road, Banasankari 2nd Stage, Bengaluru 560 070, Karnataka, India
  Ph: +91-80-26771678/79 Fax: +91-80-26771680 e-mail: bangalore@cbspd.com
- **Chennai:** 18/8B, Subbarayan Street, Shenoy Nagar, Chennai 600 030, Tamil Nadu, India
  Ph: +91-44-42032115, 26681266 e-mail: chennai@cbspd.com
- **Kochi:** 42/1325, 1326, Power House Road, Opposite KSEB, Power House, Ernakulam 682 018, Kochi, Kerala, India
  Ph: +91-484-4059061–65 Fax: +91-484-4059065 e-mail: kochi@cbspd.com
- **Kolkata:** 147 Hind Ceramics Compound, 1st Floor, Nilgunj Road, Belghoria, Kolkata 700 056, West Bengal, India
  Ph: +91-33-25633055/56 e-mail: kolkata@cbspd.com
- **Lucknow:** Basement, Khushnuma Complex, 7-Meerabai Marg (Behind Jawahar Bhawan), Lucknow 226 001, Uttar Pradesh, India
  Ph: +91-522-4000032 e-mail:tiwari.lucknow@cbspd.com
- **Mumbai:** PWD Shed, Gala No. 25/26, Ramchandra Bhatt Marg, Next to JJ Hospital, Gate No. 2, Opp Union Bank of India, Noorbaug, Mumbai 400009, Maharashtra, India
  Ph: +91-22-66661880, 66661889 e-mail: mumbai@cbspd.com

Representatives

- **Gujarat** 0-9879558667
- **Hyderabad** 0-9885175004
- **Jharkhand** 0-9811541605
- **Nagpur** 0-8692091830
- **Patna** 0-9334159340
- **Pune** 0-9664372571
- **Uttarakhand** 0-9716462459

Printed at: SRK Graphics, Delhi, India

Preface

Medicinal chemistry is an exciting and dynamic field that plays a crucial role in drug discovery and development. It integrates various scientific disciplines, including biology, toxicology, pharmacology, theoretical chemistry, microbiology, and biopharmacy. This book, *Medicinal Chemistry I*, is the result of 30 years of teaching and engaging with graduate students across multiple universities. The encouragement from faculty and students for our earlier works, including *Textbook of Medicinal Chemistry,* Volumes I & II and *Medicinal Chemistry for Pharm D* has motivated us to present this new edition. Designed as a comprehensive yet accessible resource, this book aligns with the latest syllabus set forth by the Pharmacy Council of India, catering specifically to undergraduate students preparing for Medicinal Chemistry I. This volume comprises 12 chapters covering essential topics such as the history and development of medicinal chemistry, physicochemical properties, metabolism, and various classes of drugs, including adrenergic, cholinergic, sedatives, antipsychotics, anticonvulsants, narcotics, and anti-inflammatory agents. Each chapter provides a clear introduction, classification with examples, structure-activity relationships (SAR), detailed information on individual drugs including structure, IUPAC names, mechanisms of action, uses, and selected synthesis to facilitate student understanding. We gratefully acknowledge the support of colleagues, family, and friends who contributed to the creation of this book. We also extend our heartfelt thanks to the faculty and student community for their ongoing encouragement, which has inspired this new edition. We welcome suggestions for improvement and hope that students and faculty will continue to engage with us.

K Ilango
P Valentina

Contents

Syllabus

BP402T Medicinal Chemistry I (Theory)

Unit I **10 hrs**

Introduction to Medicinal Chemistry

History and Development of Medicinal Chemistry

Physicochemical Properties in Relation to Biological Action

Ionization, Solubility, Partition coefficient, Hydrogen bonding, Protein binding, Chelation, Bioisosterism, Optical and Geometrical isomerism.

Drug Metabolism

Drug Metabolism Principles: Phase I and Phase II

Factors Affecting Drug Metabolism including Stereo Chemical Aspects

Unit II **10 hrs**

Drugs acting on Autonomic Nervous System

Adrenergic Neurotransmitters:

Biosynthesis and Catabolism of Catechol amines.

Adrenergic Receptors (Alpha and Beta) and their Distribution.

Sympathomimetic Agents: SAR

Direct acting: Norepinephrine, Epinephrine, Phenyl ephedrine* Dopamine, Methyl dopa, Clonidine, Dobutamine, Isoproterenol, Terbutaline, Phenylephrine, Salbutamol*, Bitoterol, Naphazoline, Oxymetazoline and Xylometazoline.

Indirect acting Agents: Hydroxy Amphetamine, Pseudoephedrine, Propylhexedrine.

Agents with Mixed Mechanism: Ephedrine, Metaraminol

Adrenergic Antagonists:

Alpha Adrenergic Blockers: Tolazoline*, Phentolamine, Phenoxybenzamine, Prazosin, Dihydroergotamine, Methysergide.

Beta Adrenergic Blockers: SAR of β-blockers, Propranolol*, Metipranolol, Atenolol, Betazolol, Bisoprolol, Esmolol, Metoprolol, Labetolol, Carvediol.

Unit III **10 hrs**

Cholinergic Neurotransmitters: Biosynthesis and catabolism of Acetyl choline,

Cholinergic Receptors (Muscarnic & Nicotinic) and their distribution.

Parasympathomimetic Agents: SAR

Direct Acting Agents: Acetylcholine, Carbachol*, Bethanechol, Methacholine, Pilocrapine.

Indirect Acting/Cholinesterase Inhibitors (Reversible & Irreversible)

Physostigmine, Neostigmine*, Pyridostigmine, Edrophonium chloride, Tacrine hydrochloride, Ambenonium chloride, Isoflurophate, Echothiophate iodide, Parathione, Malthione.

Cholinesterase Reactivator: Pralidoxime chloride

Cholinergic Blocking Agents: SAR of Cholinolytic agents.

Solanaceous Alkaloids and Analogues: Atropine sulphate, Hyoscyamine sulphate, Scopolmaine hydrobromide, Homatropine hydrobromide, Ipratropium bromide.

Synthetic Cholinergic Blocking Agents: Tropicamide, Cyclopentolate hydrochloride, Clidinium bromide, Dicyclomine hydrochloride*, Glycopyrrolate, Methantheline bromide, Propantheline bromide, Benxtropine mesylate, Orphenadrine citrate, Biperidine hydrochloride, Procyclidine hydrochloride*, Tridihexethyl chloride, Isopropamide iodide, Ethopropazine hydrochlioride.

Unit IV **08 hrs**

Drugs acting on Central Nervous System

A. Sedative and Hypnotics

Benzodiazepines: SAR, Chlordiazepoxide, Diazepam*, Oxazeoam, Clorazepate, Lorazepam, Alprazolam, Zolpidem

Barbiturates: SAR, Barbital*, Phenobarbital, Mephobarbital, Amobarbital, Butabarbital, Pentobarbital, Secobarbital

Miscellanous:

Amide and Imide: Glutethimide

Alcohols and their **Carmbamate Derivatives:** Meprobamate, Ethchlorvynol

Aldehyde and their Derivatives: Triclofos sodium, Paraldehyde.

B. Antipsychotics

Phenothiazines: SAR, Promazine hydrochloride, Chlorpromazine hydrochloride*, Triflupromazine, Thioridazine hydrochloride, Piperacetazine hydrochloride, Prochlorperazine maleate, Trifluperazine hydrochloride.

Ring Analogue of Phenothiazines: Chlorprothiexene, Thiothixene, Laoxpine succinate, Clozaoine.

Flurobutyrophenone: Haloperidol, Droperidol, Risperidone.

Beta amino Ketone: Moilndone hydrochloride

Benzamide: Sulpiride

C. Anticonvulsants: SAR and Mechanism of Action

Barbiturates: Phenobarbitone, Methabarbital.

Hydantoins: Phenytoin*, Mepheytoin, Ethotoin.

Oxazolidine dione: Trimetahdione, Paramethadione.

Succinimides: Phensuximide, Methsuximide, Ethosuximide

Urea and Monoacyl Ureas: Phenacemide, Carbamazepine*.

Benzodiazepine: Clonazepam

Miscellaneous: Primidone, Valproic acid, Gabapentin, Felbamate.

Unit V **07 hrs**

Drugs acting on Central Nervous System

General Anaesthetics

Inhalation Anaesthetics: Halothane*, Methoxyflurane, Enflurane, Sevoflurane, Isoflurane, Desflurane.

Ultra Short acting Barbiturates: Methohexital sodium*, Thiamylal sodium, Thiopental sodium,

Dissociative anaesthetics: Ketamine hydrochloride*

Narcotics and Non-narcotic Anaethtetics

Morphine and Related Drugs: SAR of Morphine analogues, Morphine sulphate, Codeine, Meperidine hydrochloride, Anileridine hydrochloride, Diphenoxylate hydrochloride, Loperamide hydrochloride, Fentanyl citrate*, Methadone hydrochloride, Propoxyphene hydrochloride, Pentazocine, Levorphanol tartarate.

Narcotic Antagonists: Nalorphine hydrochloride, Levallorphan tatarate, Naloxone hydrochloride.

Anti-inflammatory Agents: Sodium salicylate, Aspirin, Mefenamic acid*, Neclofenamate, Indomethacin, Sulindac, Tolmetin, Zomepirac, Diclofenac, Ketorolac, Ibuprofen*, Naproxen, Piroxicam, Phenacetin, Acetaminophen, Antipyrine, Phenylbutazone.

Chapter 1

INTRODUCTION TO MEDICINAL CHEMISTRY

Medicinal and Pharmaceutical Chemistry is a chemistry-based scientific discipline, with an interaction of chemistry and pharmacology. Medicinal Chemistry also involves the aspects of biological, medical and pharmaceutical sciences. It is concerned with the invention, discovery, design, identification and preparation of biologically active compounds, the study of their metabolism, the interpretation of their mode of action at the molecular level and the construction of structure-activity relationships.

The process of drug discovery involves the identification of candidates, synthesis, characterization, screening and assays for therapeutic activity. Once a compound has shown its value in these tests, it will begin the process of drug development prior to clinical trials. Pharmaceutical chemistry is focused on quality aspects of medicines and aims to assure fitness for the purpose of medicinal products. The science of medicinal chemistry involves the design and synthesis of novel drugs based on an understanding of how drugs work in the body at the molecular level. Medicinal Chemistry is a multifaceted discipline that encompasses synthetic organic chemistry, natural products chemistry, enzymology, chemical biology, structural biology and computational methods, all of which is aimed at the discovery and development of new therapeutic agents. It is a multidisciplinary subject involving Organic chemistry, Biochemistry, Physiology, Microbiology, Pharmacology, Toxicology, Genetics and Computer modeling. It explains the design and production of compounds, which can be used for prevention and treatment of human or animal diseases. It also includes the study of existing drugs, their biological properties and Quantitative Structure Activity Relationship (QSAR).

In 1948 the term **'Division of Pharmaceutical Chemistry'** founded by the American Chemical Society was renamed as 'Division of Medicinal Chemistry.' A new discipline was born, but it took quite a time before it was accepted as such. Medicinal chemistry meanwhile found a place within the pharmaceutical industry and at universities. In 1970 a Section Medicinal Chemistry was started by the Organic Chemistry Division of the IUPAC, followed by the founding of the European Federation of Medicinal Chemistry in 1972. These developments in the framework and the organizational structures have not helped to arrive an internationally accepted definition for this branch of science and also difficulty in deciding the name of the field: Medicinal chemistry (English), Chimie therapeutique (French), Wikstofforschung (German), Chimica Farmaceutica (Italian), and Farmacochemie (Dutch). The use of the term 'Pharmaceutical Chemistry' when medicinal chemistry is meant is especially confusing as Pharmaceutical Chemistry is the established term for chemistry related to finished medicinal products.

In textbooks dating from the early 1970s several definitions could be found and IUPAC published a comprehensive definition of Medicinal chemistry as

"Medicinal Chemistry concerns the discovery, the development, the identification and the interpretation of the mode of action of biologically active compounds at the molecular level. Emphasis is put on drugs, but the interest of the medicinal chemist is not restricted to drugs but include bioactive compounds in general. Medicinal chemistry is also concerned with the study, identification and synthesis of the metabolic products of these drugs and related compounds"

Medicinal chemistry includes:

- The process of drug discovery: The process of drug discovery includes the identification and production of new active compounds. The use of plants, minerals, and animal parts as medicines has been recorded since the most ancient civilizations. With the evolution of the knowledge, the means for drug discovery also evolved. New molecules with potential pharmaceutical interest, "hits" are obtained from either natural products or synthetic compounds generated by computational chemistry, like screening of chemical libraries, combinatorial chemistry, pharmaceutical biotechnology etc.
- Optimization process: The "hit" compound is improved for its pharmacologic, pharmacodynamic and pharmacokinetic properties by chemical or functional group modifications, transforming it into a more effective, selective and less toxic lead compound. The pharmacokinetic phase is usually identified with the ADME

(absorption, distribution, metabolism, elimination), while the safety of a drug is a matter of toxicology: both are crucial for a bioactive molecule to be used as a drug.

- Development process: Optimization of synthetic lead compound molecule for mass production and modification of its pharmacokinetic properties so that it is safe to use in human clinical trials.
- Evaluation of the properties of existing drugs is also part of medicinal chemistry.

Modern drug research and development (R&D) has experienced remarkable changes as technological and scientific developments in the past years have dramatically changed the pharmaceutical innovation process. Well-established strategies, such as high-throughput screening (HTS), have progressively been applied in association with novel techniques founded on genomics, molecular and structural biology and molecular modeling. More efficient organic synthesis methods, chemical biology approaches and bio- and chemo informatics strategies have intensely changed the process by which an initial hit is converted into a marketable drug. In fact, this endeavor has become more challenging and more complex. In part, this can be attributed to the expansion of the field towards novel therapeutic areas that are at the limits of the science and technology available today.

Chapter 2

HISTORY OF MEDICINAL CHEMISTRY

The ancient folk medicine and early natural-product emerged the field of medicinal chemistry about 150 years ago. The oldest record (~ 5100 years ago) of the use of medicinal plants are from the ancient civilization of the Greek, the Romans, Galenic medicine in Europe, Chinese, Mayans of Central America and Ayurvedic Medicine in India. The therapeutic uses of plants are recorded in the writings of Hippocrates, Dioscorides, Pliny and Galenus by the Ancient Greeks and Romans. Some of these herbal drugs are still in use today; for example, Coca leaves containing Cocaine and Mushroom containing Methylated tryptamine were chewed by South American for hallucination; Ipecacuanha containing emetine for the treatment of dysentery was used by ancient people of Brazil; the ancient Greeks used opium, squill, hyoscyamus, reserpine and ephedrine. In the Middle Age various “Materia Medica” and “Pharmacopoeias” brought together traditional uses of plants. The Pharmaceutical years before 1800s are called the age of botanicals.

Late 18th or early 19th centuries may be viewed as the birth period of modern medicinal chemistry with the introduction of side chain theory of drug action in 1885 by Berlin immunologist Ehrlich, who coined the term chemotherapy and defined it as “the chemical entities exhibiting selective toxicities against particular infectious agent”. At the beginning of the 19th century, the development of modern organic chemistry and medicinal chemistry focused on finding active ingredients present in medicinal plants and certain animals. The isolation of pure substances from plants namely Morphine, Quinine, Atropine, Emetine, Caffeine, Colchicines etc., from crude medicinal plant extracts contributed to the increased use of pure substance as therapeutic agents.

Many of the developments after 1860s arose from the synthesis of compounds specifically for their medicinal properties. For example, even though the use of willow bark as a pain-killer was known, the analgesic activity of its constituent Salicin and salicylic acid were developed in the 1860s and 1870s; Paracetamol and Phenacetin (1886) were also known as pain-killers. The end of the 19th century also saw the development of several important vaccines, including those for tetanus and diphtheria. As a result of these discoveries and the progress made in organic chemistry, the pharmaceutical industry came into existence at the end of the nineteenth century.

At the turn of the 20th century, Medicinal Chemist Paul Ehrlich (who synthesized Salvarsan, the first chemical treatment for syphilis) initiated the transition from the study of plants or their extracts with specified therapeutic activities towards the synthesis of a specific drug substance in the laboratory. Antibacterial sulphonamides were developed, after the identification of antibacterial activity of Prontosil red by Domagk in 1930s. The activity of these compounds as inhibitors of folic acid biosynthesis and as anti-metabolites of p-aminobenzoic acid was identified later by Woods (1940). The synthesis of the first synthetic pharmaceutical drug, Aspirin, occurred in this period which was later on recognized as universal pain reliever and this discovery spawned the era of therapeutic agents

Together with the discovery of Penicillin in 1929 by Sir Alexander Fleming and its subsequent examination by Florey and Chain in 1941 led to a water-soluble powder of much higher antibacterial potency and lower toxicity than those of previously known synthetic chemotherapeutic agents. It is the best example of serendipitous discovery which is called as Golden Age of Antibiotics a new era in medicine. The relatively easy bio-assays for anti-bacterial and anti-fungal activity led to the isolation of a number of antibiotics including Streptomycin (1944), Chloramphenicol (1949) and the Tetracyclines such as Aureomycin (1949).

The middle third of the 20th century witnessed a blossoming of pharmaceutical invention, with breakthroughs in the development of synthetic vitamins, hormones (Thyroxine, Oxytocin, Corticosteroids etc.,) anticonvulsant, psychotropics, antihistamines and new vaccines. Several of these constituted entirely new classes of medicines. Illness such as tuberculosis, diphtheria and pneumonia could be treated and cured for the first time in human history. The structures of the steroid hormones were established in the 1930s and 1940s. The discovery of Cortisone as anti-inflammatory agent in 1949 motivated the synthesis of number of anti-inflammatory semi-synthetic steroids such as Prednisolone, Betamethasone, Triamcinolone, Ethinylestradiol and Progestogens. Problems associated with separating the anti-inflammatory activity from the mineralocorticoid activity of the cortical steroids led to interest in the development of non-steroidal anti-inflammatory agents (NSAIDs). Major innovations were made in cardiovascular drugs starting with anti-hypertensive and β-blockers in the 1960s, followed by calcium-channel blockers, ACE inhibitors and cholesterol-reducing drugs. The successes of 1950s and 1960s were leading light by the work of Gertrude Elion and George Hitchings (1988 Nobel Laureates) who introduced Azathioprine, the first immunosuppressive agent, Allopurinol for gout, Acyclovir the first useful antiviral compound against herpes and other DNA viruses.

Early 20th century also proposed that drugs might elicit therapeutic and pharmacological actions via interactions with discrete membrane-associated recognition sites, on target organs called receptor turned out as new target in the field of drug research. The pharmacological characterization of receptors in almost all organs, including the brain, provided the basis for a large number of benzodiazepines, β-blockers γ -amino butyric acid and introduction of monoclonal antibodies, which block receptors of growth on tumor cells. The enhancement of instrumentation and the introduction of powerful technology also facilitated laboratory automation and aided the discovery and development of new drugs. Drug companies attempted to develop more useful tools to facilitate the drug discovery process. This caused a significant shift away from the serendipitous approach towards rational drug design. The development of *in vitro* assays using animal tissues became an essential support tool for tracking Structure Activity Relationship (SAR) and allowing chemist to optimize structures before animal testing. This allowed a wide range of compounds to be made around a SAR hypothesis. Rational design of drugs based on knowledge of the biological system being investigated allowed highly specific selective antagonists and agonists to be developed

Other notable advancements in drug design made in the mid to late 20th century include: intervention of charge transfer (Kosower, 1955); induced-fit theory of drug action (Koshland, 1958); concepts of drug latentiation (Harper, 1959) and prodrug (Albert, 1960); concepts of isosterism and bioisosterism (Grimm's and Erlenmeyer's, 1929-1931) had a tremendous impact on the understanding of structure activity relationship (SAR) of drugs ;application of mathematical methods to medicinal chemistry and transformation of SAR studies into quantitative SAR (QSAR) (Hansch and others, 1960s); and application of artificial intelligence to drug research (Chu, 1974). Significant advancements in the discovery process were seen with the advances in molecular and cellular biology. This technology allowed *in vitro* optimization of lead molecules against the human version of receptor or enzyme and allowed a deeper analysis of their physiological nature.

Simultaneous advances in analytical technology viz. detection systems and data capture systems, laboratory automation etc., and in molecular biology viz. *in vitro* introduction of bioassay design techniques and microplate technology etc., allowed biological targets to be screened that had proven to be intractable before. With all these essential technology ingredients in place, the pharmaceutical laboratory in the early 1990s was set for the first real version of High Throughput Screening (HTS). HTS is a highly automated robotic system that tests small amounts of large numbers of compounds against potential targets. In 1990s, when Combinatorial chemistry mushroomed it provides very large numbers of new chemical entities to be screened for biological activity through HTS. It is a novel approach to chemical synthesis that enables the creation of large numbers of organic compounds by linking chemical building blocks in all possible combinations. The objective of both approaches is to provide very large numbers of new chemical entities to be screened for biological activity *in vitro*. Since the mid-1980s, the geometrical aspects of molecular structures were also taken into account leading to the development of the 3D-QSAR, which exploits information on the molecular geometry.

In spite of the significant advances in biological screening of large number of compounds by using HTS techniques, the screening of many millions of chemicals against hundreds of biological targets are too expensive. Virtual screening of chemical libraries has emerged as a complementary approach to HTS. Molecular graphics added a new dimension to computational chemistry and opened up the field of molecular modeling. Advances in the field of NMR and X-ray crystallography gave scientists the means for determining the three-dimensional (3-D) structure of larger and more complicated protein structures. Molecular modeling advanced beyond the capabilities of physical molecular models and it became possible to develop sophisticated molecular graphics for the use in chemical design and computer-aided drug discovery (CADD). In this new world, Medicinal Chemists identify and optimize lead compounds not only for potency, but also with a strong emphasis on avoiding potential side effects (for drug safety) and on controlling *in vivo* absorption, distribution, metabolism and excretion properties.

During the early stages of medicinal chemistry development, Chemists were primarily concerned with the isolation of medicinal agents found in plants. Presently, the advent of genomics, proteomics, bioinformatics and efficient technologies like, combinatorial chemistry, high throughput screening (HTS), virtual screening, *de novo* design, *in vitro, in silico,* ADMET screening and structure-based drug design has revolutionized the process of modern drug discovery. Genomic technology also brings the potential to clone and express human receptors for HTS. Availability of huge database of drugs from drug bank, protein data bank coupled with recent advances in technology further fuel the use of *in silico* techniques to increase the chance of success in many stages of the discovery process.

Despite so many advances, the therapeutic treasury is still lacking of drugs and there remains an increasing need for novel, innovative therapeutic agents not only in area that are historically well served, but also for the diseases associated with environmental, occupational, aging and lifestyle factors for which there is no effective medicine available and considerable demand exists in market. Therefore, the quest for newer and potent therapeutic agents is never ending. Medicinal chemistry continues to play a major role in drug research and development, taking advantage of newer techniques and increased knowledge of different branches of related sciences.

PHYSICOCHEMICAL PARAMETERS IN RELATION TO BIOLOGICAL ACTIVITY

Chapter 3

1. INTRODUCTION

The pharmacological/therapeutic activity of the drugs solely depends on its physicochemical properties and on the biochemical interaction with it. Following introduction into the body; the drug must pass through many barriers before it reaches the site of action usually a receptor or cell. A good understanding is required how the drug is transported, distributed throughout the body compartment, metabolic alteration and excretion along with structural characteristic of the receptor. So, physical and chemical properties of the drug play a vital role in its Pharmacokinetic parameters.

2. PHYSICOCHEMICAL PROPERTIES

2.1 Ionization and pk$_a$ value

Ionization is an important physiochemical property for a drug molecule. Most of the drugs are either weak acid or base and can exist in either ionized or unionized state. The ionization of the drug depends on its pk$_a$ and pH. The pk$_a$ value is important for its pharmacological activity, as it influences both absorption and the passage of the drug through cell membrane. The rate of drug absorption in the biological fluids is not proportional to the concentration of the drug at the absorption site but the concentration of the absorbable form of the drug.

For example, Aspirin in stomach will be more than 99% unionized and hence it gets more readily absorbed in the stomach. Same way, barbituric acid is inactive because it is a strong acid (unionized form). But 5, 5' – disubstituted barbituric acid has CNS depression action as it is weak acid and exist in ionized form.

Using drug pk$_a$, the formulation can be adjusted to pH to ensure maximum solubility in water (ionic form) or maximum solubility in non-polar solvent (unionized form).

The pH of a substance can be adjusted to maintain water solubility and complete ionization. For example Phenytoin injection adjusted to pH 12 with sodium hydroxide to obtain 99.98% of the drug in ionized form. Tropicamide eye drops, an anticholinergic drug has a pk_a of 5.2, and the drug has to be buffered to pH 4 to obtain more than 90% ionization.

Those drugs in an ionized form will tend to distribute throughout the body more than the unionized molecule. In general drug pass through the non-polar membranes of capillary walls, cell membranes and blood brain barrier in unionized form. A drug must cross many lipid barriers as it travel to the receptor that is its site of action. Cell membranes contain many ionic species (phospholipid, protein) that can repel/or bind ionic drugs. The ion channel receptor is usually lined with polar functional groups can act in an analogue manner. Ionic drugs are also more hydrated; therefore they are more bulky than non-ionic drugs.

According to the rule of Thumb, the unionized form of drug pass through membranes, but act as ions if ionization possible. A pKa in the range of 6 to 8 would therefore be most advantageous, because the non-ionized species that pass through then lipid membrane have good probability of becoming ionized and active within this pKa range. A high degree of ionization can prevent drugs from being absorbed from the GI tract and thus decreases systemic toxicity. This is advantage for externally applied disinfectant or antibacterial sulfanilamide which is meant to remain in the intestinal tract to fight infection. Therefore, when conducting experiments on drug-receptor binding, protein dissociation must be regulated using buffer.

Ionization also plays an important role in the electrostatic interaction between ionic drugs and ionized protein side chain in cell surface or receptors. The changes in pH may affect the reactivity of acidic and basic groups on the cell surface or within the cell. At isoelectric point, anion and cation in protein exist as Zwitter ions; increasing the pH of the medium will increase the concentration of the anion on the cell thereby increasing the activity of biologically active cation. Similarly decrease in pH, increase the concentration of cation and the activity of anion.

2.2 Solubility

The solubility of the drug is important since our body contains normally 65% water. Water acts as an inert solvent, a dispersing medium for colloidal solutions and a nucleophilic reagent in numerous biological reactions in living matter. So, it is necessary to assess the water solubility of the drug. Solubility and membrane permeability are an important factor for any drug. Only in the solution form, drug can interact with the cellular structure that carries the receptor and so solubility is highly significant physical property. Solubility is expressed in terms of its affinity/philicity or repulsion/phobicity for either an aqueous (hydro) or lipid (lipo) solvents. To reach the target site, drugs require both aqueous (plasma, extracellular fluids, cytoplasm etc.,) and lipid (biological membrane) solubility. Most of the drugs possess balanced solubility-having same degree of solubility in both aqueous and lipid layer. The most important intramolecular attractive forces (bonds) that governs solubility are

- Vander Waals forces of attraction
- Dipole-dipole bonding
- Ionic bonding
- Ion-dipole bonding

2.2.1 Importance of Solubility

- Orally administered drug either in solid or suspension form have to dissolve in gastric fluid (dissolution) before absorption and distribution to their site of action. The dissolution depends on drug solubility. The rate and extent of dissolution is the major factor in controlling the absorption of the drug. Once the drug enters the systemic circulation water solubility influences its transport to the body compartments available for that drug.

- Drugs that are sparingly soluble in water may deposit on route to their site of action which can clog up blood vessels and damage organs. For example. Crystallization of sulfonamides in the kidney.
- Sometime poor solubility is also essential in delivering the drug to the site of action, drug depots and chewable dosage form and to mask bitter taste of the drug. For example,
    a) Converting Pyrantel to water insoluble salt Pyrantel embonate deposit more drug in the site of action (ie.GI).
    b) Penicillin G procaine is converted to its salt form, which act as a slow releasing penicillin.
    c) Chlorpromazine hydrochloride is water soluble but has a bitter taste that is unacceptable to some patients. This is overcome by converting it to tasteless water insoluble embonate salt.
- Hydrolysis by water is main routes for the metabolism of the drug containing hydrolysable functional groups like ester or amine. For example, Local anaesthetics Lignocaine on hydrolysis gives 2, 6-dimethyl amine as a metabolite.
- Although successful drug exhibit solubility in both aqueous and lipid layer, there are few examples with solubility is only one of these phases correlates with pharmacological activity. For example, in a series of esters of p-amino benzoic acid, the length of the alkyl chain i.e., lipid solubility is proportional to local anaesthetics activity.

The water solubility of the lead compound can be improved by three general methods.

a) Salt formation
b) Incorporation of water solubilizing groups in a structure.
c) Use of special dosage form.

2.3 Partition co-efficient

The ability of a drug to dissolve in lipid phase is referred as lipophilicity. Highly water-soluble drug cannot penetrate organs rich in lipid such as brain and other neural tissue. On the other hand, compound that is very lipophilic will be trapped in the first "site of loss" like fat tissues and will be unable to leave this site quickly to reach the target.

Partition coefficient is one of the several physio-chemical parameters influencing the drug transport and distribution; the way in which the drug reaches the site of action from the site of application. Since the blood distributes the drug they must penetrate and transverse many cells to reach the site of action.

Partition coefficient can be defined as equilibrium constant of drug concentration for a molecule in lipid and aqueous phases. It is defined as a ratio of unionized drug distributed between aqueous phase and organic (lipid) phase at equilibrium.

$$P_{\left[\text{Unionized molecule}\right]} = \frac{\left[\text{drug}\right]_{\text{lipid}}}{[\text{drug}]_{\text{water}}}$$

$$P_{\left[\text{Ionized molecule}\right]} = \frac{\left[\text{drug}\right]_{\text{lipid}}}{[1 - \alpha]\,[\text{drug}]_{\text{water}}}$$

$\alpha \rightarrow$ degree of ionization in aqueous solution

Since partition coefficient are difficult to measure in living system, they are usually determined *in vitro* using 1-octanol as a lipid phase and phosphate buffer of pH 7.4 as the aqueous phase. The n-octanol/water system is frequently chosen, because it appears to be a good mimic of lipid polarity; however more accurate results may be obtained if the organic phase is matched to the area of biological activity being studied. For example, n-octanol usually gives more consistent result for drugs absorbed in GI tract while less polar solvents such as olive oil give more consistent correlation for drugs crossing the blood-brain barrier. More polar solvents such as chloroform give more consistent value for buccal absorption. n-octanol/ water system has more advantages over other systems:

- It is a suitable model of the lipid constituents of biological membrane due to its long alkyl chain and the polar hydroxyl group.

- n-octanol has a low vapor pressure, allowing reproducible measurements
- n-octanol is UV transparent over a large range, making the quantitative determination of a compound is relatively easy.

The partition coefficient, P is dimensionless and its logarithm (log P) is widely used as the measure of lipophilicity. Compounds with lop P value between 0 to 0.1 are poorly absorbed in lipophilic medium. It is widely used in QSAR.

Partition coefficient is measured by the following methods.

(i) Shake Flask Method

(ii) Chromatographic Method

(iii)Computational Method

(i) Shake Flask Method

Weighed amount of the substance is shaken in a flask containing a measured amount of buffer pH - 7.4 or water and n-octanol. The amount of chemical in one or both the phase is determined by appropriate analytical technique and the partition coefficient is calculated. The method is tedious, time consuming, messy and smelly. Advantage of this methods are that can be used in case of very low log P value, simple, lab operative and accurate for broadest range of solute.

(ii) Chromatographic Method

Compounds with known log P values are injected into a C_{18} reverse phase high performance liquid chromatography (RPHPLC) column to create a calibration curve. Unknown compound are then injected to predict log P. The chromatographic method suffers the disadvantage that the retention time is linearly related to partition coefficient ie. for doubling of log P, there is a tenfold increase in the retention. This often requires different length column to be used, short one for high log P and long ones for low values.

(iii) Computational Method

In this method log p values are predicted to using software packages. In software packages log P are generally calculated on the hydrophobic fragmentation constant of the molecule. Computational determination of log P value is very convenient, more reliable and accurate.

2.3.1 Importance of Partition coefficient

- It is helpful in the prediction of distribution of drug in biological system
- Bioavailability of the drug can be determined for new compounds in drug design. According to Lipinski rule of 5 the compound having log P value less than 5 have a good bioavailability.

2.4 Hydrogen Bonding

Hydrogen bonding is a type of dipole-dipole interaction between non-bonding electron pairs of hetero atoms like N, S, O and electron deficient hydrogen atom in polar bonds such as OH, NH, F etc., these are weak bonds (10kcal/mol.) and denoted as dotted lines. eg.

$$\overset{\delta^-}{O}-\overset{\delta^+}{H} \cdots\cdots \overset{\delta^-}{O}\ ; \quad HN-\overset{\delta^+}{H} \cdots\cdots \overset{\delta^-}{O}\ ; \quad R-\underset{|\atop H}{\overset{\delta^-}{O}} \cdots\cdots \overset{\delta^+}{H}-\underset{|\atop H}{\overset{\delta^-}{O}}$$

The compounds that are capable, of forming hydrogen bonding are only soluble in water. Proteins are held in specific configuration by hydrogen bonds and denaturation of protein involves the breaking up of the same bond. Generally hydrogen bonding is classified into two types.

(i) Intermolecular hydrogen bonding

(ii) Intramolecular hydrogen bonding

i) Intermolecular Hydrogen Bonding

Hydrogen bonding occurs between two or more molecules.

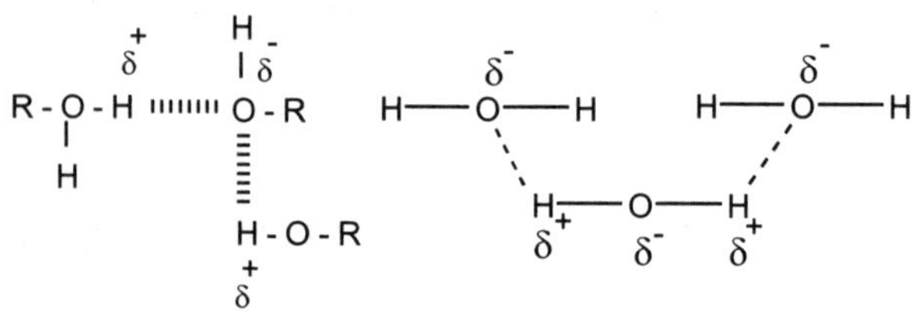

ii) Intramolecular Hydrogen Bonding

Hydrogen bonding occurs within the molecules

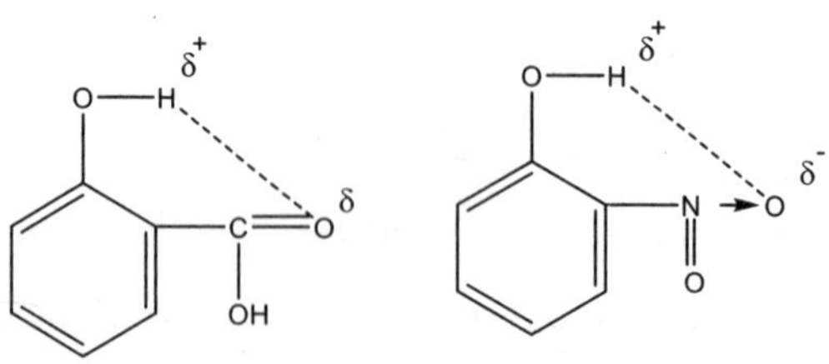

Salicylic acid   o - Nitrophenol

2.4.1 Hydrogen Bonding and Biological Action

Hydrogen bonding is an important parameter in chemical process. It is responsible for water unique solvent capabilities. Hydrogen bonds hold the two strands of DNA helix together and in protein they hold α-helix and β-sheet together. It is responsible for the determination of three dimensional structure of folded protein including enzymes and antibodies.

Antibodies produced in the body binds to antigen through a series of interaction including hydrogen bonds. The presence or absence of hydrogen bond is very important in designing a drug. For example,

(i) Antipyrine, 1- Phenyl - 2, 3 - dimethyl - 5 - pyrazolone has analgesic activity but 1- Phenyl - 3 - methyl - 5 - pyrazolone is inactive. This is due the formation of hydrogen bonding in the 1 - Phenyl - 3 - methyl - 5 - pyrazolone, gives rise to linear polymer which cannot pass through membrane.

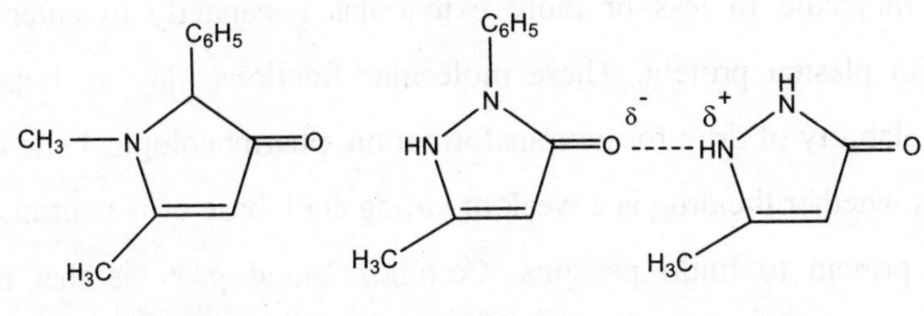

Antipyrine

1 - Phenyl - 3 - methyl- 5 - pyrazolone

(ii) Salicylic acid (o - Hydroxy benzoic acid) has antibacterial activity but not the p-isomer and m-isomers ie. *p* and *m* - Hydroxy benzoic acids are inactive. This is because, salicylic acid forms intra molecular hydrogen bonding, so it is less water-soluble and its partition coefficient is also greater.

The *m* and the *p* isomer can form intermolecular H-bonds, results in dimer and does not easily pass through the bio membranes. The partition co-efficient of it is also less and hence low antibacterial action.

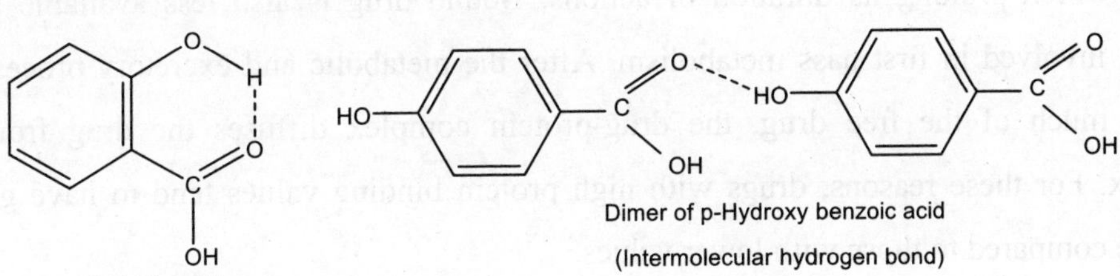

Salicylic acid

Dimer of p-Hydroxy benzoic acid
(Intermolecular hydrogen bond)

2.5 Protein Binding

The reversible binding of drug with non-specific and non-functional site on the body protein without showing any biological effect is called as protein binding. A drug's efficiency may be affected by the degree to which it binds. The less bound a drug is, the more efficiently it can traverse cell membranes or diffuse.

$$\text{Drug} + \text{Protein} \rightleftharpoons \text{Drug} + \text{Protein complex}$$

A drug molecule to less or more extent has a capacity to enter into specific combination with plasma protein. These molecular fractions play an important role in deciding the availability of drug for biotransformation, pharmacological site and excretion. Depending upon whether the drug is a weak or strong acid, base or is neutral, it can bind to a single blood protein to multi proteins. Common blood proteins that drugs bind to are albumin, lipoprotein, glycoprotein, and α, β, and γ globulins.

The most significant protein involved in the binding of drug is albumin, which comprises more than half of blood volume. Albumin interacts with acidic or basic drugs in the plasma by Vander - Waal's force, hydrophobic binding, hydrogen bonding and ionic interaction. Acid – glycoprotein interacts with basic entities and lipoproteins bind with both basic and neutral drugs.

The drug-protein complex is large, hence cannot pass through phospholipid bilayers including capillary membranes, glomerular membrane in the nephrons and the blood brain barrier, which prolong its duration of actions. Bound drug is also less available to the enzyme involved in first pass metabolism. After the metabolic and excretory process has cleared much of the free drug, the drug-protein complex diffuses the drug from the complex. For these reasons, drugs with high protein binding values tend to have greater half-life compared to those with lower values.

2.5.1 Factor Affecting Protein Binding

- Lipophilicity is the most desirable physiochemical parameters that favour protein binding to occur. Also, an increase in the lipid content of drug moiety eventually enhances the rate as well as extends of protein binding process. For example, intramuscular Injection of Cloxacillin displays 95% protein binding due to its greater lipophilicity.
- Alteration in the concentration of drug substance as well as the protein molecules or surfaces subsequently brings alteration in the protein binding process.
- Drug's affinity towards specific protein/tissue is also an important factor for activity of the drug. For example, Digoxin has more affinity for cardiac muscles proteins as compared to that of proteins of skeletal muscles or those in the plasma.

2.6 Chelation/Complexation

Complexes or co-ordination results from a donor-acceptor mechanism (donating accepting electron or rather an electron pair) or Lewis acid-base reaction (donating accepting protons). Since complex drug cannot cross the natural membranous barriers, they reduce the rate of absorption of the drug. The compounds that are obtained by donating electrons to metal ion with the formation of a ring structure are called chelates. The compounds capable of forming a ring structure with a metal atom are termed as ligands.

2.6.1 Importance of Chelates in Medicine

(a) Antidote for metal poisoning

(i) Dimercaprol is a chelating agent. It is an effective antidote for organic arsenical and also used to treat poisoning by Gold and Arsenic.

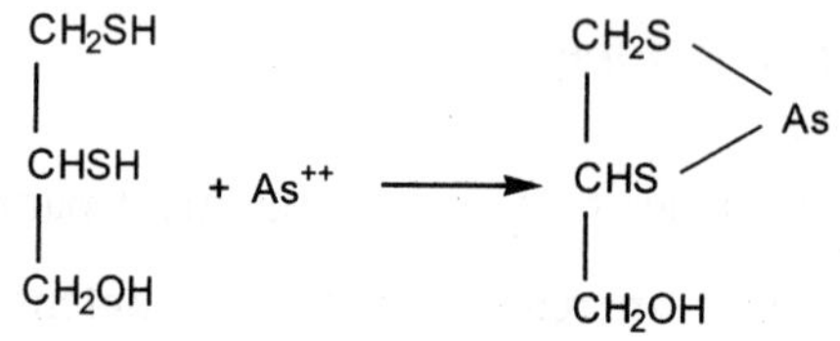

(ii) Penicillamine used in Wilson's disease because it forms water soluble chelates with copper.

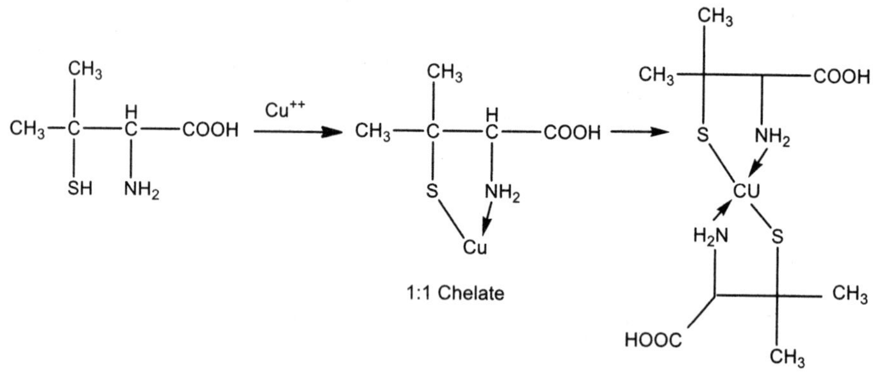

(b) Removal of metals causing deterioration in pharmaceuticals

Water-soluble ligands are referred as sequestering agents. Certain drug, eg. Epinephrine and ascorbic acid are destroyed by oxidation and metals catalyze this oxidation. Common sequestering agents EDTA is used which forms a water-soluble ligand.

(c) Undesirable side effects caused by drugs, which chelates with metals

A side effect of Hydralazine an antihypertensive agent is formation of anemia and this is due to chelation of the drug with iron.

(d) 8-Hydroxy quinoline and its analogs act as antibacterial and antifungal agent by complexing with iron or copper.

2.7 Bioisosterism

Bioisosterism is a strategy applied in the rational design of new drugs in a lead compound as a special process of molecular modification. In 1919, Longmuir introduced the term isosterism, which postulated that two molecules or molecular fragments containing an identical number and arrangement of electron should have similar properties and termed as isosteres. Isosteres should be isoelectric i.e. they should possess same total charge. For example CO and NO_2; $CO_2$and N_2O; N_3 and NCO; CH_2 N_2 and $CH_2 = CO$

Bioisosterism is defined by Burger as "*Compounds or groups that possess near-equal molecular shapes and volumes, approximately the same distribution of electrons and which exhibit similar physical properties.*"

Drug design with isosteric modification involves the replacement of an atom or group of atoms in a molecule by another group with similar electronic and stearic configuration. To apply bioisosteric group, a complete well-known chemical structure, mechanism of action, topographic interaction with the receptor, the pathways of metabolic inactivation, the bioavailability and side effects, of the lead compound should be known. They are classified into two types:

a. **Classical isosteres**

- Monovalent atoms or groups.
- Divalent atoms or groups
- Trivalent atoms or groups
- Tetravalent atoms
- Ring equivalents

b. **Non-classical isosteres**

- Cyclic vs. Non cyclic
- Non-classic bioisosterism of functional groups

- Carbonyl group bioisosteres
- Carboxylic group bioisosteres
- Ester group bioisosteres
- Catechol group bioisosteres
- Hydroxyl group bioisosteres
- Amide group bioisosteres
- Halogen bioisosteres
- Spacer group bioisosteres

2.7.1 Classical Bioisosteres

Classical bioisosteres have similarities of shape and electronic configuration of atoms, groups and molecules, which they replace. The classical bioisosteres atoms and groups are:

Classical bioisosteres	
Univalent atoms and groups ▪ Cl, Br, I, F ▪ -CH3. NH2, -OH, -OR,–SH ▪ -Si3, -SR	**Tetrasubstituted atoms** = C = ; = N = ; = P =;
Bivalent atoms and groups ▪ C=C, C=N, C=O, C=S ▪ –CH2–, –NH–, –O–, –S–	**Ring equivalents** (i) – CH = CH - ; - S – (benzene, thiophene) (ii) – CH =; -N = (benzene, pyridine) (iii) – O -; - S -; - CH2; - NH - (tetrahydrofuran, tetrahydrothiophene, cyclopentane, pyrrolidine)
Trivalent atoms or groups –CH=, –N=-,- P =,-As =,-Sb=	

2.7.2 Non-classical Bioisosteres

Non-classical bioisosteres do not obey the stearic and electronic definition of classical bioisosteres. Also, they do not have the same number of atoms as a replacement. These isosteres retain activity by the retention of their properties such as pKa, electrostatic potentials, which can alter selective enzyme processes. For which modern computational analysis methodology can aid in rationalization.

Non Classical bioisosteres

- **Cyclic vs Noncyclic bioisosteres**
- **Functional groups bioisosteres**

Functional group		Bioisosteres
Carbonyl group	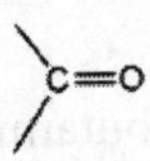	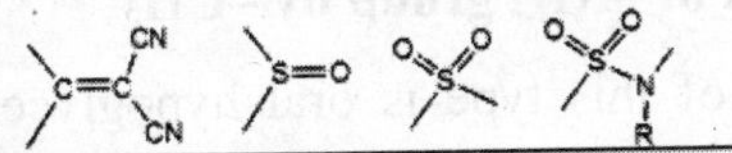
Carboxylic acid group	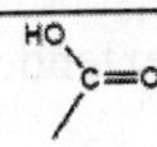	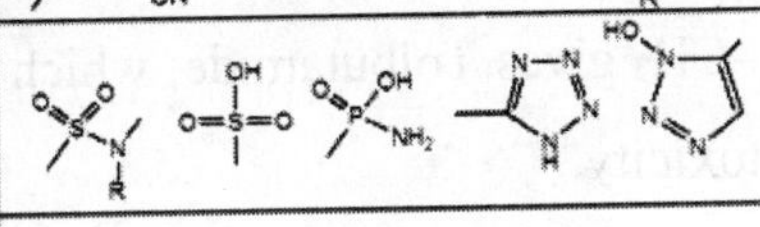
Amide	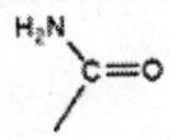	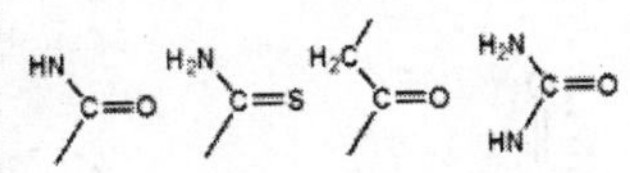
Ester	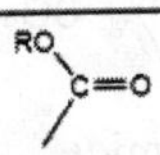	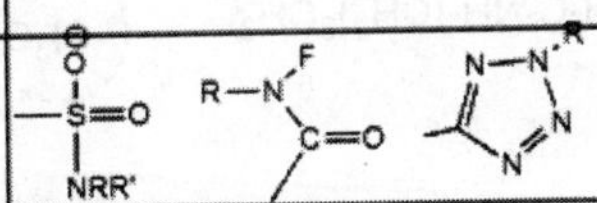
Hydroxyl group	—OH	$-CH_2OH$ —NHCOR $-NHSO_2R$ $-NHCONH_2$
Catechol	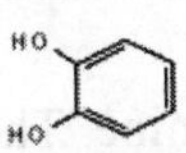	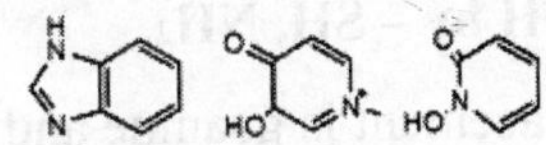
Halogens X (Cl, Br,F)		—CN $-N(CN)_2$ $-N(CN)_3$
Spacer group	$-(CH_2)_3-$	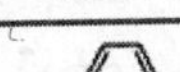

2.7.3 Applications of Classical Bioisosteres in Drug Design

a. Replacement of Fluorine atoms for Hydrogen

Fluorine is most commonly employed as monovalent bioisosteric replacement for hydrogen. Stearic parameter for hydrogen and fluorine are similar, their Vander Waal's radii being 1.2 and 1.35A° respectively. The anti-neoplastic agent 5-fluorouracil is a classical example, in which the fluorine replaced with hydrogen in 5th position of Uracil a normal substrate, result in a derivative, which can alter, selected enzymatic derivative. Fluorine in fluorouracil forms a covalent binding with the enzyme and inhibits it.

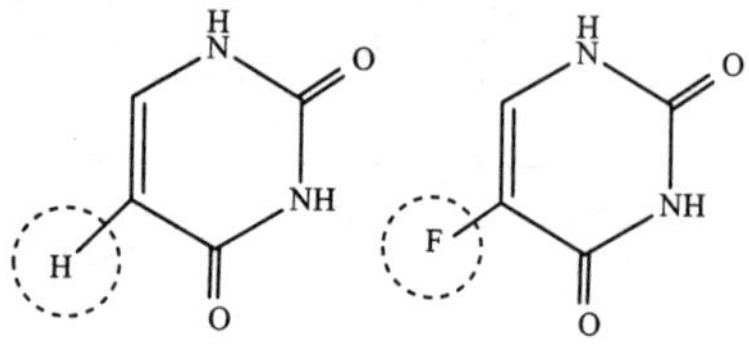

Uracil 5 - Fluorouracil

b. **Replacement of $-NH_2$ group by $-CH_3$**

An example of this type is oral hypoglycemic Carbutamide, the $-NH_2$ group is replaced by $-CH_3$ gives Tolbutamide, which possess extended biological half-lives and reduces toxicity.

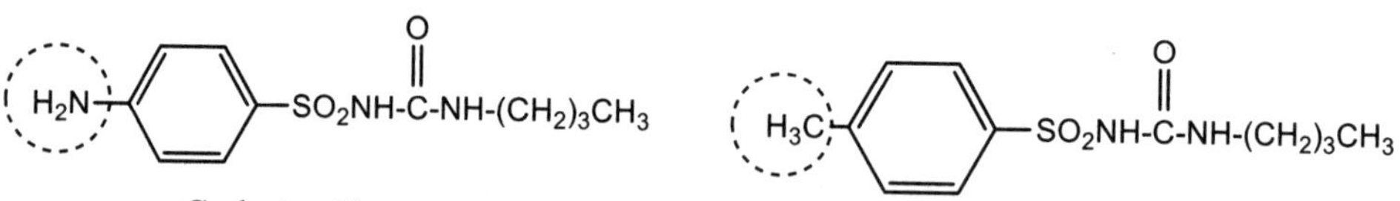

Carbutamide Tolbutamide

c. **Replacement of– OH by – SH, NH2**

Example of this replacement is guanine and 6-thioguanine. The antineoplastic agent 6-thioguanine inhibits the enzyme hypoxanthine-*guanine phosphoribosyl transferase* and blocks the synthesis of DNA.

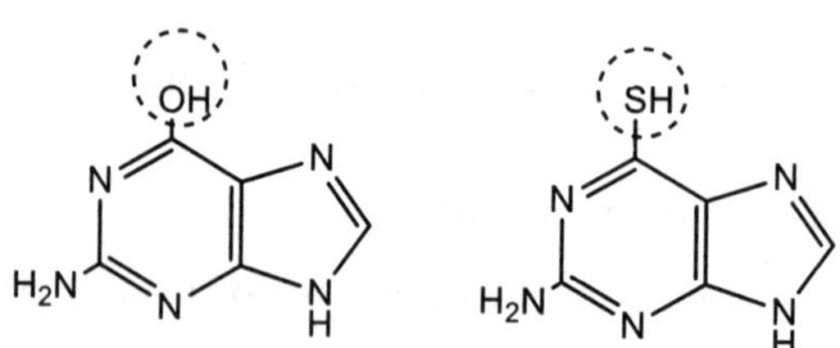

Guanine 6 - Thioguanine

Another example is Calcium channel blockers dihydro pyrimidine. Substitution of the hydroxyl with thiol group resulted in enhanced potency.

d. **Replacement of - O - group by NH group**

The replacement of - O - group by NH group in Procaine gives Procainamide. The local anesthetic activity of Procaine is more than Procainamide due to difference in lipid solubility.

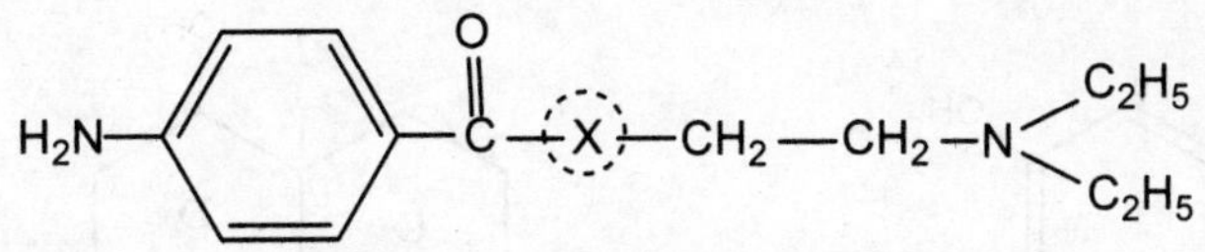

Name	X
Procaine	—O—
Pracainamide	—NH—

e. Replacement of - CH - for - N =

The trivalent substitution of - CH - with - N = is commonly used in modern drug design. Substitution of the pyridinyl amino – N = in Mepyramine by – CH - produces Chlorpheniramine with less sedative effect an undesirable side effect of antihistaminic.

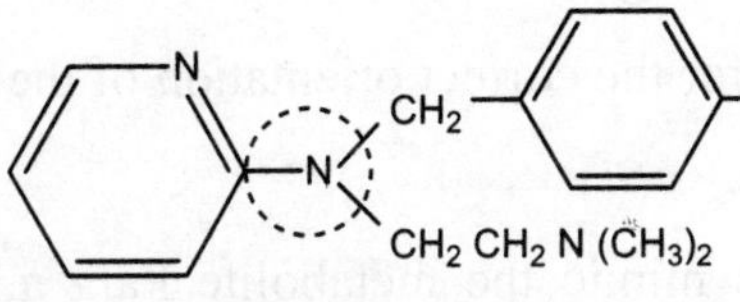

Mepyramine

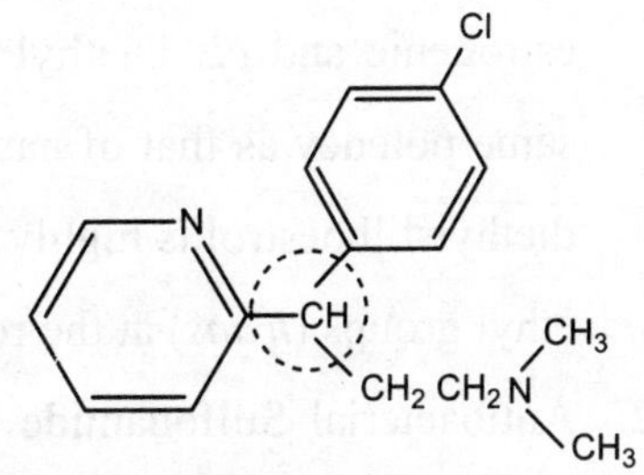

Chlorpheniramine

f. Ring replacements

The phenyl group of antibacterial Sulfonamide is replaced by various heterocyclic aromatics which resulted in more active compounds.

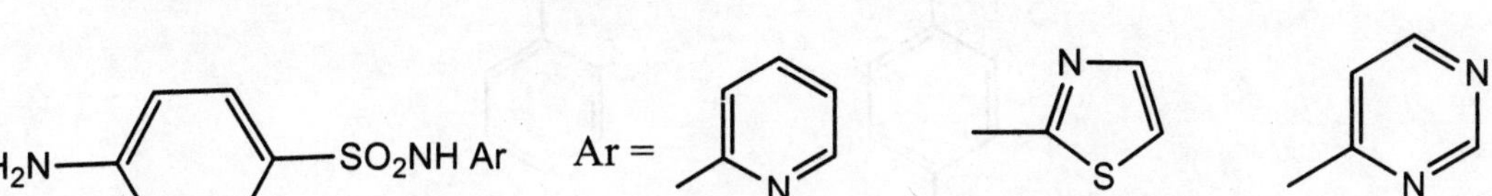

Sulfapyridine Sulfathiazole Sulfapyrimidine

2.7.4 Applications of Non-classical Bioisosteres in Drug Design

1. A classic example of ring versus non-cyclic structure is Diethyl stilboestrol and 17β-oestradiol.

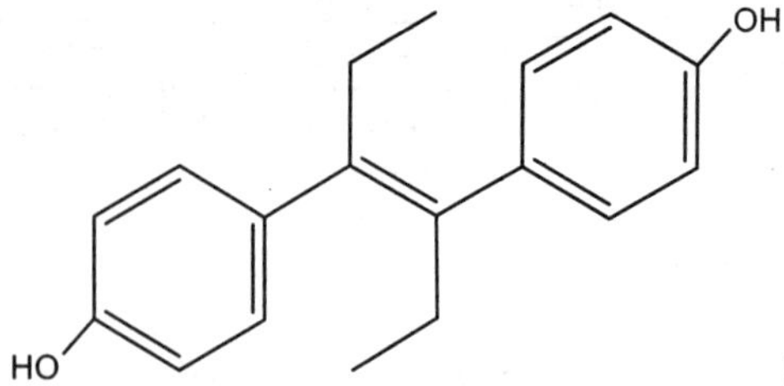

Trans - Diethylstilboestrol

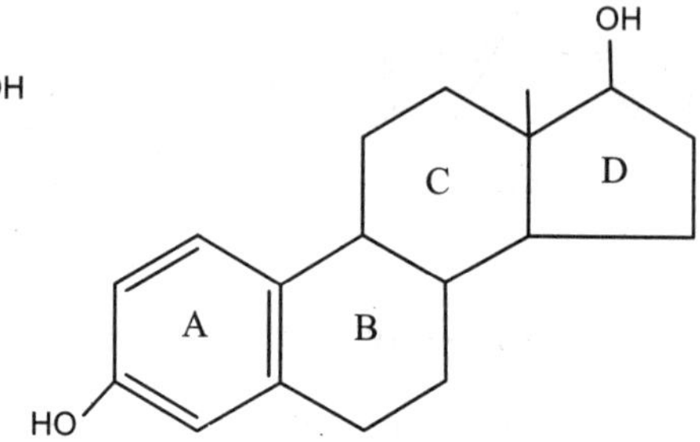

17β - oestradiol

The molecular design of Diethylstilboestrol was carried out by opening the B and C of steroidal nucleus of oestradiol. Due to the presence of double bond Diethyl stilboesterol exist in two fixed stereo isomeric forms; *trans*-Diethyl stilboesterol estrogenic and *cis* Diethyl stilboestrol (7% as active).Trans isomer has about the same potency as that of naturally occurring Oestradiol. The central double bond of diethylstilboestrol is highly important for the correct orientation of the phenolic and ethyl groups (*trans*) at the receptor site.

2. Antibacterial Sulfonamide derivatives mimic the metabolite Para amino benzoic acid was found during elucidation of its mechanism of action. This similarity was based on electronic and conformational aspects as well as the physicochemical properties such as pKa and log P.

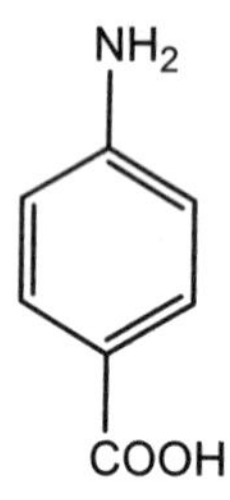

Para amino benzoic acid

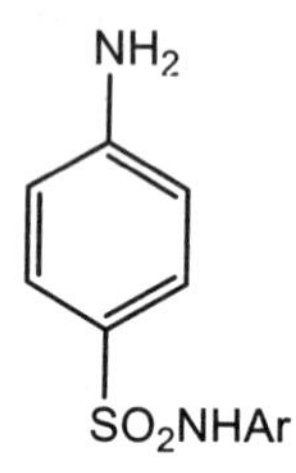

Sulphonamdes

3. The 3-hydroxyl group *of β*-adrenoceptor agonists Isoproterenol, has been replaced with bioisosteric groups $-CH_2OH$, $-NHSO_2CH_3$ and $-NHCONH_2$ gives Salbutamol, Sternal and Carbuterol respectively. This results in agents with potent and selective activities.

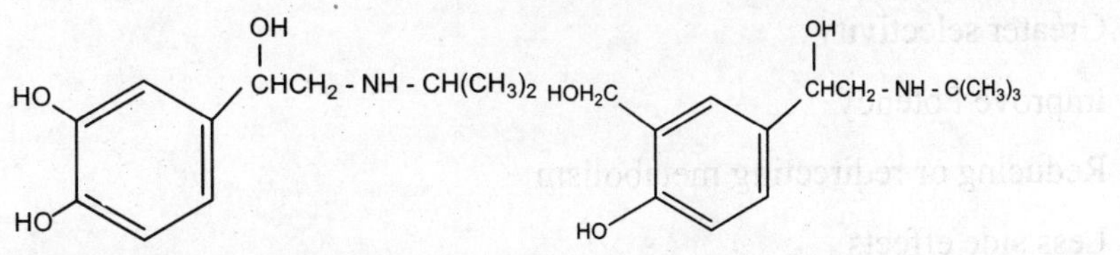

Isoproterenol Salbutamol

4. Trimaperidine is the propanoate ester of a piperidyl alcohol, while Pethidine, Meperidine, is an ethyl ester of a piperidyl carboxylic acid a reversal of an ester group.

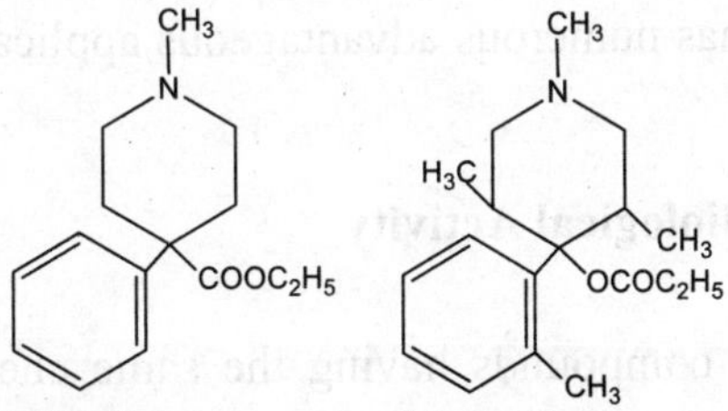

Pethidine Trimaperidine

5. Isosteric modification of the imidazole nucleus in Cimetidine is Ranitidine without side effects associated with Cimetidine.

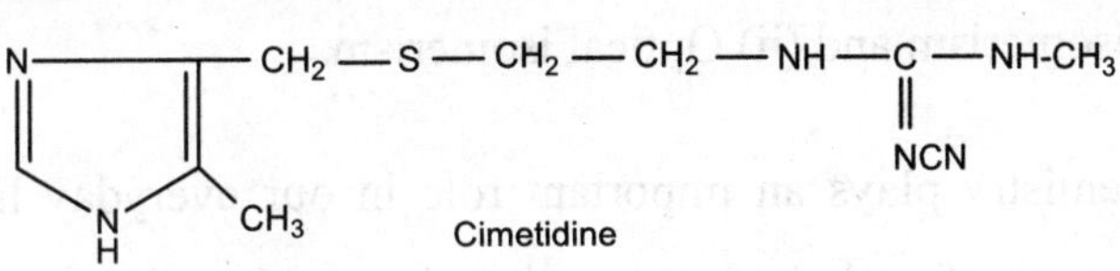

Cimetidine

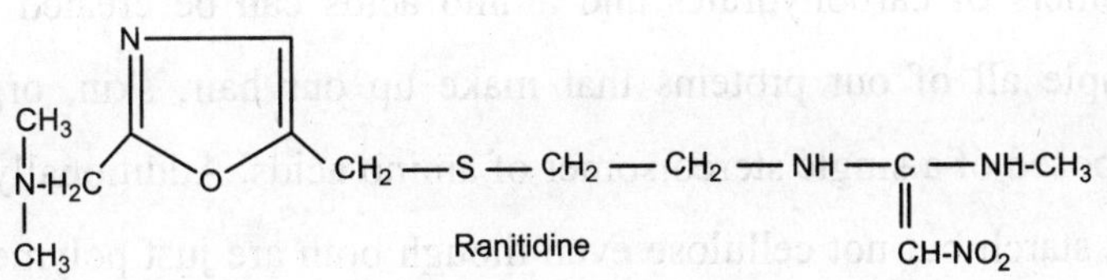

Ranitidine

Bioisosterism represents one approach used by the Medicinal Chemists for the rational modification of lead compounds into safer and more clinically effective agents. The design of bioisosteres introduces structural changes that can be beneficial or toxic depending upon the size, shape, electronic distribution, polarizability, dipole, polarity, lipophilicity, pKa etc., the development and application of bioisosteres have been adopted as a fundamental approach for number of aspects associated with the design and development. The following properties can be modulated with appropriate bioisosteres

- Greater selectivity
- Improve Potency
- Reducing or redirecting metabolism
- Less side effects
- Decreased toxicity
- Increased stability
- Simplified synthesis
- Patented lead compounds

Thus bioisosterism has numerous advantageous applications in resolving biological problems effectively.

2.8 Stereoisomerism and Biological Activity

Isomerism arises in compounds having the same chemical formula but different orientations of the atoms belonging to the molecule in three-dimensional space is known as Stereoisomerism. The compounds that exhibit stereoisomerism are often referred to as stereoisomers. This phenomenon can be further categorized into two subtypes. (i) Geometrical isomerism and (ii) Optical isomerism.

Stereochemistry plays an important role in our everyday live in our body. Only certain stereoisomers of carbohydrates and amino acids can be created and digested by body. For example all of our proteins that make up our hair, skin, organs, brain, and tissues, are composed of a single stereoisomer of amino acids. Additionally, our bodies can make and digest starch but not cellulose even though both are just polymers of glucose of different stereochemistry.

Because living systems are themselves stereo selective, each stereo isomeric drug can behave very differently *in vivo*. The drug must approach and fit closely to the receptor surface to evoke the pharmacological action. Hence the drug must possess a high degree of structural specificity or stereo selectivity. Many drugs show stereo selectivity because mostly receptor binds are optically active biological macromolecules such as protein, polynucleotide or glycolipids.

2.8.1 Geometrical Isomerism

The isomers which possess the same structural formula but differ in the spatial arrangement of the groups around the double bond are known as geometrical isomers and the phenomenon is known as geometrical isomerism. This isomerism is shown by alkenes or their derivatives. When similar groups lie on the same side, it is the *cis* isomer; while when the similar groups lie on opposite sides, the isomer is *trans*. In geometric isomers, *cis* and *trans* isomers differ in their physical and chemical properties. Therefore, their distribution in the biological medium is different.

For example, Diethyl stilboesterol exist in two fixed stereo isomeric forms; *trans*-Diethyl stilboestrol *cis* oestrogenic, whereas *cis* isomer is only 7% as active. In *trans*-Diethyl stilboestrol, resonance interaction and minimal stearic interference tend to hold the two aromatic ring and connecting ethylene carbon atom in the same plane.

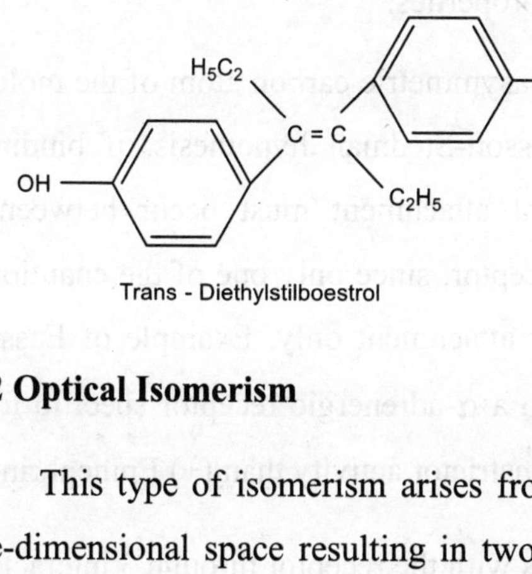

Trans - Diethylstilboestrol

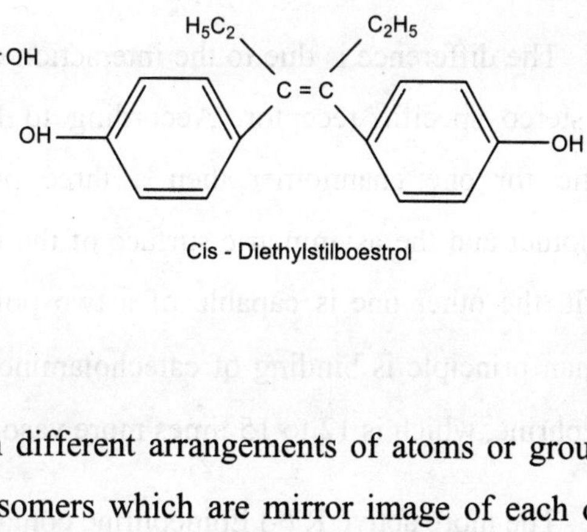

Cis - Diethylstilboestrol

2.8.2 Optical Isomerism

This type of isomerism arises from different arrangements of atoms or groups in three-dimensional space resulting in two isomers which are mirror image of each other. Optical isomers contain an asymmetric (chiral) carbon atom (a carbon atom attached to four different atoms or groups) in their molecules

A chiral compound containing one asymmetric center has two enantiomers. Optical isomers or enantiomers have same physical and chemical properties like identical melting points, pKa, solubility, etc. But the important difference between two is that each member rotates the plane of polarized light to the same degree, in opposite directions. Enantiomer rotates the plane of polarization in a clockwise direction is known as the (+) form and anti-clockwise is known as (-) form. Enantiomers of a chiral drug have identical physical and chemical properties in an achiral environment. In a chiral environment, they may have different physiological activities like the protein binding, bioavailability, rate of metabolism, metabolites, excretion, potency and selectivity for receptors, transporters and/or enzymes, and toxicity. Because living systems are themselves chiral, each of the enantiomers of a chiral drug can behave very differently *in vivo.*

For example,

- (-) Hyoscyamine, which exhibits 15 to 20 times more mydriatic activity than (+) Hyoscyamine.
- (-) Ephedrine is 3 times more active than (+) Ephedrine, 5 times more active than Pseudoephedrine and 36 times more active than (-) Pseudoephedrine.
- (+) Ascorbic acid has more anti scorbutic properties.

The difference is due to the interaction of asymmetric carbon atom of the molecule with stereo specific receptor. According to Easson-Stedman hypothesis, if binding is specific for one enantiomer then a three point attachment must occur between the enantiomer and the asymmetric surface of the receptor, since only one of the enantiomers will fit, the other one is capable of a two point attachment only. Example of Easson – Stedman principle is binding of catecholamine to a α-adrenergic receptor specific for (-) Epinephrine, which is 12 to 15 times more vasoconstrictor activity than (+) Epinephrine.

The more active R (-) Epinephrine contacts with the receptor through 3 interactions as given in the Fig. 3.1.

A- Acceptor or donor or hydrophobic interaction between aromatic ring of epinephrine and aromatic ring of the receptor.

B- A hydrogen bonding with alcoholic hydroxyl group

C- An ionic bond between protonated amino group and specific glutamic carboxylic group in the receptor.

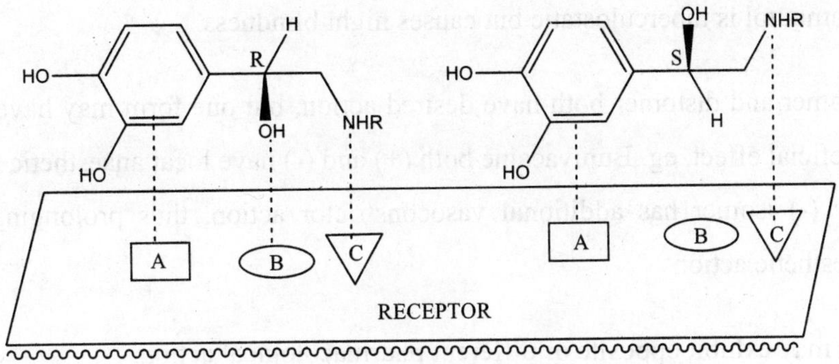

Fig. 3.1 Epinephrine and Receptor Binding

S (+) Epinephrine can make contact through only two groups.

The enantiomer, which has high affinity for receptor, is called eutomer, whereas the one with lower affinity called distomer. The ratio of activity of eutomer and distomer is called eudismic ratio, the expression of the eudismic index is

$$EI = \log \text{affinity}_{Eu} - \log \text{affinity}_{Dis}.$$

The enantiomeric pair differs in their pharmacodynamics profile and pharmacological effect.

Few examples are listed below:

- Both enantiomers have same pharmacological profile eg. Cyclophosphamide.
- One enantiomeric form is more active than the other. S (-) Warfarin is 5 times more active, than R (+) Warfarin; (-) Propranolol is more active than (+) Propranolol.
- One enantiomer may be inactive (s) α-methyldopa is active and used as antihypertensive but (R) form is inactive.
- Any one enantiomer may be toxic. eg. Thalidomide a sedative drug, the (S) Thalidomide is teratogenic effect leading to phocomelia in many newborns; (S)

Naproxen has anti-inflammatory activity and (R) Naproxen is toxic; (RR) Ethambutol is tuberculostatic but causes night blindness.

- Eutomer and distomer both have desired action, but one form may have additional beneficial effect. eg. Bupivacaine both (+) and (-) have local anaesthetic activity but only (-) isomer has additional vasoconstrictor action, thus prolonging the local anaesthetic action.

- One may exhibit opposite or different pharmacological action.

  - Quinine is used as antimalarial and Quinidine is anti-arrhythmic agent; 2R, 3S-Propoxyphene is used as analgesic and 2S, 3R is used as antitussive;

  - (S)-Thyroxine is thyroid hormone and (R)-Thyroxine is used as anti-hyperlipoproteinemic;

  - (S)-Timolol is an antihypertensive, whereas the (R)-Timolol is prescribed for glaucoma;

  - (-) Sotalol is adrenergic blocker and (+) Sotalol is antiarrhythmic agent;

  - (-) Indacrinone is an diuretic and (+) Indacrinone is Uricosuric agent;

  - L-Asparagine has sweet taste while the R - Asparagine is tasteless;

  - (R) - Carvone has caraway odor while (S) - Carvone has spearmint odor.

- Sometimes metabolic inversion to the active isomer occurs for example, anti-inflammatory drug Ibuprofen sold as racemic mixture. The S enantiomer shows anti-inflammatory by inhibiting cyclooxygenase. The R isomer gets converted to the S form *in vivo*.

$$\text{S - Ibuprofen} \underset{\text{inversion}}{\overset{\text{metabolic}}{\rightleftharpoons}} \text{R - Ibuprofen}$$

Single enatiomers have less complex and more selective pharmacodynamics profile as compared to racemic mixture, so have lesser adverse drug reactions, improved therapeutic profile, less chance of drug interactions than racemic mixtures.

Chapter 4

DRUG METABOLISM

1. INTRODUCTION

Metabolism is a pharmacokinetic process which converts non-polar compounds to water soluble polar compounds so that they are excreted easily from the body. All the chemical substances that are not nutrients, which enter the body through ingestion, inhalation (or) absorption is called as xenobiotics (or) exogenous compounds. Drug metabolism or Biotransformation refers to modification of xenobiotic in the biological system. Water-soluble agents undergo renal excretion whereas lipid soluble substances are passively reabsorbed from the renal tubule into the blood after glomerular filtration. Thus if such phenomenon continues, drug would accumulate in the body and precipitate toxic reaction. However, to prevent such a consequence, the body is armed with the metabolic system which transforms the water insoluble lipophilic non-polar drug into polar and water soluble product that can be easily excreted by the kidney. This enzymatic biotransformation is known as drug metabolism. *"Drug biotransformation is thus a detoxification process"*.

Drug metabolism is defined as enzymatic chemical reactions that are responsible for the conversion of drugs into metabolites within the body. The reactions involved are classified into Phase I and Phase II reactions.

Biotransformation of drug may result in any of the following conversion

i) Pharmacologically inactive metabolite: An active drug converted into inactive metabolite. Example: Phenytoin to *p*- Hydroxy phenytoin

ii) Bioactive metabolite: An active drug to more active metabolite. Example: Codeine to Morphine.

iii) Pharmacologically active metabolite: An inactive drug (Prodrug) converted to active metabolites. Example: Enalapril to Enalaprilat.

iv) Equally active metabolite: An active drug converted to equally active metabolite.

Example: Phenylbutazone to Oxyphenbutazone.

1.1 Sites of Bio-transformation

Drug metabolism occurs in all the tissues, but the principle site of drug metabolism is the liver. The other sites include kidney, lungs, GI tract, brain, placenta and skin. Orally administered drugs are absorbed through mucous membrane of the small intestine or from the stomach. Once out of GI tract it is carried by the blood stream to the liver, where it is usually first metabolized.

Metabolism by liver enzyme prior to the drug reaching the systemic circulation is called the first-pass metabolism or presystemic metabolism or first pass effect, which may result in complete deactivation of drug. Drugs that experience a significant first-pass effect are Imipramine, Morphine, Propranolol, Diazepam, Midazolam, Cimetidine and Lidocaine.

1.2 Pathways of Drug Metabolism

Drug metabolism has been divided into two phase viz: Phase I and Phase II transformation.

Phase I: They are enzyme biotransformation reaction, in which drug may undergo a wide variety of oxidation, reduction and hydrolysis, resulting in introduction or unmasking of functional group, which increases the polarity of the molecule and serve as a centre for the second phase of metabolic reaction. It is also called as functionalization reaction. These transformations are also called as synthetic reactions, opposite to synthetic phase II reactions.

Phase II: The original unaltered drug or polar metabolite is conjugated to glucuronic acid, sulfate, amino acid, acetyl (or) methyl group making the molecule more water soluble and therefore it is readily excreted.

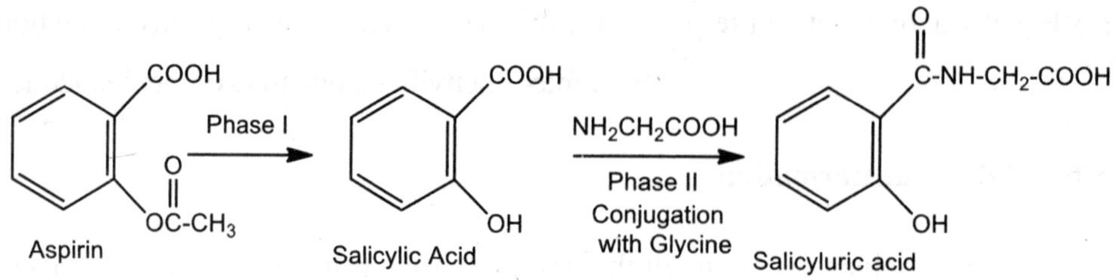

1.3 Phase I and Phase II Metabolic pathway

1.3.1 Phase I Reactions

(I) Oxidative Reactions

i) Oxidation of aromatic moieties

ii) Oxidation of Olefins

iii) Oxidation at benzylic, allylic carbon atoms and carbon atoms α to carbonyl and imines

iv) Oxidation at aliphatic and alicyclic carbon atoms

v) Oxidation involving carbon - heteroatom system

vi) Carbon - nitrogen systems (oxidative deamination, N-oxide formation, N-hydroxylation)

vii) Carbon- Oxygen system (O-dealkylation)

viii) Carbon- Sulfur systems (S-dealkylation, S-oxidation and Desulfuration)

ix) Oxidation of alcohols and aldehydes

x) Other miscellaneous oxidative reactions

(II) Reductive Reactions

i) Reduction of aldehydes and ketones

ii) Reduction of nitro and azo compounds

iii) Miscellaneous reduction reactions

(III) Hydrolytic Reactions

i) Hydrolysis of esters and amides

ii) Hydration of epoxides and arene oxides by *epoxide hydrase*

1.3.2 Phase II Reactions
i) Glucuronic acid conjugation
ii) Sulfate conjugation
iii) Conjugation with glycine, glutamine and other amino acids
iv) Glutathione or mercapturic acid conjugation
v) Acetylation
vi) Methylation

1.4 Enzymes Involved in Drug Metabolism

Enzymes involved in drug metabolism are either microsomal or non-microsomal enzymes.

i) **Microsomal enzymes**: Found in endoplasmic reticulum of liver cells. *Cytochrome P450s*, *Flavin containing monooxygenase* (FMOs), *Monooxygenase,* etc., are microsomal enzymes.

ii) **Non-microsomal enzymes:** Found in cytoplasm and mitochondria of liver cells. *Monoamine oxidases* (MAOs), *alcohol dehydrogenases* (ADHs), *Aldehyde dehydrogenases etc.,* are some non-microsomal enzymes.

(a) Oxidative enzymes

Oxidative reactions are catalyzed by *Cytochrome P450s*, *Flavin containing monooxygenase* (FMOs), *Monoamine oxidases* (MAOs), A*lcohol dehydrogenases* (ADHs), A*ldehyde dehydrogenases* (ALDHs) and P*rostaglandin H synthase* (PHS). These enzymes are responsible for the metabolism of the majority of the marketed drugs.

(b) Reductive enzymes

Reductive reactions are catalyzed by A*ldo-keto reductases*, A*zo-reductases*, N*itro reductases*, Q*uinone reductases*, P450s, ADH and NADPH-P_{450} *reductase. Aldo-keto* *reductases* are involved in metabolism of synthetic hormones, chemotherapeutic agents, CNS drugs, sugar, steroids and prostaglandins.

(c) Hydrolytic enzymes

Hydrolytic reactions are catalyzed by hydrolytic enzymes that include *esterases, proteases, dehalogenases*, *lipases* and e*poxide hydrolases.*

(d) Conjugative (Phase II) enzymes

Conjugative enzymes include phase II enzymes such as *Uridine diphosphate glucuronyl transferase* (UGTs), *Sulfotransferase*, *N-acyl transferase, Glutathione-S-transferase,* γ*- glutamyl transpeptidase, N-acetyl transferase* and *Methyl transferases.*

2. PHASE I REACTIONS

2.1 Oxidative Reactions

Oxidation reaction increases the hydrophilicity of the xenobiotics by introducing the polar functional group such as OH. This reaction is catalyzed by a group of membrane *bound mono-oxygenase* found in the smooth endoplasmic reticulum of liver and other hepatic tissue called the cytochrome P_{450} *mono-oxygenase* enzyme system (CYP_{450}). These enzymes require both molecular oxygen (O_2) and the reducing agent NADPH to effect reaction. They are therefore referred as mixed function oxidase. The catalytic reaction is

$$RH + O_2 + 2H^+ + 2e^- \longrightarrow \underset{\text{Product}}{ROH} + H_2O$$

Since only one oxygen atom from the molecular oxygen is incorporated in the product formed, the mixed function oxidase is also called as mono-oxygenase (or) microsomal hydroxylase. The multi enzyme mixed function oxidase system consists of 3 components- a haem protein known as cytochrome P_{450}, the flavo protein known as *cytochrome* P_{450} *reductase* and a heat stable lipid component known as phosphotidyl choline.

Cytochrome P_{450} oxidation- reduction cycle

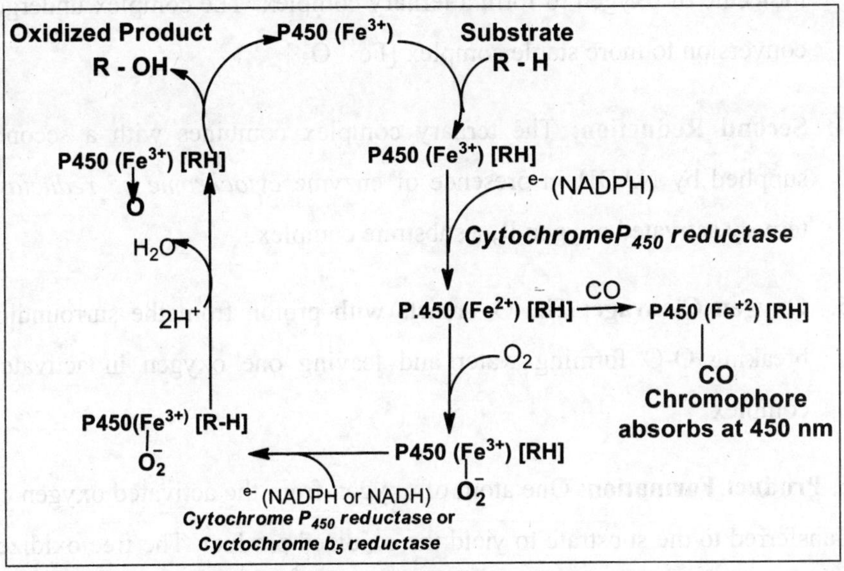

Fig. 4.1 **Cytochrome P_{450} oxidation- reduction cycle**

The various steps involved in the mechanism of cytochrome P_{450} catalyzed metabolism of xenobiotics (Fig. **4.1**) are:

1. **Substrate Binding**: Binding of the substrate (RH) to the oxidized form of the cytochrome P_{450} (Fe^{+3}) to form a complex.

2. **First Reduction**: A one electron transfer from NADPH to the complex by *cytochrome P450 reductase*, to form reduced (Fe^{+2}) P450 substrate complex; this step is considered as the rate-limiting step in the overall oxidation of xenobiotics.

The reduced form (Fe^{+2}) of this enzyme binds with carbon monoxide to form a complex that shows maximum absorption at 450nm hence the name cytochrome P_{450}.

3. **Oxygen Binding:** The reduced enzyme substrate complex combines with a molecule of oxygen to form a ternary complex. The complex undergoes a slow conversion to more stable complex [Fe^{3+} O_2^-]

4. **Second Reduction**: The ternary complex combines with a second electron supplied by NADH in presence of enzyme *cytochrome b5 reductase* to form ternary activated oxygen P_{450} substrate complex.

5. **Oxygen Cleavage**: The O_2^- reacts with proton from the surrounding solvent breaking O-O forming water and leaving one oxygen in activated oxygen complex

6. **Product Formation**: One atom of oxygen from the activated oxygen complex is transferred to the substrate to yield the oxidized product. The free oxidized form of cytochrome P_{450} is now ready to attach another molecule of substrate.

2.1.1 Oxidation of Aromatic Carbon Atom

(i) Oxidation of aromatic carbon gives corresponding phenols (arenol). The reaction proceeds via formation of reactive intermediate arene oxide or arene epoxide, which results in multiple reactions like Arene oxide rearrangement, *trans* dihydrodiol formation or formation of toxic glutathione adduct

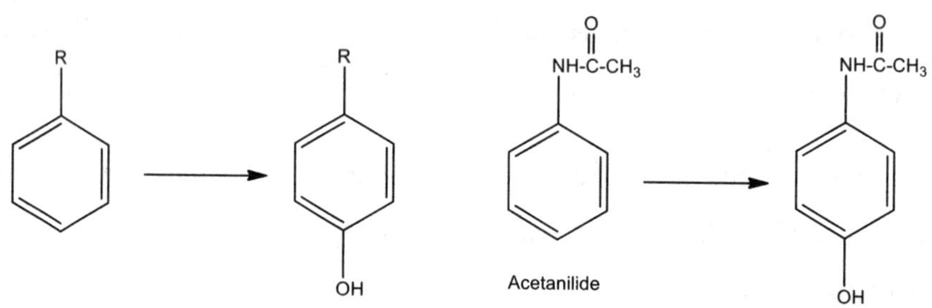

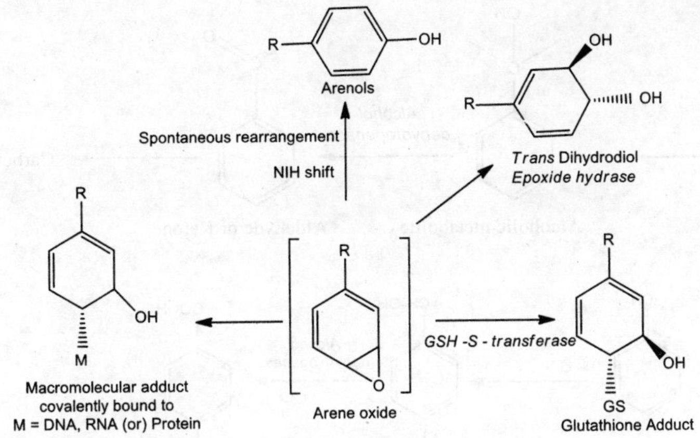

Fig. 4.2 Possible Reaction Pathways of Arene Oxides

2.1.2 Oxidation of Olefins

Oxidation of non-aromatic C-C double bond is analogue to aromatic hydroxylation; it proceeds via epoxide to yield 1, 2 - dihydrodiol. The epoxide is not very reactive like aromatic epoxide.

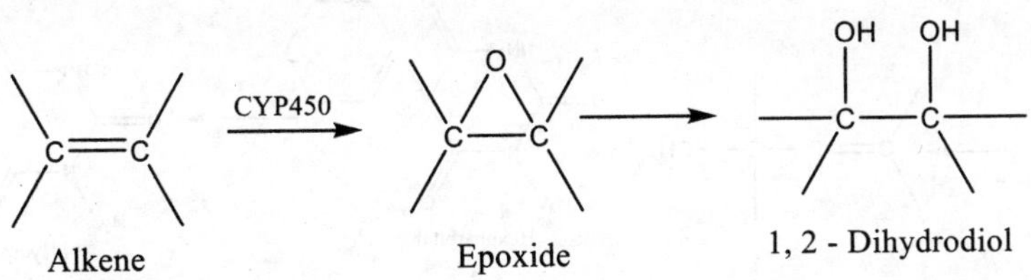

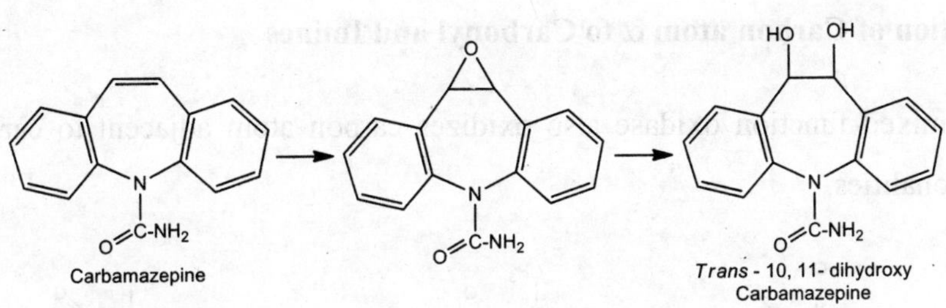

2.1.3 Oxidation at Benzylic Carbon

Carbon atom attached directly to the aromatic ring (benzylic carbon) is hydroxylated to corresponding carbinols or alcoholic metabolite. The alcoholic metabolite is further oxidized to aldehyde and further to carboxylic acid by *dehydrogenases*.

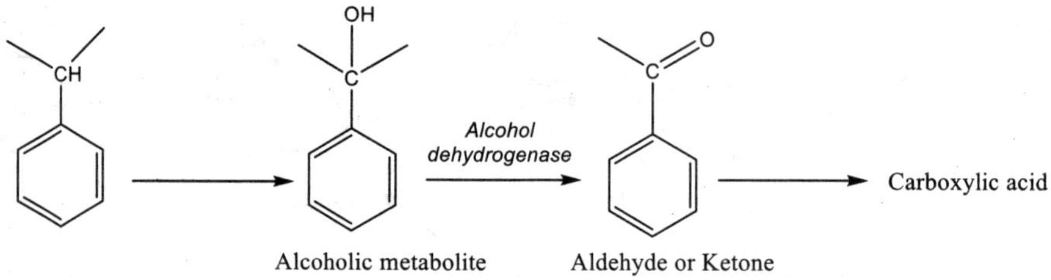

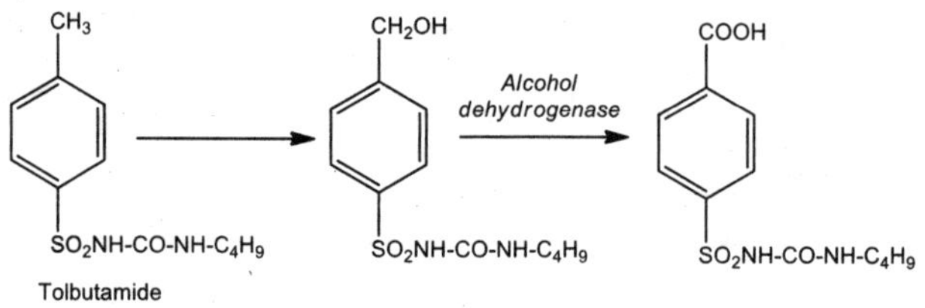

2.1.4 Oxidation of Allylic Carbon

Carbon atom adjacent to olefinic double bonds undergoes hydroxylation similar to benzylic carbon. eg. Hexobarbital on oxidation gives 3'- hydroxy hexobarbital.

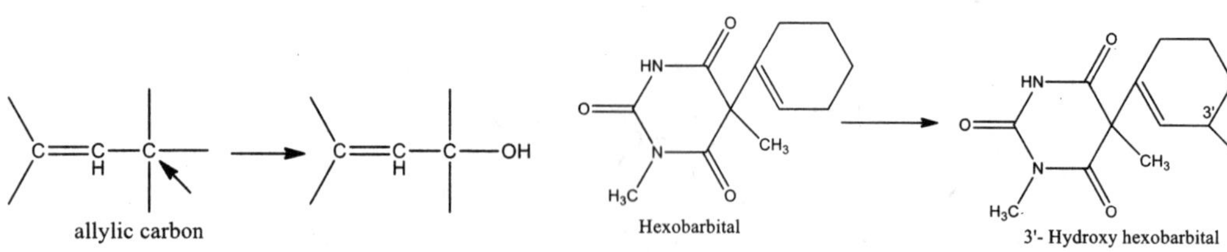

2.1.5 Oxidation of Carbon atom α to Carbonyl and Imines

The mixed function oxidase also oxidizes carbon atom adjacent to carbonyl and imino functionalities.

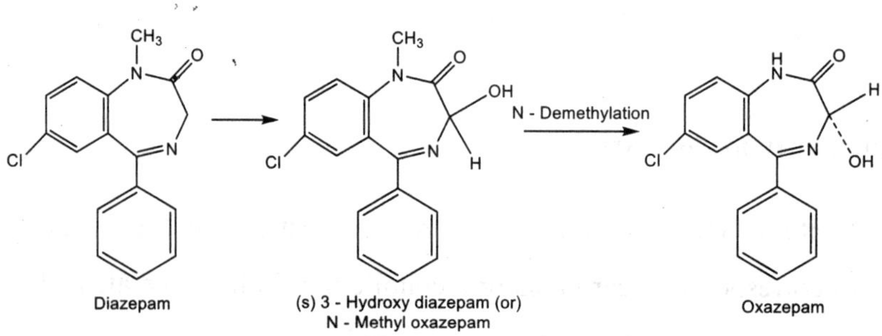

2.1.6 Oxidation of Aliphatic Carbon Atom (Aliphatic Hydroxylation)

Alkyl or aliphatic carbon atom can be hydroxylated at two positions, terminal methyl group is often referred as ω oxidation and oxidation at penultimate carbon atom (ie. next to the last carbon) is called ω-1 oxidation. Commonly ω and ω-1 oxidation takes place in drug molecule with straight or branched alkyl chains.

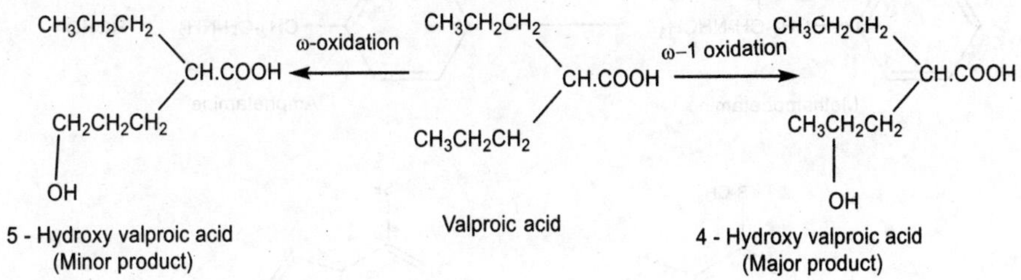

2.1.7 Oxidation of Alicyclic Carbon Atom

The cyclo hexyl group is also susceptible to mixed function oxidation. The enzymatic hydroxylation occurs in C-3 or C-4 and leads to *cis* and *trans* conformational stereoisomer.

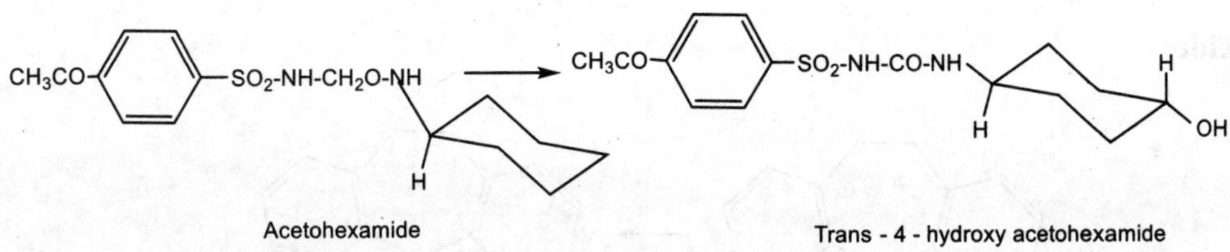

2.1.8 Oxidation of Carbon-Hetero Atoms

Biotransformation of C-N, C-O and C-S system proceed in one of the two ways.

(i) Hydroxylation of the α carbon atom attached directly to the heteroatom. The resulting compound is unstable and decomposes with the cleavage of carbon hetero system. Example - Oxidative, N, O, and S dealkylation, Oxidative deamination.

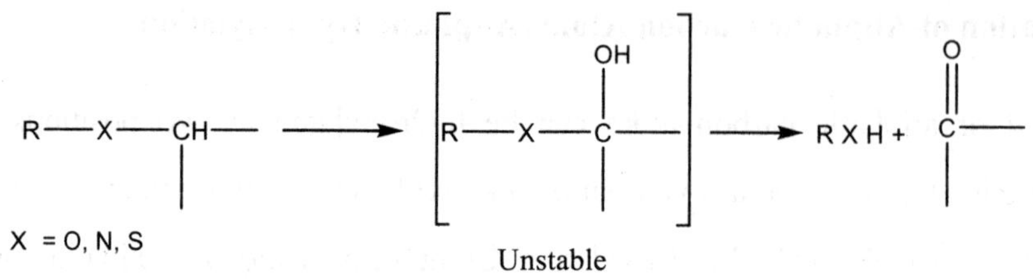

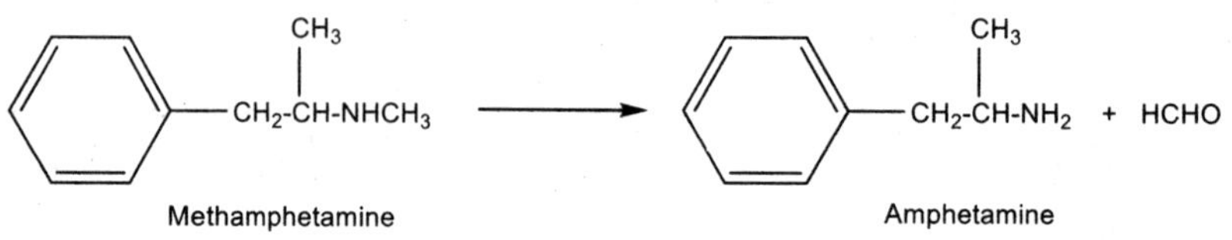

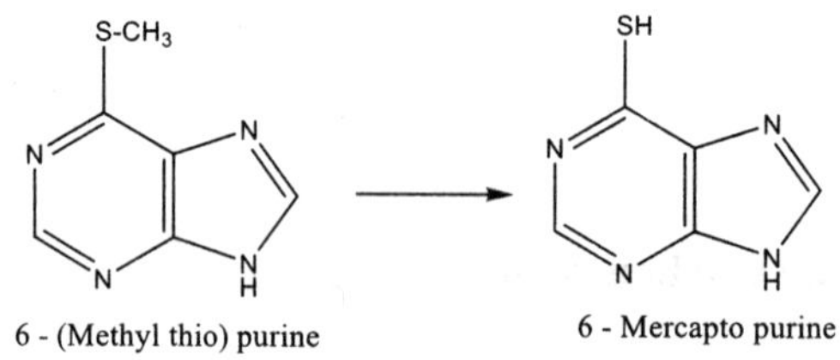

(ii) Oxidation or hydroxylation of hetero atom itself N and S only

Example N- Hydroxylation, N-Oxide, Sulfoxide, Sulfone formation

N-oxide

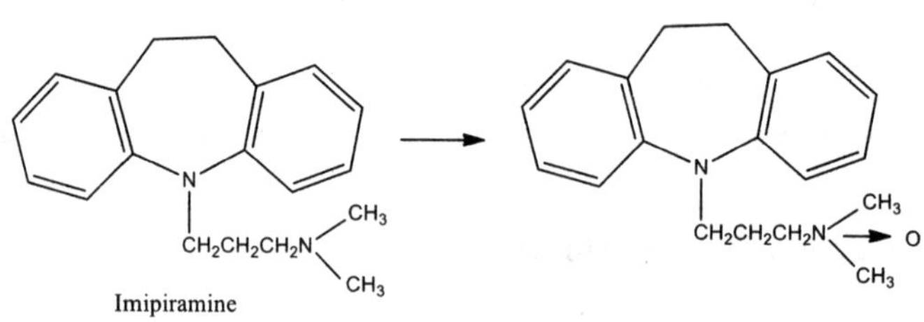

S-Oxidation

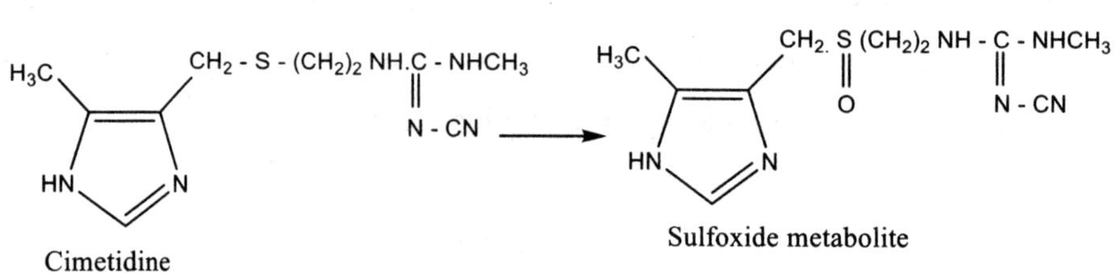

N-Hydroxylation

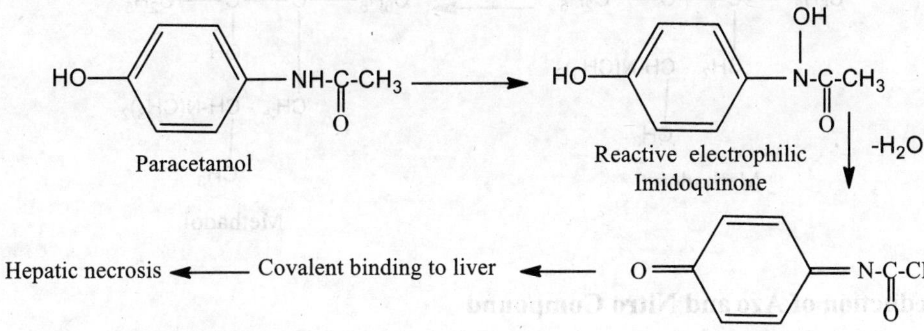

Methemoglobinemia toxicity is caused by several aromatic amines, including aniline and Dapsone is due to the bioconversion of aromatic amine to its N-hydroxy derivative. N-hydroxyl amine oxidizes the Fe^{2+} form hemoglobin to Fe^{3+} state (called methemoglobinemia).

2.2 Reduction Reactions

Reductive reaction plays an important role in metabolism of many compounds containing carbonyl, nitro and azo group. Bio-reduction of carbonyl group results in alcohol whereas nitro and azo group give rise to amino group. The amino group and hydroxyl group are more susceptible to conjugation.

2.2.1 Reduction of Aldehyde and Ketone

Metabolites containing carbonyl moiety frequently occur in many drugs as well as from oxidative deamination of xenobiotics. Aldehydes are usually metabolized to carboxylic acid, but occasionally reduced to primary alcohol. Bio-reduction of ketone leads to asymmetric center and thereby two stereo isomeric alcohols are produced. Diverse soluble enzyme called *aldo-keto reductase* carry out bio-reduction of aldehyde and ketones. When chiral ketone is reduced, they yield two possible diastereomeric or epimeric alcohols.

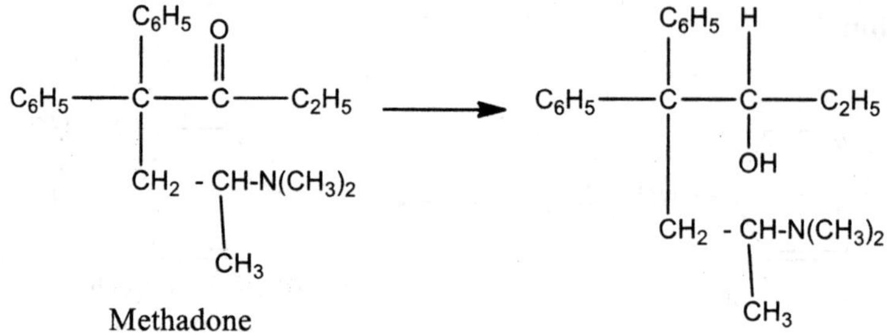

Methadone → Methadol

2.2.2 Reduction of Azo and Nitro Compound

Reduction of aromatic nitro and azo-xenobiotics leads to aromatic 1° amino metabolite. Reduction of nitro group proceeds via formation of nitroso and hydroxylamine intermediates to yield amines.

$$\underset{\text{Nitro}}{RNO_2} \longrightarrow \underset{\text{Nitroso}}{R-N=O} \longrightarrow \underset{\text{Hydroxylamine}}{RNH.OH} \longrightarrow \underset{1^{\circ}\text{Amine}}{RNH_2}$$

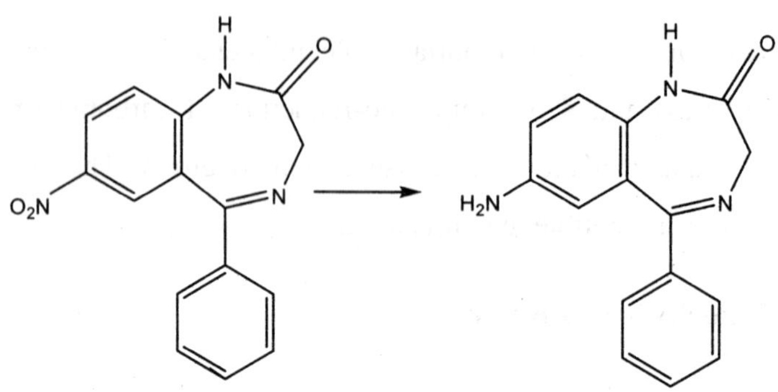

Nitrazepam → 7 - Amino metabolite

Azo reduction proceeds via hydrazo intermediate (-NH-NH-) that is subsequently cleaved reductively to yield corresponding amines.

$$Ar\,N=N-Ar' \longrightarrow Ar\,NH-NH-Ar' \longrightarrow Ar\,NH_2 + Ar'NH_2$$

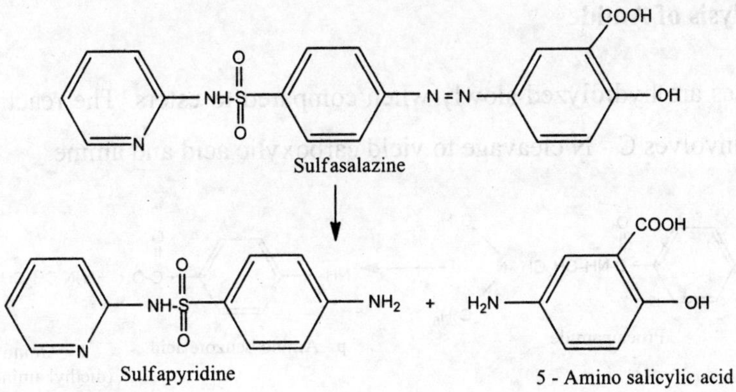

2.3 Hydrolytic Reactions

2.3.1 Hydrolysis of Esters

The metabolisms of ester and amide linkages in many drugs are catalyzed by hydrolytic enzyme present in various tissues and plasma. The metabolic products formed (carboxylic acid, phenol, alcohol and amines) are generally polar and more susceptible to conjugation. Aromatic esters are hydrolyzed by *aryl esterase* and aliphatic esters by *carboxyl esterase*.

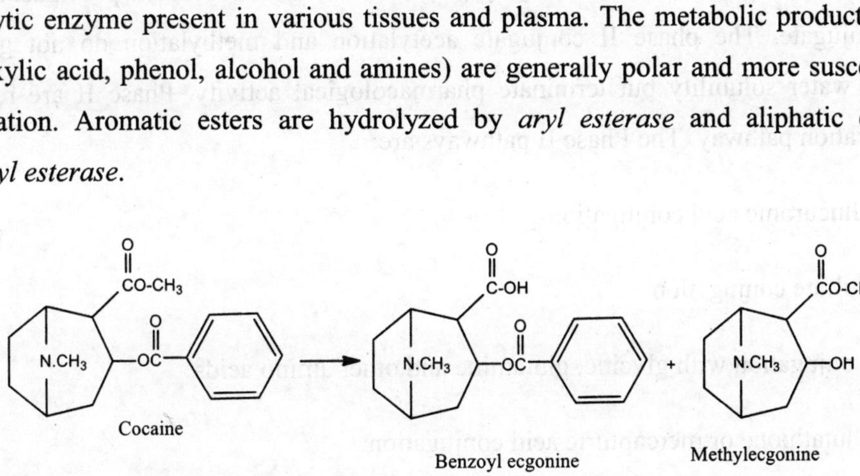

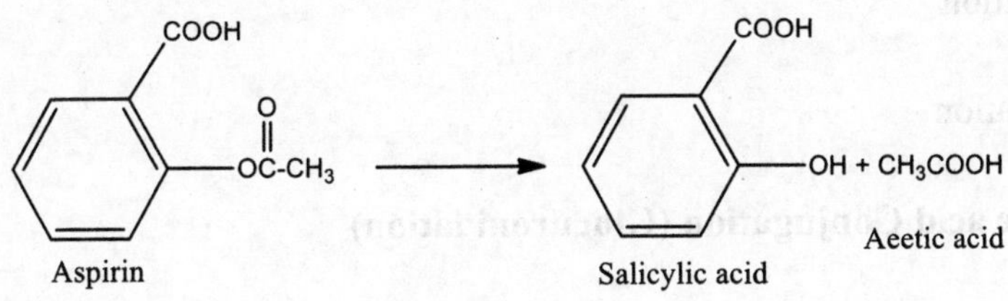

2.3.2 Hydrolysis of Amide

Amides are hydrolyzed slowly when compared to esters. The reaction is catalyzed by *amidase*, involves C - N cleavage to yield carboxylic acid and amine.

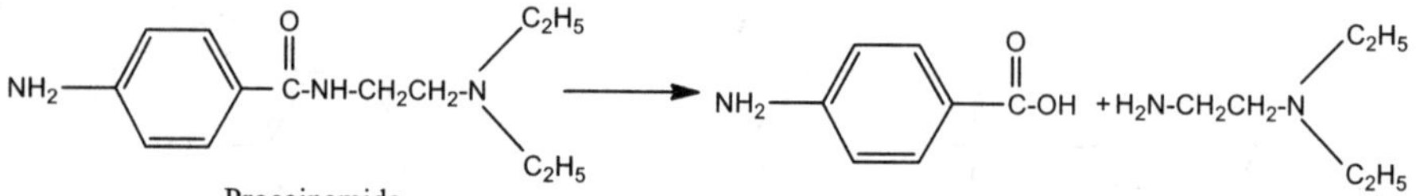

Procainamide p - Amino benzoic acid 1 - Amino - 2, 2 - (diethyl amino) ethanol

3. PHASE II (OR) CONJUGATION REACTIONS

Phase II involve transfer of suitable moiety such as glucuronic acid, sulfate, glycinate in the presence of enzyme *transferase* to drug or metabolites of phase - I having suitable functional group to form highly polar, readily excretable and pharmacologically inert conjugate. The phase II conjugate acetylation and methylation do not generally increase water solubility but terminate pharmacological activity. Phase II are real drug detoxification pathway. The Phase II pathways are:

- ✓ Glucuronic acid conjugation
- ✓ Sulfate conjugation
- ✓ Conjugation with glycine, glutamine and other amino acids
- ✓ Glutathione or mercapturic acid conjugation
- ✓ Acetylation
- ✓ Methylation

3.1 Glucuronic acid Conjugation (Glucuronidation)

Glucuronic acid conjugation or Glucuronidation is a most common and important Phase II reaction. In this reaction glucuronide acts as a conjugation molecule and binds to a substrate via the catalysis of Uridine diphosphate (UDP) *glucuronyl transferase* or *glucuronosyltransferases (*UGTs). Uridine diphosphate (UDP) *glucuronyl transferase* located predominantly in the endoplasmic reticulum of liver, kidney, intestine, lungs, prostate, mammary glands, skin, brain, spleen and nasal mucosa.

First, in a series of reactions

- The co-substrate uridine diphosphate glucuronic acid (UDPGA) act as a donor of Glucuronic acid to the substrate.
- The glucuronosyltransferases (UGTs) then catalyze the transfer of glucuronic acid from UDPGA to a substrate containing suitable functional groups (- OH, - COOH, - NH2, -SH) resulting in a glucuronidated substrate and leaving uridine 5'-diphosphate.
- The resulting water-soluble β- glucuronide easily excreted in urine or bile.
- The pKa value of glucuronic acid is in the range of 3.5 to 4 and hence ionisable at both plasma and urine pH, thereby increasing the water solubility of the conjugated, substrate.

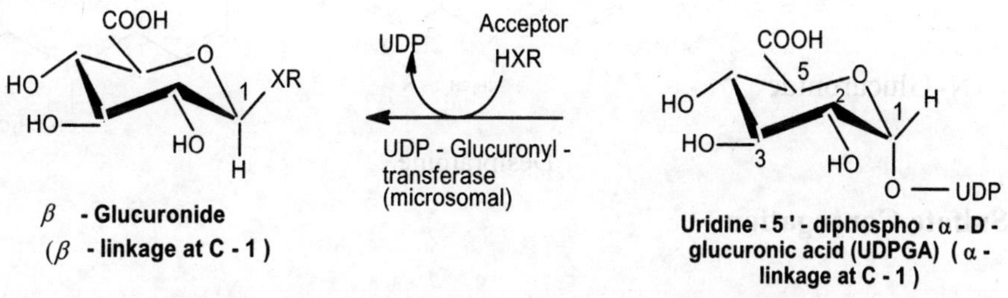

β - glucuronide conjugates.

Fig . 4.3 Formation of UDPGA and Beta - glucuronide conjugates

Glucuronide conjugation can take place in most body tissues because the UDPGA the glucuronic acid donor (derived from D-glucose) is present in abundant in body. A large number of drugs and endogenous substances such as steroids, bilirubin, catechols and thyroxine undergo glucuronidation. In neonate and children glucuronide conjugation are not developed fully. In such subject, the compound that is metabolized normally by glucuronidation may accumulate and causes toxicity. For example, inability of newborn to conjugate with bilirubin cause neonatal hyperbilirubinemia and with Chloramphenicol cause grey baby syndrome respectively. It forms O- glucuronides with phenol, alcohol, hydroxyl amine and carboxylic acid, N-glucuronides with sulfonamides, amines and amides and S-glucuronides with thiols

	Compound	**Metabolite**
O- Glucuronide	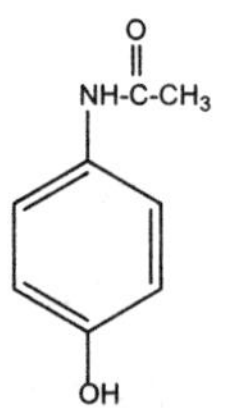 Paracetamol	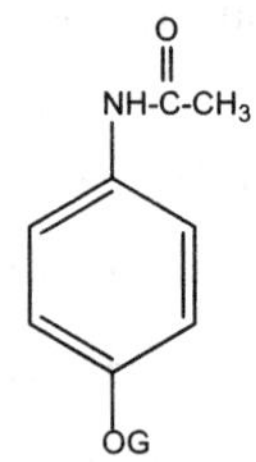
S- Glucuronide	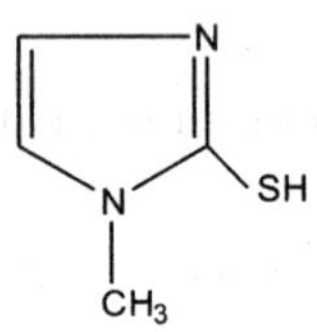 Methimazole	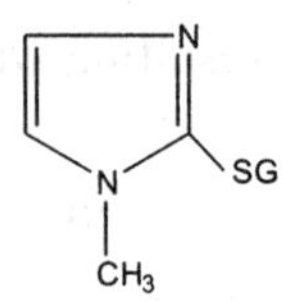
N- Glucuronide	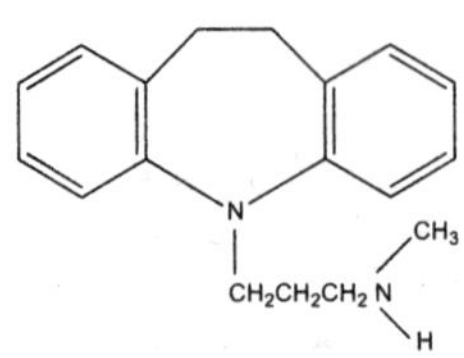 Desipramine	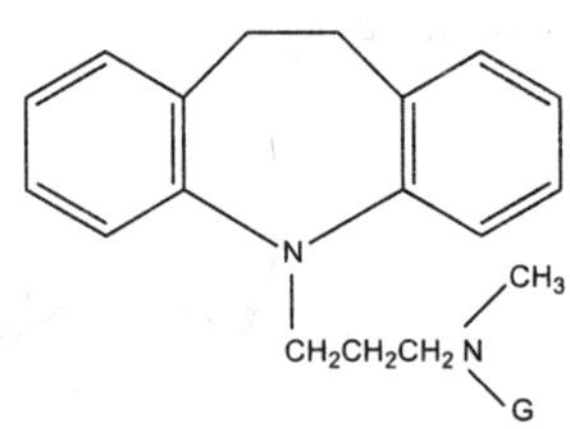

3.2 Sulfate Conjugation

The body uses sulfate to conjugate numerous endogenous compounds such as steroids, catecholamines and thyroxine. Sulfonation is similar to glucuronidation but it is catalyzed by *sulfotransferase* a large multigene family, found primarily in the liver, kidney, intestine, lung, platelets and brain. This process is predominant at low substrate concentration and glucuronidation is predominant at high concentration. Conjugation of xenobiotics with sulfate occurs with phenol, alcohol, aromatic amine and N-hydroxy compound.

Sulfonation occurs in two steps

(i) The interaction between sulfate and adenosine triphosphate (ATP) yield adenosine 5' phosphosulfate (APS). Activation of APS synthesizes activated coenzyme 3'-phosphoadenosine-5'-phosphosulfate (PAPS), which acts as a donor of sulfate to the substrate.

(ii) Transfer of sulfate group from PAPS to the substrate RHX in the presence of enzyme *sulfotransferase.* The sequence of events involved in sulfate conjugation is given below.

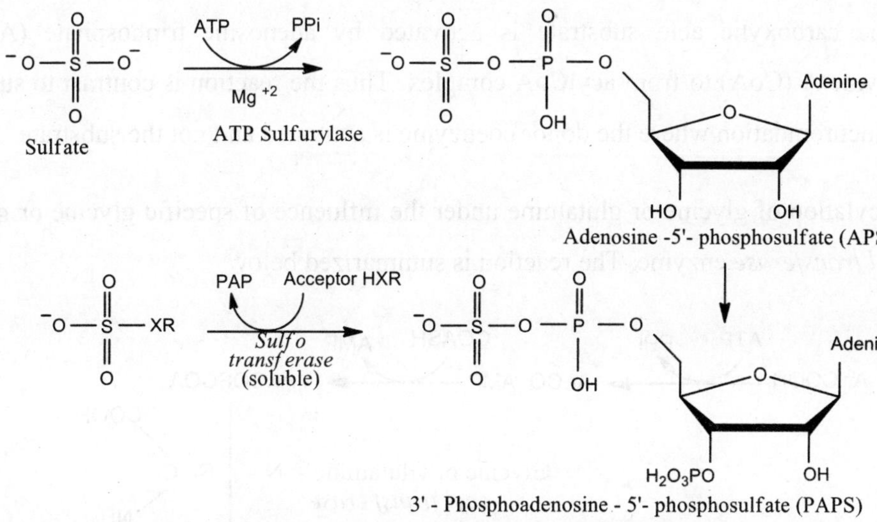

Fig. 4.4 Formation of PAPS and Sulfate Conjugates

Examples of Sulfate Conjugates

Compound **Metabolite**

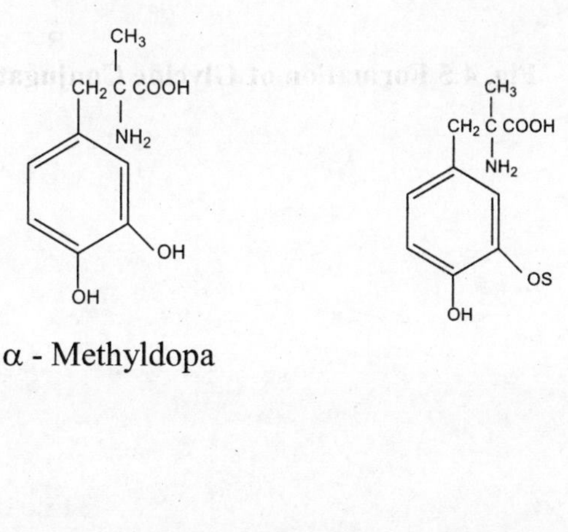

α - Methyldopa

$CH_3(CH_2)_4OH$ $CH_3(CH_2)_4OS$

N - Pentanol

3.3 Conjugation with α-Amino Acids

The amino acid glycine and glutamine are used to conjugate aromatic and aryl alkyl acids. This reaction occurs to a minute extend because of limited availability of amino acids.

The reaction occurs in two-step:

(i) The carboxylic acid substrate is activated by adenosine triphosphate (ATP) and coenzyme A (CoA) to from acylCoA complex. Thus the reaction is contrast to sulfonation and glucuronidation where the donor coenzyme is activated and not the substrate.

(ii) Acylation of glycine or glutamine under the influence of specific glycine or *glutamine N-acyl transferase* enzyme. The reaction is summarized below

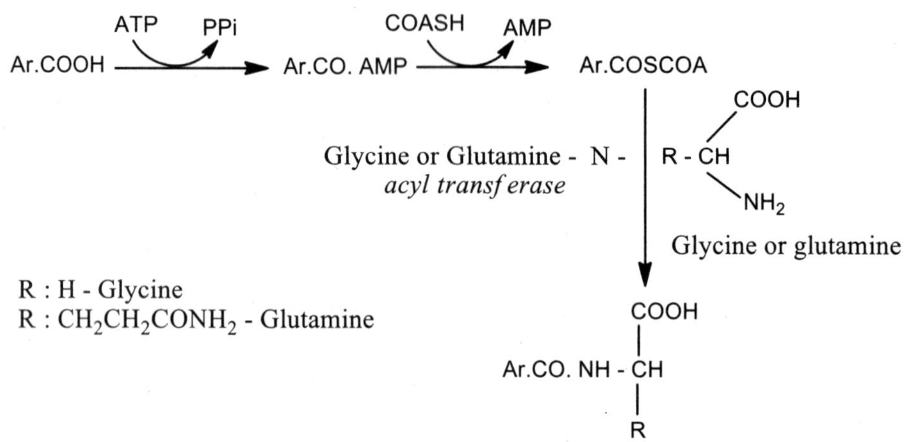

Fig. 4.5 Formation of Glycine Conjugate

Examples of Glycine and Glutamine Conjugates

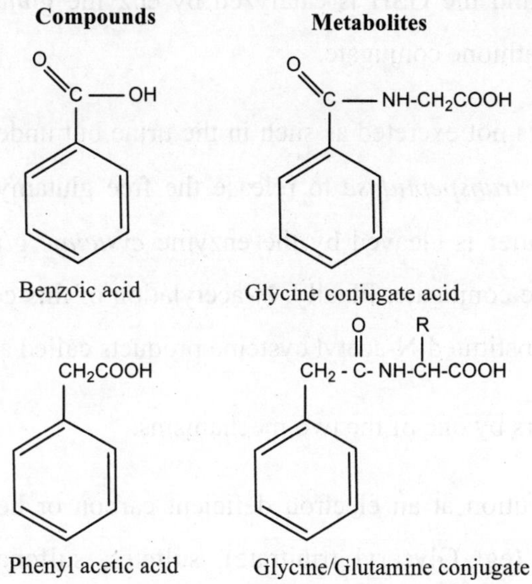

3.4 Conjugation with Glutathione

Glutathione (γ – glutamyl cysteinyl glycine or GSH) is a tripeptide with a strongly nucleophilic character due to the presence of a -SH (thiol) group in its structure.

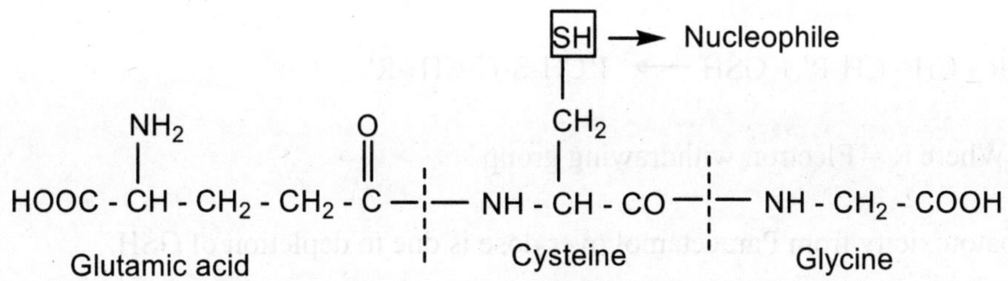

Highly electrophilic metabolite has a tendency to react with tissue nucleophilic groups such as -OH, $-NH_2$ and -SH and precipitate toxicities such as tissue necrosis, carcinogenesis, mutagenesis, teratogenesis, etc. Conjugation with glutathione protects the tissue from such reactive moieties and thus the reaction is an important detoxication route.

GSH conjugation differs from other conjugation reactions because it does not require initial activation of the coenzyme or the substrate since the GSH, which is a nucleophile itself, is highly reactive towards an electrophilic substrate. The interaction between the substrate and the GSH is catalyzed by enzyme *glutathione-S-transferase* to form S-substituted glutathione conjugate.

This conjugate is not excreted as such in the urine but undergoes cleavage, first by the enzyme *γ-glutamyl transpeptidase* to release the free glutamyl residue and cysteinyl glycine derivate; the latter is cleaved by the enzyme *cysteinyl glycinase* to produce free glycine and the cysteine conjugate. Finally, N-acetylation of this conjugate by the enzyme *N-acetylase* yields S-substituted-N-acetyl cysteine products called as mercapturic acids.

GSH Conjugation occurs by one of the two mechanisms:

(i) Nucleophilic substitution at an electron deficient carbon or heteroatom such as alkyl halides, alkyl nitrates (eg. Glyceryl trinitrate), sulfates, sulfonates, organophosphates, epoxides, lactones, etc.,

$$RX + GSH \longrightarrow R\text{-}S\text{-}G + H^+ + X^-$$

(ii) Nucleophilic addition at the electron deficient double bond such as the α, β-unsaturated carbonyl compounds, eg. Ethacrynic acid

$$R\text{ - }CH{=}\ CH\text{-}R' + GSH \longrightarrow RCH\text{-}S\text{-}G\text{-}CH_2\text{-}R'$$

Where R = Electron withdrawing group.

The hepatotoxicity from Paracetamol over dose is due to depletion of GSH.

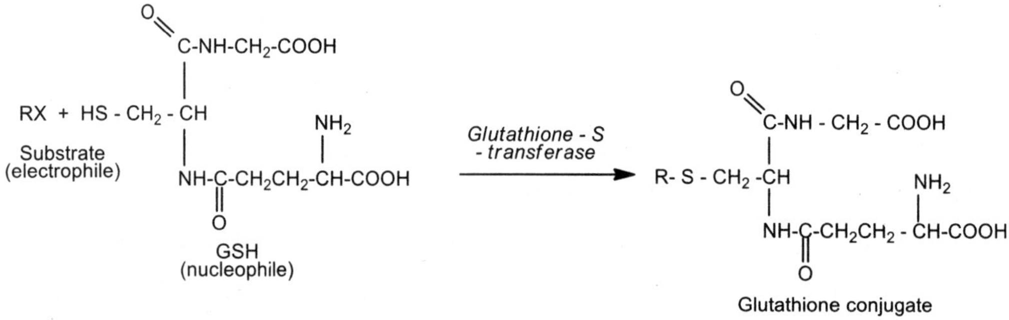

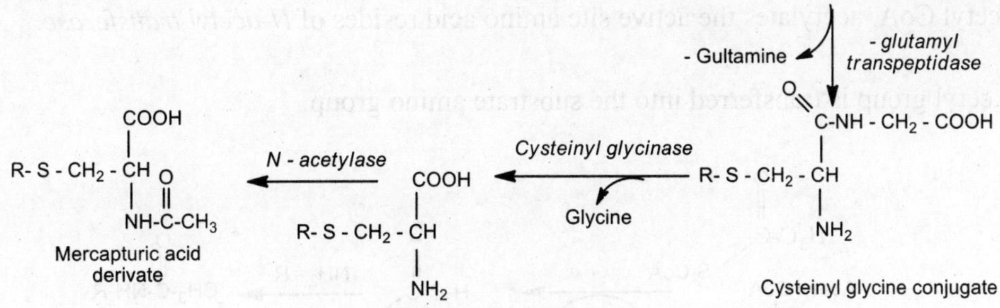

Fig.4.6 Formation of Glutathione Conjugates

Example of Glutathione Conjugates

Compound	Metabolite
CH_3I Methyl iodide	CH_3SG
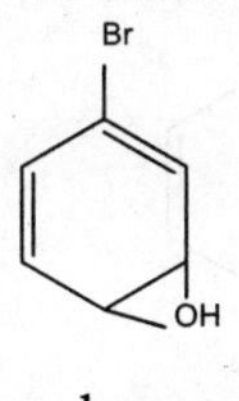 4 - Bromo benzene oxide	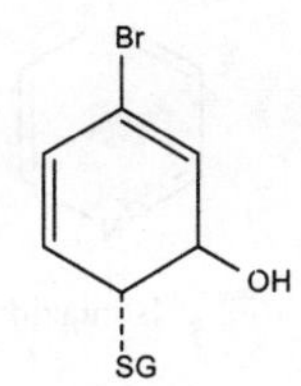

3.5 Acetyl Conjugation

Acetylation is an important route of metabolism for xenobiotics containing a primary amino group, including aliphatic and aromatic amine, amino acids, sulfonamides, hydrazines and hydrazides. This reaction is similar to conjugation with α – amino acid, because both the reactions yield amide product. The enzyme involved is the non-microsomal *N- acetyl transferase*. The acetyl group used in N-acetylation is supplied by acetyl CoA.

The amide formed are generally inactive, non-toxic and less water-soluble. The function of acetylation may be to deactivate the drug. Acetylation is a two-step process.

(i) Acetyl CoA, acetylates the active site amino acid resides of *N-acetyl transferase.*

(ii) Acetyl group is transferred into the substrate amino group.

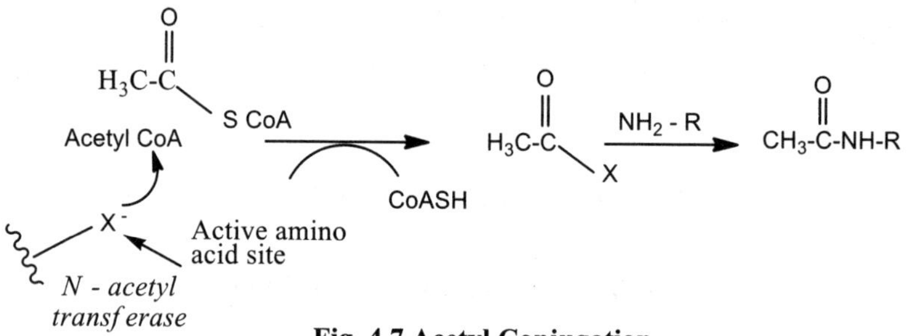

Fig. 4.7 Acetyl Conjugation

Examples of Conjugates of Acetylation

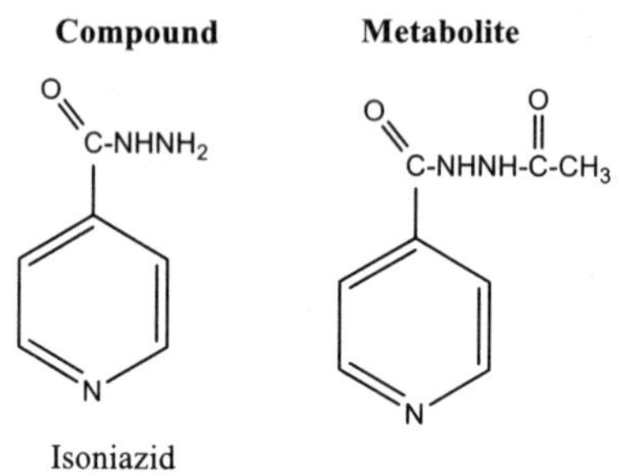

3.6 Methylation

Although methylation is an important route in the biosynthesis of many endogenous compounds (Epinephrine, Melatonin) it is only a minor pathway of xenobiotics. Methylation does not lead to highly water-soluble compounds except when methylation produces quaternary ammonium compounds. For example Nicotine to quaternary ammonium compounds.

Compounds undergoing methylation includes phenols, amine, the nitrogen atom of certain heterocyclic compounds and thiols. In case of aromatic compounds containing two vicinal hydroxy groups ie. catechol on monomethylation with the assistance of the enzyme *Catechol - o - methyl transferase* (COMT)

Methylation of substrate proceeds

(i) Synthesis of activated methyl transferring coenzyme S - adenosyl methionine (SAM) from L - Methionine and ATP in the presence of the enzyme *methionine adenosyl transferase*. (MAT)

(ii) Transfer of methyl group from SAM to the substrate in presence of non-microsomal enzyme *methyl transferase*.

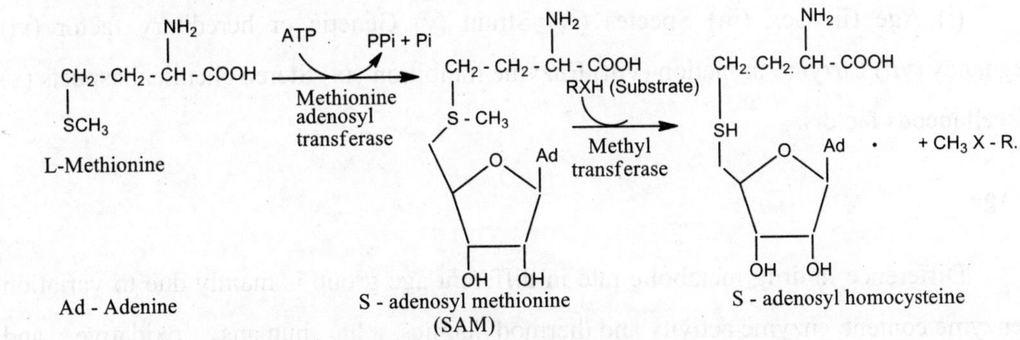

Fig. 4.8 Formation of S-adenosyl Homocysteine and Methylation

Examples of Conjugates of Methylation

Compound **Metabolite**

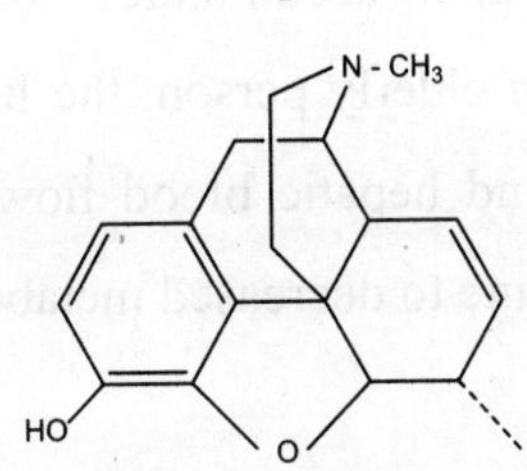

Morphine

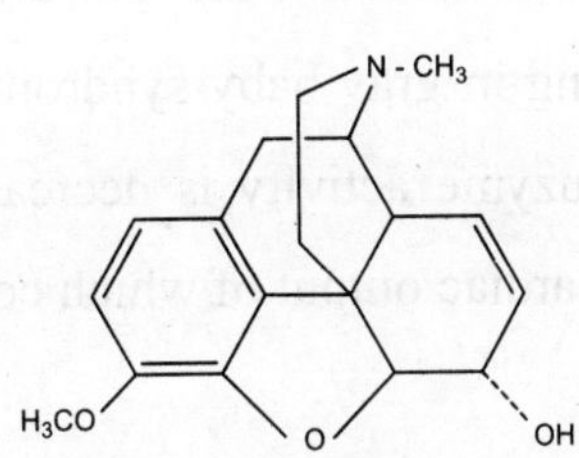

Codeine

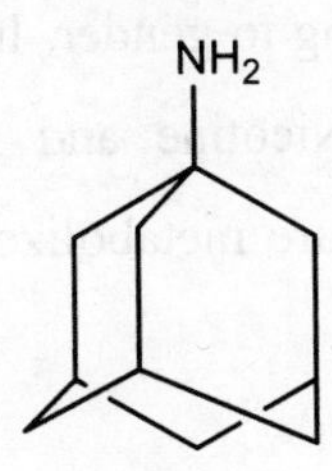

Amantadine

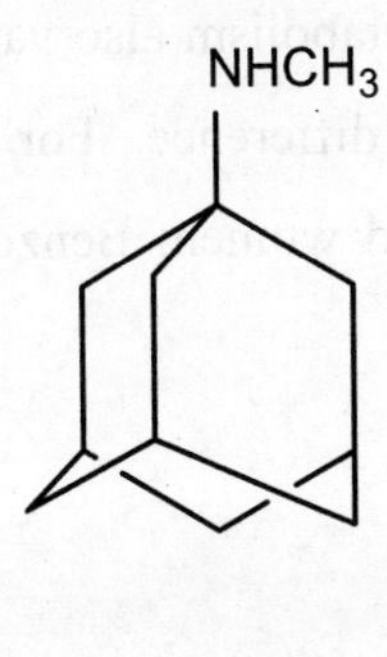

4. FACTORS AFFECTING DRUG METABOLISM

The rate of drug metabolism is important for its pharmacological action of the drug. The increase in the rate of drug metabolism will decrease the intensity, duration of action and efficacy of the drug. But the decrease in the rate of drug metabolism may lead to the accumulation of drug to toxicity level.

The various factors that may affect drug metabolism are:

(i) Age (ii) Sex (iii) Species (iv) Strain (v) Genetic or hereditary factor (vi) Pregnancy (vii) Enzyme induction (viii) Enzyme inhibition (ix) Stereo chemical aspects (x) Miscellaneous factors.

(i) Age

Difference in drug metabolic rate in different age group is mainly due to variation in enzyme content, enzyme activity and thermodynamics. In humans, oxidative and conjugative capabilities of newborn are low compared with those of adults. So in neonates (up to 2 months) many drugs are bio transformed slowly. For example, caffeine has a half-life of 4 days in neonates in comparison to 4 hours in adult. The inability of infants to conjugate Chloramphenicol with glucuronic acid accumulates toxic level of these antibiotics, resulting in gray baby syndrome. In elderly person, the liver size is reduced; the microsomal enzyme activity is decreased and hepatic blood flow also declines as a result of reduced cardiac output of which contribute to decreased metabolism of drugs.

(ii) Sex

The rate of metabolism also varies according to gender. In human, there have been few reports on sex difference. For example, Nicotine and Aspirin are metabolized differently in men and women; Benzodiazepines are metabolized slowly in women than men.

(iii) Species

Species difference has been observed in both Phase I and Phase II reaction. For example, metabolism of amphetamine occurs by two main pathways; oxidative deamination or aromatic hydroxylation. In humans, rabbits and guinea pig oxidative deamination appear to be predominant pathway; in rat aromatic hydroxylation appear to be major route. In humans, Phenytoin undergoes aromatic oxidation to give S (-) hydroxy phenytoin but in dogs it is metabolized as R (+) m - hydroxy phenytoin. Species difference in Phase II is caused by the presence or absence of the *transferase* enzyme involved in the conjugation pathway. For example, cats lack *glucuronyl transferase* enzyme and therefore tend to conjugate phenolic xenobiotic by sulfonation. In pigs it is reversed: pigs lack *sulfate transferase*, so they excrete as glucuronide conjugate. Glycine conjugation is a common conjugation pathway for benzoic acid in animals. But certain birds utilize ornithine.

(iv) Strain

Strain difference in drug metabolism exists particularly in inbred mice and rabbit. The differences apparently are caused by genetic variation in the amount of metabolizing enzyme present among the different strain. For example, *in vitro* studies indicate, cottontail rabbit liver microsome metabolizes 10 times faster than New Zealand rabbit liver microsomes.

(v) Hereditary or Genetic Factor

Many genetic factors are responsible for the large difference in the rate of metabolism of these drugs. For example, biotransformation of Isoniazid by acylation varies among different races.

(vi) Pregnancy

Studies in animals show that the maternal drug metabolizing ability is reduced during the later stage of pregnancy. This is due to high steroid hormone level during pregnancy. In women, the metabolism of Promazine and Pethidine is reduced during pregnancy or when receiving oral contraceptives.

(vii) Enzyme Induction

The activity of drug metabolizing enzyme can be increased by certain drugs, pesticides, polycyclic aromatic hydrocarbon. This process is termed as enzyme induction. Inducers may increase the rate of their own metabolism as well as those of other unrelated drugs.

For example, induction of microsomal enzyme by Phenobarbitone increases the metabolism of Warfarin, which decreases the anticoagulant activity when administered together. Long term treatment of anticonvulsant drug Phenobarbitone and Phenytoin result in osteomalacia due to enhanced metabolism of vitamin D_3. Theophylline, Pentazocine, Phenacetin and Propoxyphene are metabolized more rapidly in cigarette smokers due to the induction of microsomal enzyme cytochrome P_{450} by benzo (α) pyrene (present in cigarette smoke).

(viii) Enzyme Inhibition

Inhibitors are agents, which decrease rate of metabolism. Enzyme inhibition generally results in prolonged pharmacological action of drug. Some examples of inhibitors and drugs affected by them are given below:

Inhibitors	**Drugs which decrease metabolism**
Phenylbutazone	(S) (-) Warfarin
Allopurinol	6 - Mercapto purine
Chloramphenicol	Tolbutamide
Isoniazid	Phenytoin
Para Amino Salicylic acid	Hexobarbital

(ix) Stereochemical Aspects

Many drugs are administrated as racemic mixture. The two enantiomers present in the racemate may metabolize in different rates. For example less active (+) - Propranolol metabolizes more rapidly than the (-) enantiomer. S (-) Warfarin is 5 times more active than the R (+) - Warfarin because the latter metabolizes rapidly.

If only one stereoisomer is a substrate for the metabolizing enzyme or metabolic process, then it is termed as "substrate selective". For example, S (-) Warfarin is 7 - hydroxylated and R (+) isomer is keto reduced to R and S Warfarin.

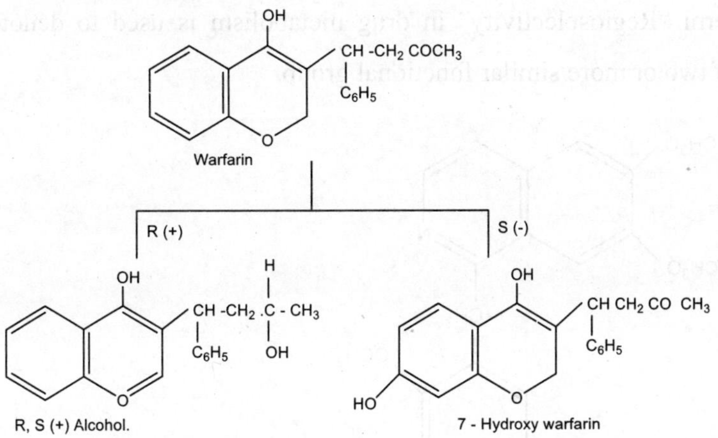

Drug biotransformation may also create a new asymmetric center in the metabolite; if one enantiomer predominates then it is termed as "stereo selective product". For example xenobiotic containing keto group predominantly gives one stereo isomeric alcohol.

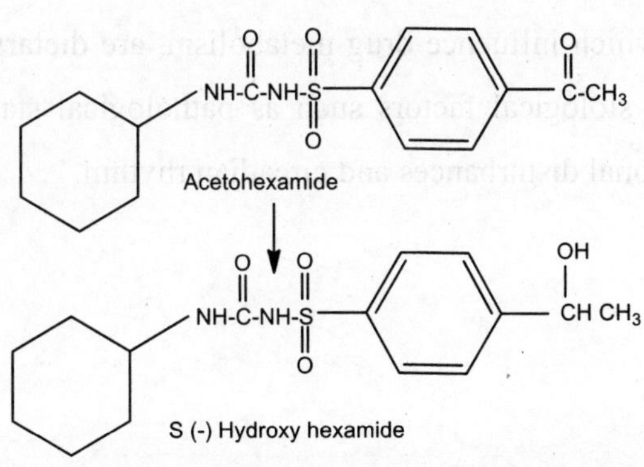

Phenytoin, the p-hydroxylation takes place predominantly in pro-(S) phenyl ring.

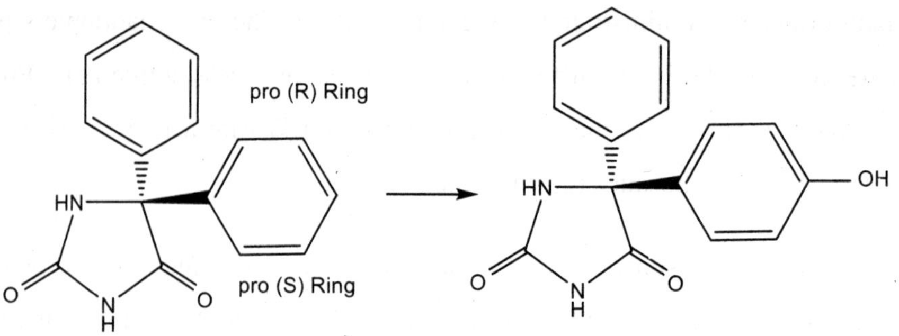

S (-) 5 - (4 - Hydroxy pheny) - 5 - phenyl hydantoin
major product

The term "Regioselectivity" in drug metabolism is used to denote the selective metabolism of two or more similar functional group.

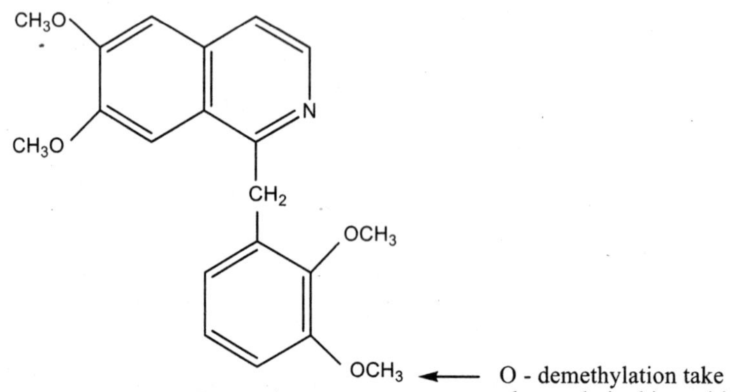

Papaverine

(x) Miscellaneous Factors

Other factors, which influence drug metabolism, are dietary factors like protein to carbohydrate ratio, Physiological factors such as pathological state of liver (eg. hepatic cancer, hepatitis) hormonal disturbances and circadian rhythm.

Chapter

5

ADRENERGIC DRUGS

1. INTRODUCTION

The adrenergic nervous system is the branch of autonomic nervous system which regulates many physiologic functions as blood pressure, heart rate, GIT motility and bronchial tone and also transport of lipid from fat depots to the liver. Adrenergic drugs are those chemical agents, which exert their pharmacological and therapeutic effects by acting at the peripheral sites of the sympathetic division of the autonomic nervous system.Adrenergic drugs, act by either enhancingor inhibiting the sympathetic nervous activity.

The drug that produces effect similar to stimulation of sympathetic nervous activity (Fight or Flight responses, e.g. an increase in heart rate, rise in blood pressure and dilated pupils of eyes) are known as sympathomimetic, adrenomimetics or adrenergic stimulants. The agents which inhibit or decrease the sympathetic nervous activity are known as sympatholytic, antiadrenergic or adrenergic blocking agents.

1.1 Adrenergic Nerve Transmission

Adrenergic nerves release the neurotransmitters namely Nor-epinephrine (Nor-adrenaline), Epinephrine and Dopamine.

(i) Norepinephrine (NE)

It is a neurotransmitter of the postganglionic sympathetic neuron. It is released from nerve ending in response to a nerve impulse or drug. It interacts with α and β-receptor site at presynaptic and postsynaptic receptors.

(ii) Epinephrine

It is not released from nerve endings, but synthesized and stored in the adrenal medulla, from which it is released into the circulation. Thus Epinephrine is often referred as a neuro-hormone.

(iii) Dopamine

It is a neurotransmitter in the basal ganglia of CNS. *Dopamine β-hydroxylase* enzyme converts Dopamine into Norepinephrine. This enzyme is not present in the dopaminergic neuron. Hence it remains in original form to carry out the function of neurotransmitter.

1.2 Biosynthesis

The endogenous catecholamines are Epinephrine, Norepinephrine (NE) and Dopamine (DA). The catecholamines are so named because they contain a catecholgroup and an aminegroup. A catechol group is a benzene ring that has hydroxyl groups on two adjacent carbons. The amine component of the catecholamine is ethylamine. Catecholamines biosynthesis takes place in adrenergic and dopaminergic neurons in the central nervous system and in sympathetic neurons in autonomic nervous system and in the adrenal medulla.

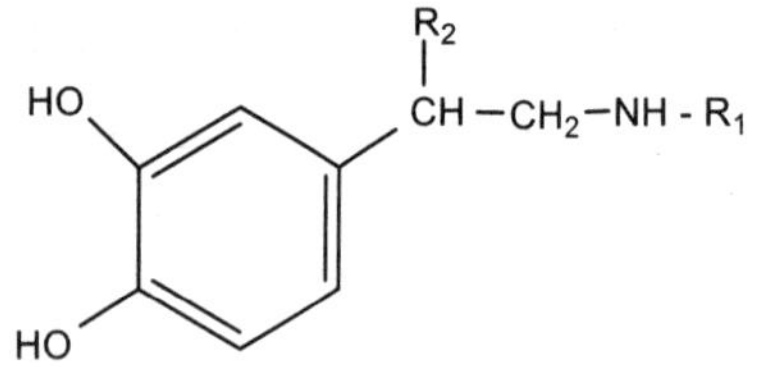

Name	R_1	R_2
Epinephrine	$-CH_3$	-OH
Norepinephrine	-H	-OH
Dopamine	-H	-H

The catecholamine biosynthesis involves the following steps (Fig. 5.1)

(i) The aromatic amino acid L-Tyrosine serves as a precursor. It is converted intoL-dihydroxy phenyl alanine (L-dopa) by *Tyrosine hydroxylase (Tyrosine-3-monooxygenase)*. This is the rate limiting step, so inhibition of *Tyrosine hydroxylase* is target for many drugs.

(ii) The second step is the decarboxylation of L-dopa by *L-aromatic amino acid decarboxylase (dopa decarboxylase)* to dopamine.

(iii) The dopamine formed in the cytoplasm of the neuron is transported into storage vesicle, where it is β-hydroxylated stereo specifically by the enzyme D*opamine β-monooxygenase* (*dopamine-β-hydroxylase*) in the side chain to Nor-epinephrine and stored in vesicles as its adenosine triphosphate complex.

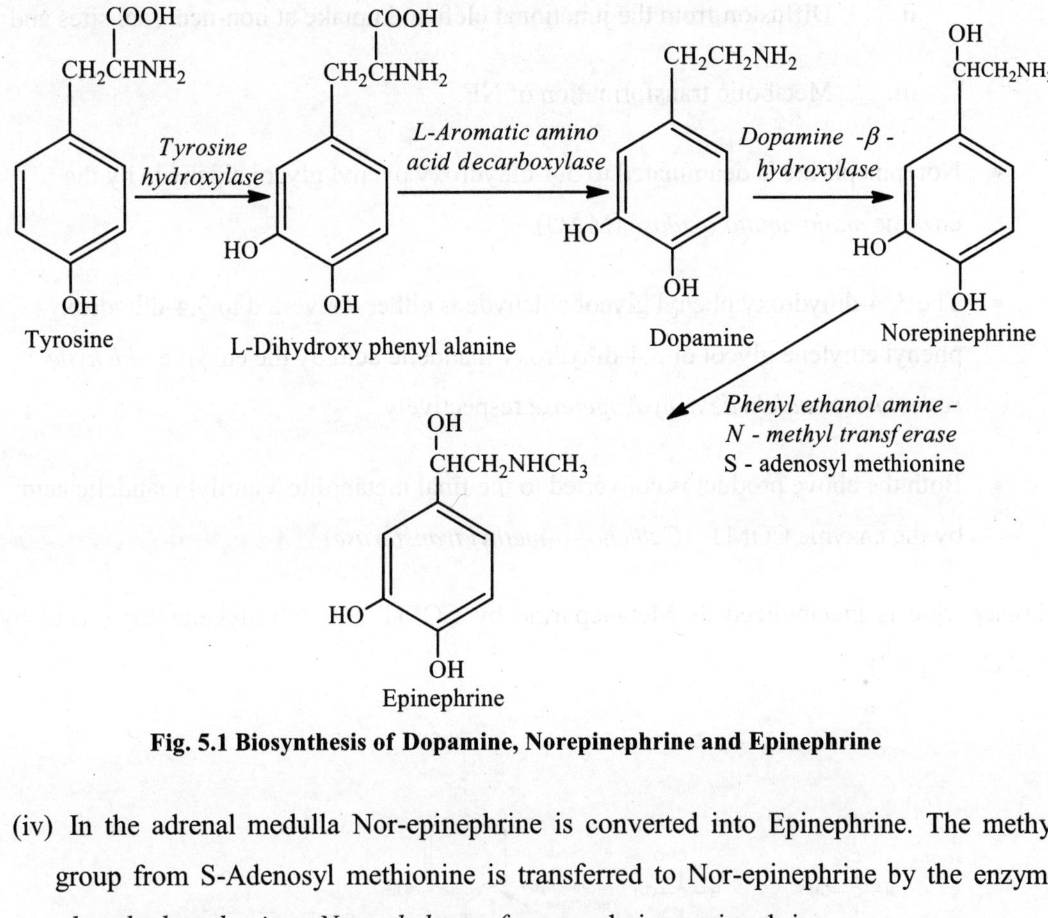

Fig. 5.1 Biosynthesis of Dopamine, Norepinephrine and Epinephrine

(iv) In the adrenal medulla Nor-epinephrine is converted into Epinephrine. The methyl group from S-Adenosyl methionine is transferred to Nor-epinephrine by the enzyme *phenyl ethanolamine - N- methyl transferase* and gives epinephrine.

Following the biosynthesis and storage in a vesicle, NE is released in the synapses due to the entrance of Ca+ into the cells. The inflow of Ca^{++} triggers the fusion of vesicle with the cell membrane resulting in exocytosis.

1.3 Metabolism of Catechol amines

The actions of Adrenaline and Noradrenaline are terminated by three processes;

i. Re-uptake into the presynaptic neuron terminal.

ii. Diffusion from the junctional cleft and uptake at non-neuronal sites and

iii. Metabolic transformation of NE.

- Norepinephrine is deaminated to 3,4-dihydroxy phenyl glycol aldehyde by the enzyme *mono amino oxidase* (MAO)
- The 3, 4-dihydroxy phenyl glycol aldehyde is either converted to 3,4-dihydroxy phenyl ethylene glycol or 3,4-dihydroxy mandelic acid by the enzyme *aldehyde reductase* or *aldehyde dehydrogenase* respectively.
- Both the above product is converted to the final metabolite Vanillyl mandelic acid by the enzyme COMT (*Catechol-o-methyl transferase*)

Epinephrine is metabolized as Metanephrine by COMT and Vanillyl mandelic acid by MAO. (Fig.5.2)

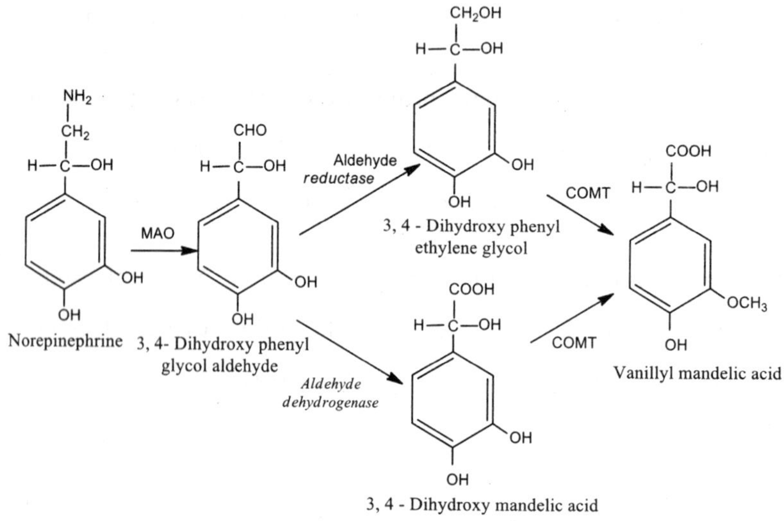

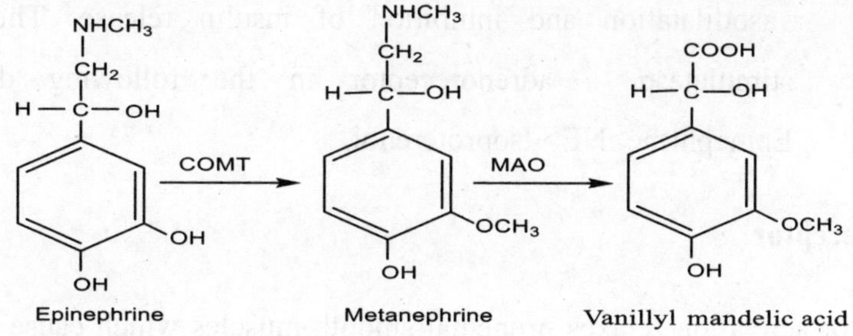

Fig. 5.2 Metabolic Pathways of Catecholamines

1.4 Adrenergic Receptors

Adrenoreceptor is a class of G protein coupled receptor.They islocated throughout the body on neuronal and non-neuronal tissues where they mediate endogenous catecholamines. They are classified into 2 major classes: α-adrenoceptors and β-adrenoceptorson the basis of their responses to the adrenergic agonists. Binding of catecholamine to the receptor is responsible for fight or flight response. All adrenoceptors contains 7-*trans* membrane alpha helical subunits, three extra cellular loops and three intracellular loops. Subtypes of both α- and β-adrenoceptors exist.

a) Alpha Receptors

The subtype of α receptors are α_1 and α_2 receptors which are furtherdivided into α_{1A}, α_{1B}, $\alpha_{1C}$and α_{1D} and into α_{2A}, α_{2B} and α_{2C}.Stimulation of α- receptors is associated with constriction of small blood vessels in the bronchial mucosa and relaxation of smooth muscles.

(i) α_1-Adrenergic receptors. They are found in the smooth muscles of iris, arteries, arterioles and veins.Agonism causes vasoconstrictionand relaxation of GIT.

(ii) α_2-Adrenergic receptors. They are found in presynaptic neurons, postsynaptic tissues (ocular, adipose, intestinal, hepatic, renal, and endocrine) pancreas and arterioles. Agonism causes sedation, analgesia, vasodilatation and inhibition of insulin release. The catechol amine stimulatesα – adrenoreceptor in the following descending order: Epinephrine>NE> Isoproterenol.

b) Beta Receptor

β-receptor activation relaxes bronchial smooth muscles which cause the bronchi of the lungs to dilate. In addition, β-receptor stimulatory effects cause an increase in the rate and force of heart contractions.

β-Adrenergic receptors are of three types. They are;

(i) β_1-Adrenergic receptors: They are found in the myocardium (heart) where their stimulation increases the force and rate of myocardial contraction.

(ii) β_2-Adrenergic receptors: These are found in uterine, skeletal, vascular and bronchial smooth muscles where their stimulation causes smooth muscle dilation or relaxation.

(iii) β_3-Adrenergic receptors: These receptors are present on fat cells and their stimulation causes lipolysis and thermogenesis.β-adrenoreceptors are stimulated by catecholamines in the following descending order:
Isoproterenol>Epinephrine>NE

1.4.1 Mechanism of Adrenergic Receptors

- α_1 - receptor is a Gq coupled receptor. Activation of α_1-receptor with agonist increases intracellular Ca^{2+} through the IP_3 signal transduction pathway and activates smooth muscle contraction. Stimulation of α_1 receptors causes vasoconstriction, pupillary dilatation (mydriasis) and sphincter contraction.
- α_2 is Gi coupled receptor. Activation of the α_2-receptor decreases production of cAMP, leading to an inhibition of further release of Norepinephrine from

the neuron. Stimulation of central α_2-receptor causes sedation, analgesia and reduced sympathetic outflow (vasodilation).

- All three β-receptors are linked to Gs proteins (although β2-also couples to Gi), which in turn are linked to *adenylate cyclase*. β-receptor couple with Gs and increases intracellular cAMP activity, resulting in heart muscle contraction, smooth muscle relaxation and glycogenolysis.

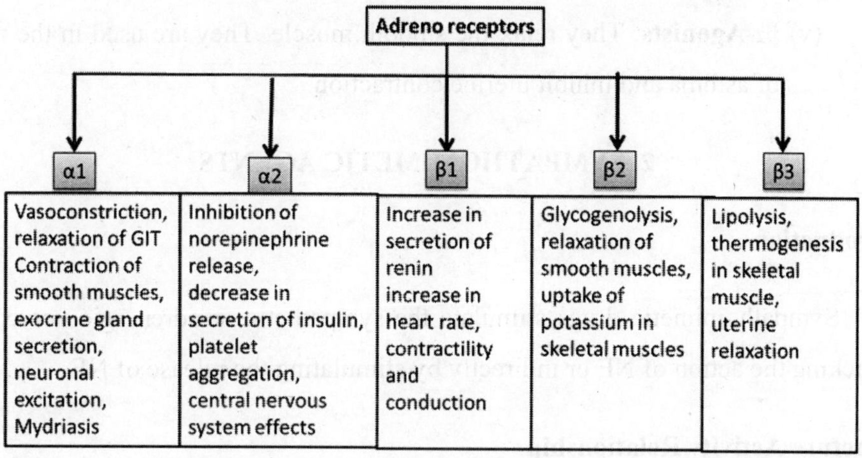

Fig. 5.3 Various Pharmacological Actions of Adrenoceptors

1.4.2 Clinical uses of Adrenergic Agents

(i) **α_1-Agonist**: Agonist act on α_1- receptor and causes vasoconstriction and so they are used along with anesthetics to prolong its duration of action. They are also used as nasal decongestant.

(ii) **α_1-Antagonist**: These agents are vasodilators, used in the treatment of hypertension. They also block α_{1A}-receptor in the smooth muscle and relax the muscle used in the treatment of benign prostatic hyperplasia (BPH)

(iii) **α_2-Agonist**: They relax the smooth muscle by decreasing the NE release at the sympathetic nerve terminal. These agent act on CNS and decreases the sympathetic out flow to the periphery. Therapeutic uses of these agents are antihypertensive, glaucoma, analgesic and sedative.

(iv) **β_1-Antagonists**: β_1-blockers slow down the heart rate and decreases the force of contraction. They are used in the treatment of hypertension, angina and cardiac arrhythmias.

(v) **β_2-Agonists**: They relax the smooth muscle. They are used in the treatment of asthma and inhibit uterine contraction.

2. SYMPATHOMIMETIC AGENTS

2.1 Introduction

Sympathomimetic drugs stimulate the sympathetic or adrenergic nerve, directly by mimicking the action of NE or indirectly by stimulating the release of NE.

2.2 Structure Activity Relationship

The sympathomimetic drugs may be divided into catechol and non-catechol amines.

- All the catechol amine possesses catechol nucleus.

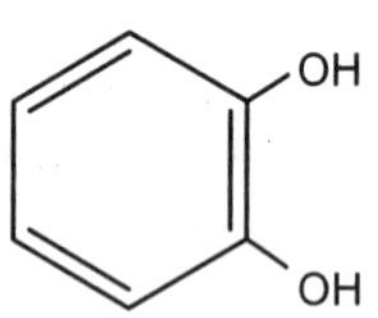

Catechol

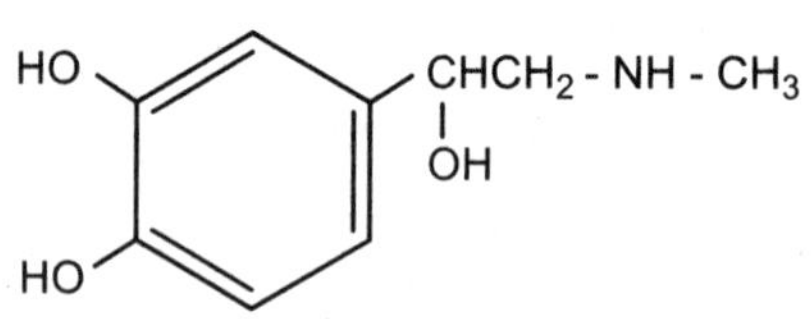

Adrenaline

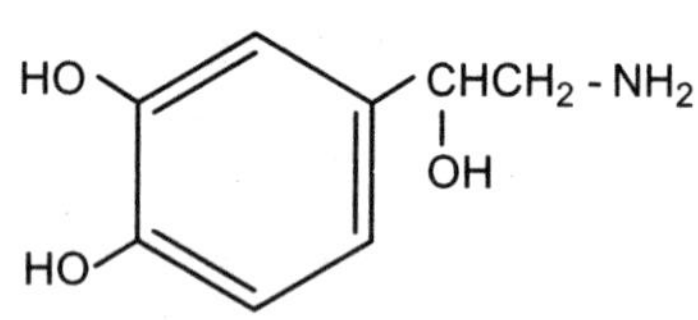

Noradrenaline

- Non catecholamine consists of a benzene ring and an ethylamine side chain.

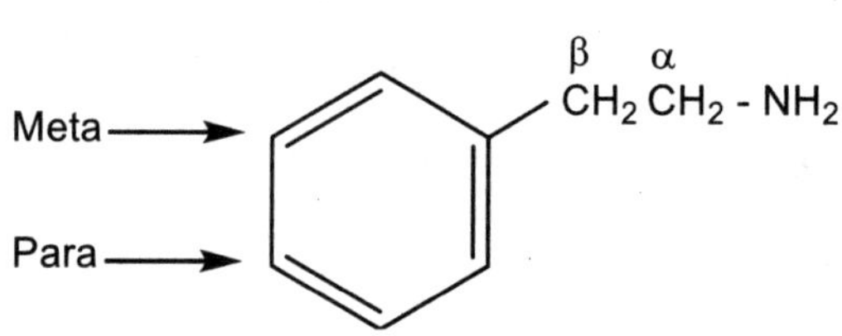

i) β-phenyl ethylamine type of Adrenergic Agonist

- β-phenyl ethylamine is the parent structure for many sympathomimetic drugs. The modifications of β-phenylethylamine influence not only the mechanism of action, receptor selectivity, but also their absorption, oral activity, metabolism and duration of action.

ii) The basic structure required for OptimalAgonist Activity

- ✓ Aromatic ring with amino side chain separated by two carbon
- ✓ Hydroxyl group at β-carbon of the side chain
- ✓ Primary or secondary amino group

iii) Aromatic Ring

- The presence of -OH group in the 3' and 4' position (Catechol) of the benzene ring show maximum α and β-adrenergic activity. But poor oral availability due to rapid metabolism by COMT.
- Removal or replacement with hydroxy methyl group of 3' and 4' -OH group increases the oral bioavailability and duration of activity. eg. Albuterol.
- The lack of -OH group in the aromatic ring and β-carbon of the side chain increases the CNS activity and decreases adrenergic activity. eg. Amphetamine, Methamphetamine.
- When both the - OH is removed potency of the compound reduces.eg. Phenyl epinephrine is less potent than adrenaline.

iv) Ethyl amine Substitution

- For optimal activity the amino group should be separated from aromatic ring by 2-carbon atom.

- The presence of -OH group in β-carbon enhances agonist activity at both α and β receptor and decreases the CNS activity.
- Substitution in C_1 and C_2results in optical isomers; 1R, 2S isomer seems to be correct configuration for direct acting agonist.
- Substitution in the β-carbon decreases CNS activity and increases adrenergic activity. For example, Epinephrine is less potent than Methamphetamine as a CNS stimulant, but more potent vasoconstrictor and bronchodilator.

v) Amino Substitution

- The presence of amino group in phenyl ethyl amine is important for direct agonist activity.
- The amine is normally ionized at physiological pH and for optimal activity the pKa should be between 8.5 -10.0.
- 1° and 2° amine have good adrenergic activity than 3° and quaternary ammonium salt.
- As the size of the alkyl group in the amino group increases, α-receptor agonist activity decreases and β-agonist activity increases

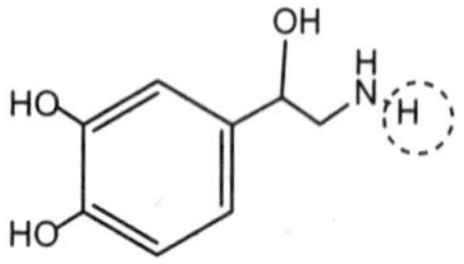

Norepinephrine
α-agonist

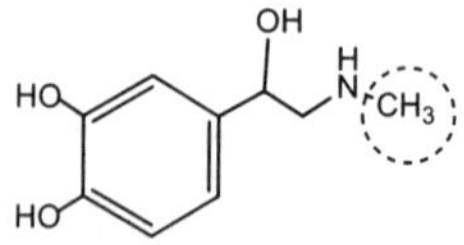

Epinephrine
non-selective α and β-agonist

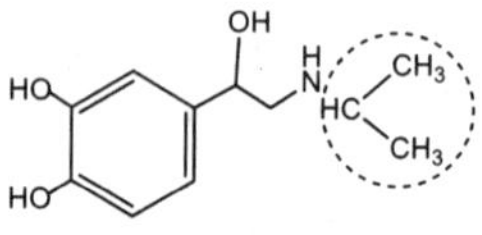

Isoproterenol
non-selective β-agonist

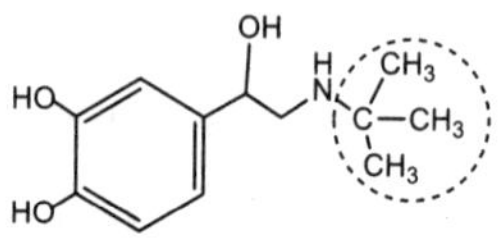

N-t-Butyl nor-epinephrine
selective β_2-agonist

Imidazoline type of α - Adrenergic Agonist

- A second chemical class of α-agonists is imidazolines. These agents are selective α-Adrenergic agonist vasoconstrictor. eg. Naphazoline,

Antazoline, Tetrahydrozoline, Xylomethazoline. They are selective for either α_1 or α_2-receptors.

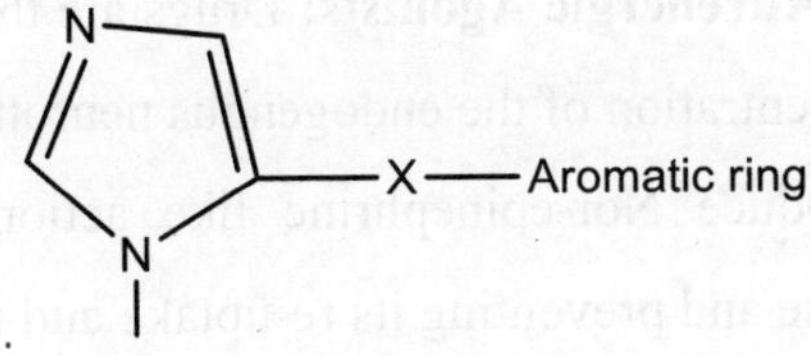

X= CH_2-, NH -

- **Structurally, most imidazolines have their heterocyclic imidazoline nucleus linked to a substituted aromatic moiety via some type of bridging unit. The optimum bridging unit (X) is usually a single methylene group or amino group.**
- Substitution in the aromatic ring enhances the agonist activity.

2.3 Classification of Adrenergic Agonists

Adrenergic agonists are sub-divided into 3 classes; direct acting, indirect-acting and dual-acting agonists. These agents act on sympathetic nervous system and activate it.

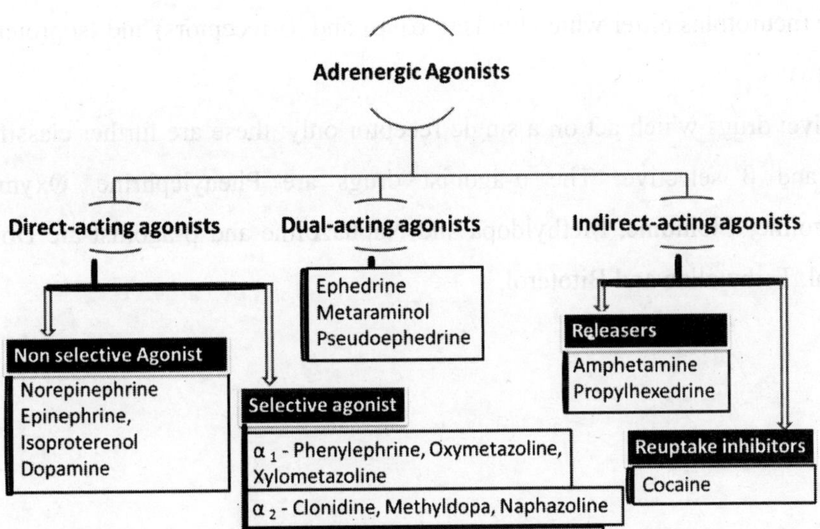

i. **Direct-acting Adrenergic Agonists**: Drugs are those that directly act on and activate the receptors to produce the desired pharmacological effects.

ii. **Indirect-acting Adrenergic Agonists:** Drugs are those that act indirectly to increase the concentration of the endogenous neurotransmitter by causing its release.They produce Nor-epinephrine like actions by stimulating Nor-epinephrinerelease and preventing its re-uptake and thus it inactivates.

iii. **Dual-acting Adrenergic Agonists:** These agents act as direct and indirect-adrenergic agonists.

2.3.1 Direct-Acting Sympathomimetics (Agonists)

These drugs act directly on one or more adrenergic receptors. According to receptor selectivity they are two types:

(i) Non-selective: drugs act on one or more receptors: Naturally occurring molecules (endogenous amines) which bind to these receptors include Nor-epinephrine (a neurotransmitter which binds to α_1, α_2 and β_1-receptors), Epinephrine (a hormone produced in and secreted from the adrenal medulla which binds to α_1, α_2, β_1 and β_2–receptors) Dopamine (neurotransmitter which binds to α_1, β_1 and β_2-receptors) and Isoproterenol (acts on β_1, β_2, β_3).

(ii) Selective: drugs which act on a single receptor only; these are further classified into α selective and β selective. The α-agonist drugs are Phenylephrine, Oxymetazoline, Xylometazoline, Clonidine, Methyldopa and Naphazoline and β-agonist are Dobutamine, Salbutamol, Terbutaline and Bitoterol.

2.3.1.1 Non-selective Agonist

A. Dopamine (Dopalim)

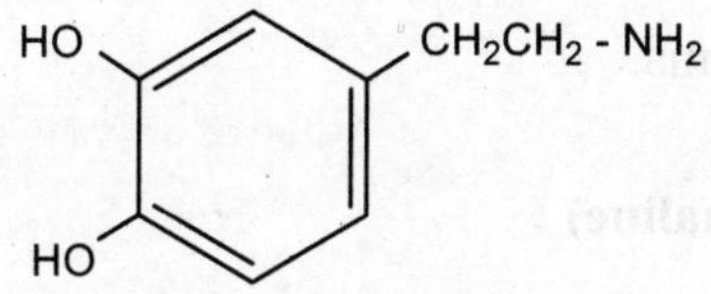

1- (3, 4 - Dihydroxy phenyl) - 2 - amino ethane

Mechanism of action: Dopamine receptor agonists can act on D1 or D2 receptors. D1 receptors activate *adenyl cyclase* and increase intracellular cAMP mainly in neurons and vascular smooth muscle. D2 receptor reduces intracellular cAMP and is found in the brain and as pre-synaptic receptors.

Use: It is used in the treatment of shock.

B. Epinephrine (Adrenaline)

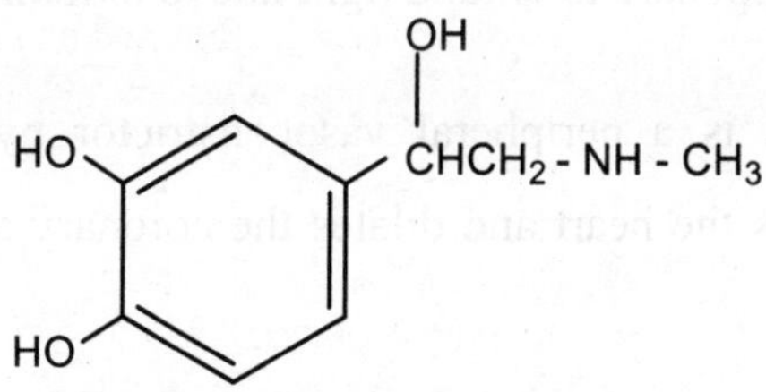

1 - (3, 4 - Dihydroxy phenyl) - 2 - methyl amino ethanol

Adrenaline is a catecholamine belongs to the family of biogenic amines.(R) Epinephrine is 12 times more active than (S) form. It has a potent stimulatory effect on both α and β-adrenergic receptors. Like other catecholamines, Epinephrine is light sensitive and easily oxidized on exposure to air because of catechol ring system.It is not effective orally because of poor absorption and rapid metabolism by MAO and COMT. Therefore, it is administered parenterally.

Mechanism of action: It acts by stimulation of α, $\beta_1$and β_2-adrenergic receptors.

Use: It is used as anti-asthmatic agent. It is used to prevent bleeding during surgery or in case of inner organ bleeding. It is also used in the treatment of heart block or circulatory collapse and open-angle glaucoma.

C. Norepinephrine (Noradrenaline)

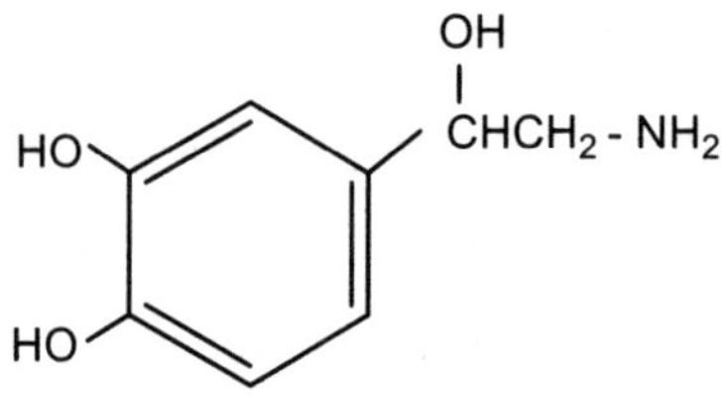

L - 1- (3, 4 - Dihydroxy phenyl) - 2 - amino ethanol

It differs from Adrenaline only by lacking the methyl substitution on the amino ethanol. L-isomer is pharmacologically active. Nor-adrenaline should be protected from air and light as it darkens on exposure to air and light due to oxidation of catechol group.

Mechanism of action: It is a peripheral vasoconstrictor by stimulating α-adrenergic receptors. It also stimulates the heart and dilates the coronary arteries byits activity at the β-adrenergic receptors.

Use: It is administered topically for the treatment of primary open angle glaucoma.

D. Isoproterenol (Isoprenaline - Saventrine)

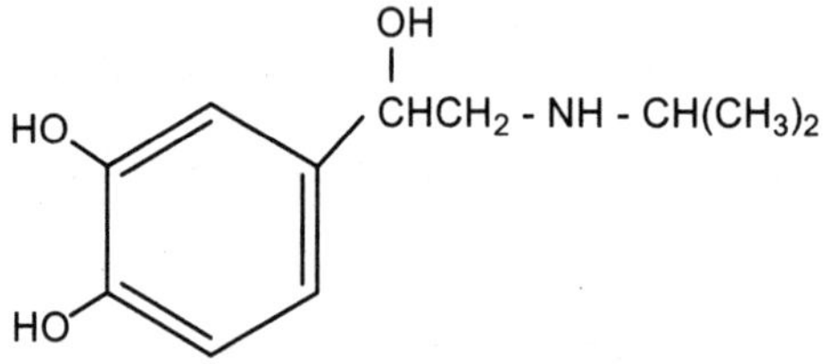

(dl) - β - (3, 4 - Dihydroxy phenyl)
isopropyl amino ethanol

It is a synthetic isopropyl analogue of Adrenaline and a non-selectiveβ-agonist. It stimulates the action of Adrenaline and has the advantage of being effective when given orally. The isopropyl amino group makes it selective for β-receptor.

Mechanism of action: It stimulates the β-adrenergic receptor and increases cAMP level associated with bronchial smooth muscle. It also acts by inhibiting the release of mediators of immediate hypersensitivity from mast cells.

Use: It is used to treat asthma, chronic bronchitis and emphysema.

2.3.1.2 Selective Agonist

A. Phenylephedrine (Ikamed)

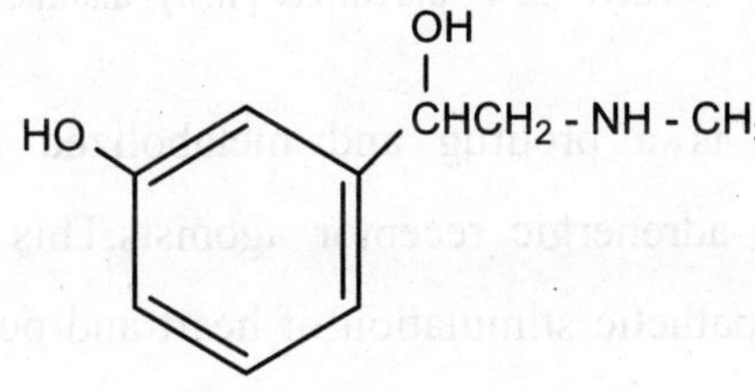

(-) - 1 - (3 - Hydroxyphenyl) - 2 - methyl amino ethanol

Phenylephrine differs from Adrenaline only by lacking 4th -OH group on the benzene ring and subsequently resistant to COMT and has predominantly α_1-agonist effect.

Synthesis

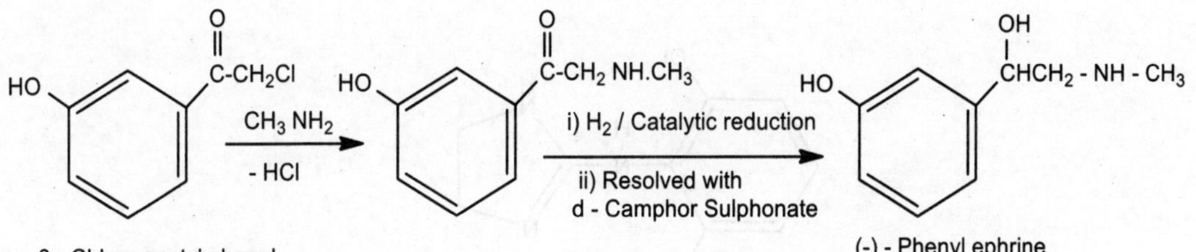

Mechanism of action: It stimulates α-adrenergic receptors causes arterial and venous constriction and increases peripheral vascular resistance and systolic blood pressure.

Intranasal use directly stimulates α-adrenergic receptors on the nasal mucosa, constricting local vessels and decreasing blood flow and mucosal edema.

Use: It is used as a nasal decongestant, mydriatic and vasopressor agent. It is also used in spinal anesthesia, to prolong the anesthesia and to prevent the drop in blood pressure during the procedure.

B. Methyldopa (Alphadopa)

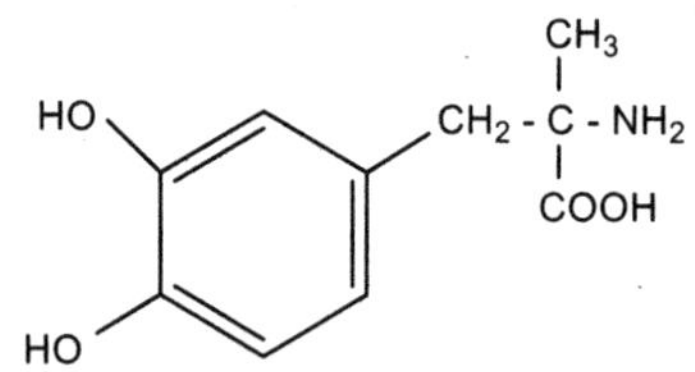

L - Methyl - 3, 4 - dihydroxy phenyl alanine

Mechanism of action: It is a prodrug and metabolized in the CNS to α-methyl norepinephrine which is α_2-adrenergic receptor agonists.This action may reduce blood pressure by decreasing sympathetic stimulation of heart and peripheral vascular system.It stimulates peripheral α-adrenergic receptors in CNS to produce transient vasoconstriction and then stimulates central α-adrenergic receptors in the brain stem to reduce peripheral vascular resistance, heart rate and systolic and diastolic blood pressure.

Use: Antihypertensive agent. It is preferred for high blood pressure in pregnancy.

C. Clonidine (Catapres)

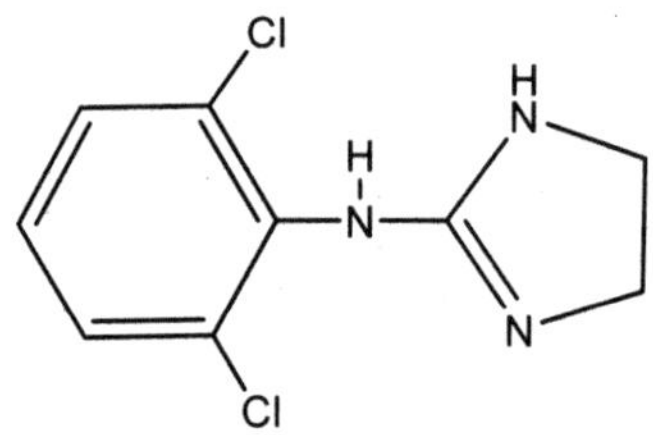

N - (2, 6 - Dichloro phenyl) - 4, 5 - dihydro -1H - imidazol - 2 - amine

Clonidine is an example of phenyl imino imidazoline derivative that possesses selective α_2-adrenergic receptor.

Mechanism of action: It stimulates peripheral α-adrenergic receptors in CNS to produce transient vasoconstriction and then stimulates central α-adrenergic receptors in the brain stem to reduce peripheral vascular resistance, heart rate and systolic and diastolic blood pressure.

Use: It is used as antihypertensive agent.

D. Dobutamine (Dobonis)

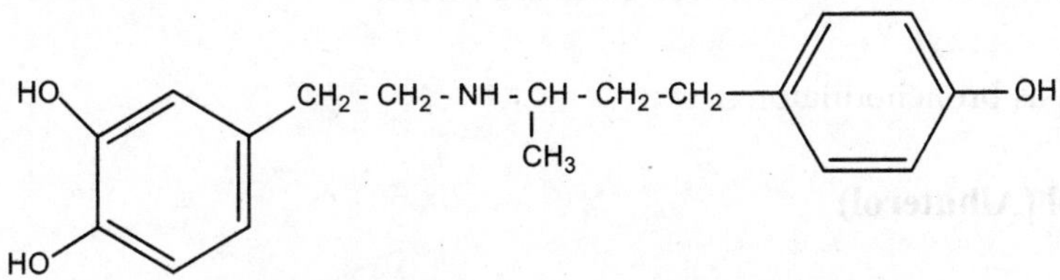

N - [1 - Methyl - 3 - (4 - hydroxyphenyl) propyl] -
3, 4 - dihydroxy phenyl ethyl amine

It resembles Dopamine chemically, but possess a bulky aromatic residue on the amino group despite the absence of a β-OH group. Racemic Dobutamine has direct activity on both α_1 and β_1-receptors. The S (-) enantiomer exhibit α_1 and β_1-agonist activity. The R (+) enantiomer is a α_1-antagonists; thus, racemates results in overall β_1-agonist activity.

Mechanism of action: It stimulates β_1, β_2 and α_1-adrenergic receptors. β_1-receptor stimulation produces a positive inotropic effect on the myocardium, increasing cardiac output by boosting myocardial contractility and stroke volume.

Use: It is used in heart failure associated with myocardial infarction, open heart surgery and cardiomyopathy.

E. Terbutaline (Bricanyl)

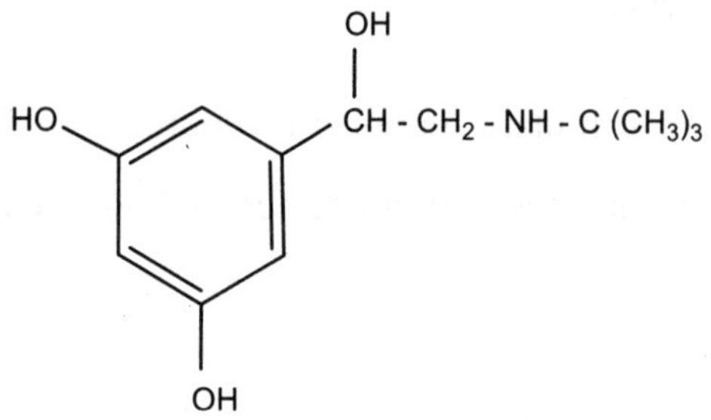

N - Tert butyl - 2 - [(3, 5 - dihydroxy phenyl) - 2 - hydroxy] ethyl amine

Mechanism of action: It stimulates β-adrenergic receptors increases c-AMP levels associated with relaxation of bronchial smooth muscle.

Use: It is used as bronchodilator.

F. Salbutamol (Albuterol)

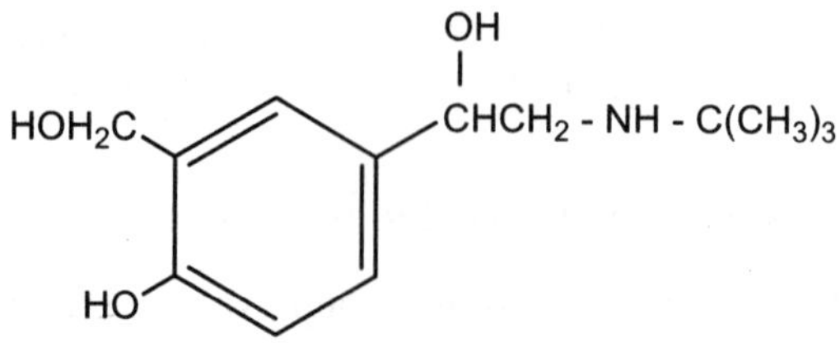

4 - Hydroxy - 3 - hydroxy methyl - α - [(tert - butyl amino) methyl] benzyl alcohol

Salbutamol is sold as racemic mixture of R and S-enantiomers. R-Salbutamol (Levalbuterol) is the active bronchodilator enantiomer whereas S-enantiomer exerts adverse effect like airway hyper reactivity and inflammation in the lungs as well as blocks the metabolic pathway.

Synthesis

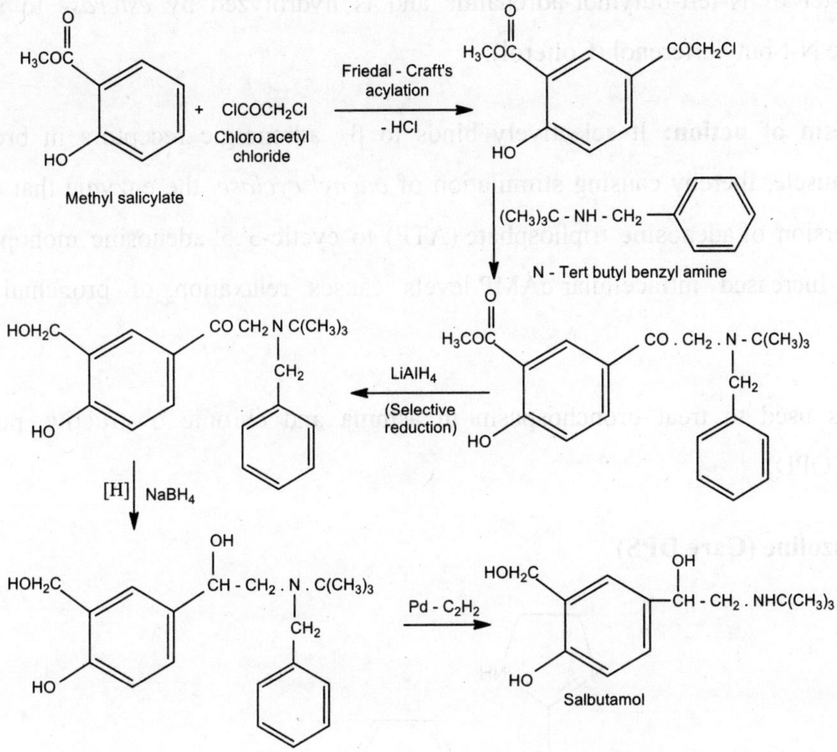

Mechanism of action: It binds to epinephrine active site in the β2-receptor and increases intracellular cyclic AMP. It inhibits the phosphorylation of myosin and lowers intracellular concentrationleads to a smooth muscle relaxation and bronchodilation.

Use: It is most widely used in the treatment of asthma and other form of reversible obstructive pulmonary disease

G. Bitoterol

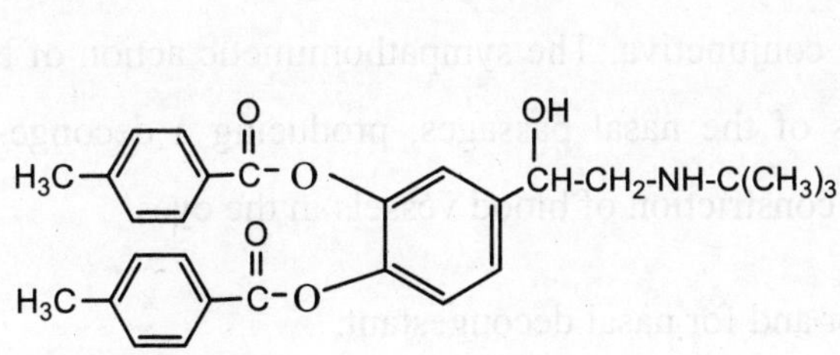

4 - (2 - (Tertbutylamino) - 1 - hydroxyethyl) - *o* - phenylene di - p - toluate

Bitoterol is a pro-drug for Colterol, a β_2-adrenergic receptor agonist. It is a di-4-toluate ester of N-tert-butylnor-adrenaline and is hydrolyzed by *esterase* to its active metabolite N-t-butylarterenol (Colterol).

Mechanism of action: It selectively binds to β_2 -adrenergic receptors in bronchiolar smooth muscle, thereby causing stimulation of *adenyl cyclase*, the enzyme that catalyzes the conversion of adenosine triphosphate (ATP) to cyclic-3',5'-adenosine monophosphate (cAMP). Increased intracellular cAMP levels causes relaxation of bronchial smooth muscle.

Use: It is used to treat bronchospasm in asthma and chronic obstructive pulmonary disease (COPD).

H. **Naphazoline (Care DPS)**

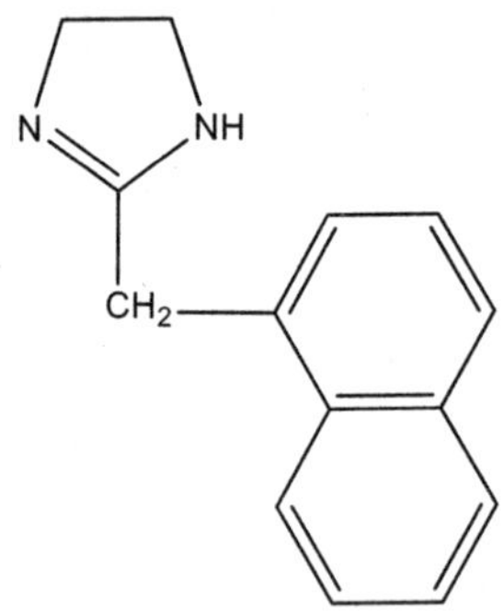

2 - (1 - Naphthyl methyl) - 2 - imidazoline

Mechanism of action: It is a direct acting sympathomimetic adrenergic α-agonist used to induce systemic vasoconstriction, thereby decreasing nasal congestion and inducingconstriction around the conjunctiva. The sympathomimetic action of Naphazoline constricts the smaller arterioles of the nasal passages, producing a decongesting effect. Naphazoline ophthalmic causes constriction of blood vessels in the eyes.

Use: It is used as vasoconstrictor and for nasal decongestant.

I. Xylometazoline (Diconal)

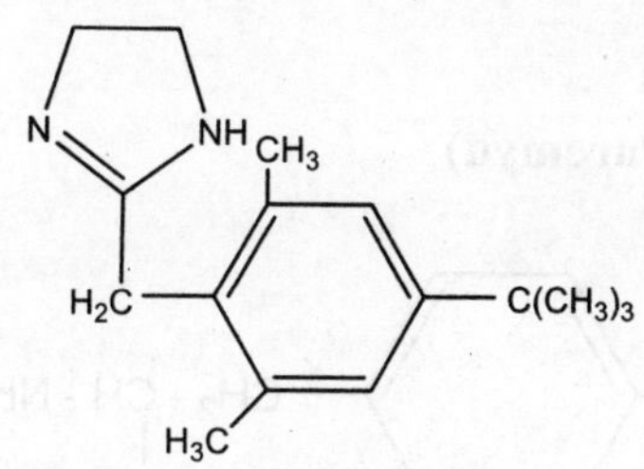

2 - [(4 - Tertbutyl) - 2, 6 - dimethyl benzyl] - 2 - imidazoline

Mechanism of action: It binds α-adrenergic receptors to activate the adrenal system which causes systemic vasoconstriction, thereby easing nasal congestion.

Use: It is a sympathomimetic decongestant. It also acts as a vasoconstrictor.

J. Oxymetazoline (Nasivion)

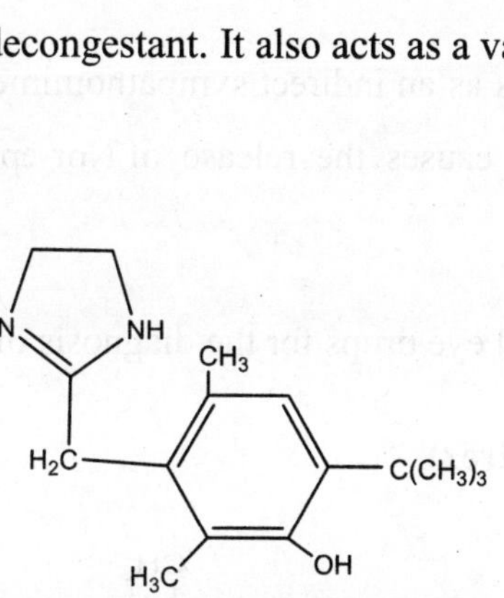

6 - Tert butyl - 3 - (4,5 - dihydro - 1H - imidazol - 2 - yl - methyl) - 2,4 - dimethyl - phenol

Mechanism of action: It is a direct acting sympathomimetic amine, which acts on α-adrenergic receptors in the arterioles of the conjunctiva and nasal mucosa.

Use: It is used topically as nasal decongestant.

2.3.2 Indirect-Acting Sympathomimetics

This class is comprised of non-catecholamines. Most of these drugs retain phenyl ethylamine skeleton. These compounds are resistant to *Catechol-o-methyltransferase* (COMT) and MAO enzymes due to lack of phenolic hydroxyl group and presence of α- methyl group. They pass more readily through blood brain barrier (BBB) because of its increased lipophilicity.

A. Hydroxyamphetamine (Paremyd)

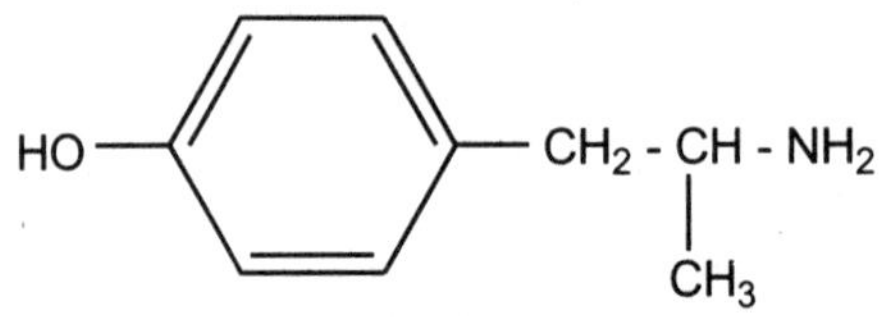

(±) - 1 - (p - Hydroxy phenyl) - 2 - amino propane

Itis a major metabolite of amphetamine, sympathomimetic amines with CNS stimulant activity.

Mechanism of action: It acts as an indirect sympathomimetic agent which causes dilation of the pupil of eyeand also causes the release of Nor-epinephrine from nerve synapses which leads to mydriasis.

Use: It is used mainly as local eye drops for the diagnosis of Horner's Syndrome.

B. Propylhexedrine (Benzedrex)

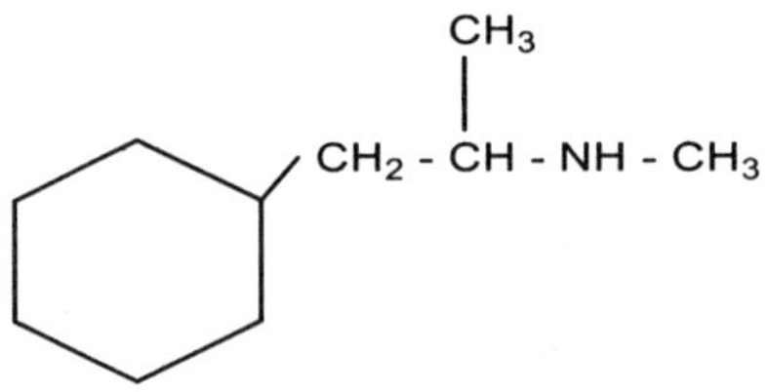

1- Cyclohexyl - 2 - methyl amino propane

Mechanism of action: It causes Nor-epinephrine, dopamine and serotonin (5HT) transporters to reverse their direction of flow. This inversion leads to the release of these transmitters from the vesicles to the cytoplasm and from the cytoplasm to the synapse.

Use: It is used as nasal decongestant and vasoconstrictor with no CNS effects.

2.3.3 Dual Acting Agonist

A. Ephedrine (Akovaz)

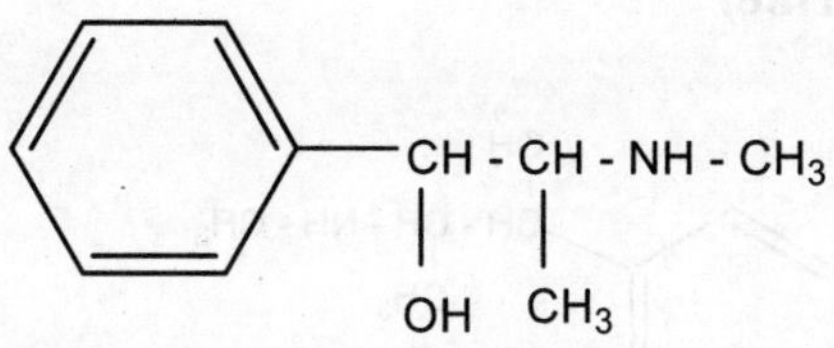

(1R, 2S) - 2 - Methyl amino - 1 - phenyl propan - 1- ol

Ephedrine is a phenyl ethyl amine alkaloid obtained from the stems of various species of *Ephedra called Ma huang* the plant containing Ephedrine. It is a synthetic non-catecholamine agonist at α_1, β_1 and β_2-receptors with both direct and indirect action. Ephedrine and pseudoephedrine are not a substrate for COMT and MAO. Therefore, these drugs have longer duration of action and excellent oral absorption. Ephedrine raises both systolic and diastolic blood pressure.

Stereochemistry

It has two asymmetric carbons, thus there are four optically active forms. The *erythro* racemate is called ephedrine and *threo* racemate is known as pseudoephedrine (Ψ ephedrine). Natural Ephedrine is D (-) isomer and is the most active of the four.

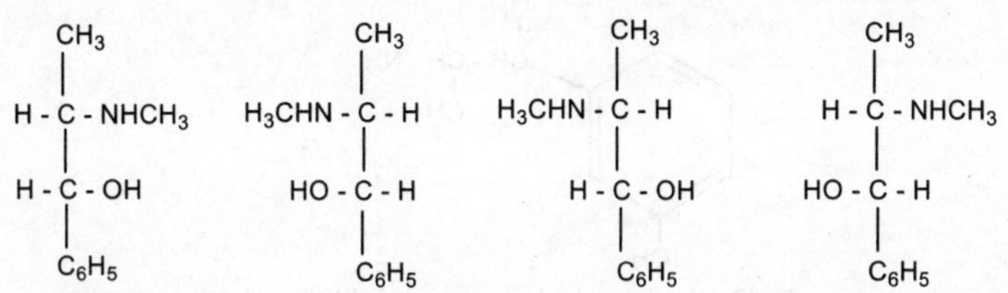

D (-) Ephedrine   L (+) Ephedrine   D (-) ψ Ephedrine   L (+) ψ Ephedrine

Mechanism of action: It has direct effect on both α and β-adrenoreceptor and inhibits MAO. It acts indirectly by releasing the stored nor-epinephrine from adrenergic neuron nerve terminal into the synaptic cleft contributing to non-specific activation. It is a mild CNS stimulant. It decreases urinary incontinence by increasing urethral sphincter.

Use: It is used in the treatment of urinary incontinence, vasoconstrictor, cardiac stimulant and nasal decongestant. It is also used as stimulant.

B. **Pseudoephedrine (Suphedrine)**

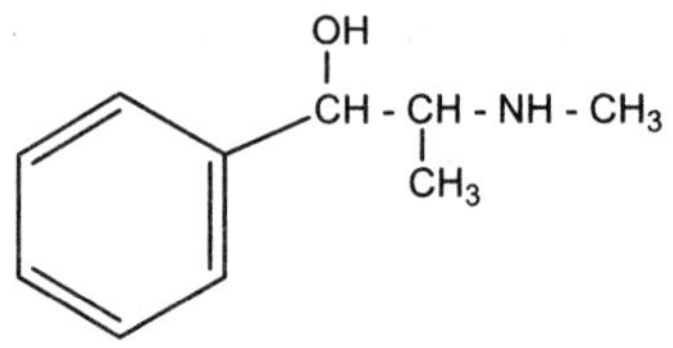

2-(Methylamino)-1-phenyl propan-1-ol

Pseudoephedrine is a diastereomer of ephedrine. It is a sympathomimetic drug of the Phenethylamine and Amphetamine chemical classes. Pseudoephedrine is a precursor of Methamphetamine and Methcathinone.

Mechanism of action: It acts directly on both α and β-adrenergic receptors. It produces vasoconstriction. It also relaxes bronchial smooth muscle by stimulating β2-adrenergic receptors.

Use: It is used as a nasal/sinus decongestant, as a stimulant or as a wakefulness-promoting agent in higher doses.

C. **Metaraminol (Pressonex)**

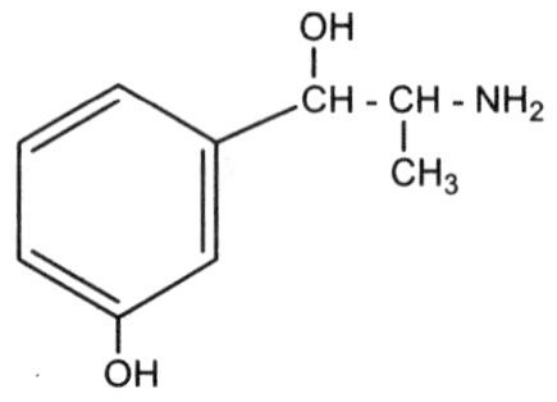

3 - (2 - Amino - 1 - hydroxypropyl) phenol

Mechanism of action: It acts through peripheral vasoconstriction by acting as α1-adrenergic agonist, which increases systemic blood pressure.

Use: It is used as a vasopressor in the treatment of hypotensive state occurring with spinal anesthesia.

3. SYMPATHOLYTICS (or) ADRENERGIC BLOCKING AGENTS

Adrenergic blocking agents refer to those drugs that reduce delivery of catecholamines to the adrenergic receptors by disrupting catecholamine synthesis, storage or release. They are called as sympatholytic because they abolish the response to stimulation of sympathetic nerves.

These agents competitively antagonize the effect of the catechol amines at α-and/ or β-adrenergic receptor.

3.1 α-Adrenergic Blocking Agents

α-blockers are employed as antihypertensive, on the chemical basis, they can be classified as:

α- Adrenergic Blocking Agents

Ergot alkaloids	Imidazolines	Quinazolines	β - Halo alkyl amines
Ergotamine Methysergide Dihydroergotamine Ergocristine	Tolazoline Phentolamine	Prazosin Tetrazosin Doxazosin	Phenoxybenzamine

3.1.1 Ergot Alkaloids

A. Methysergide (Sanserk)

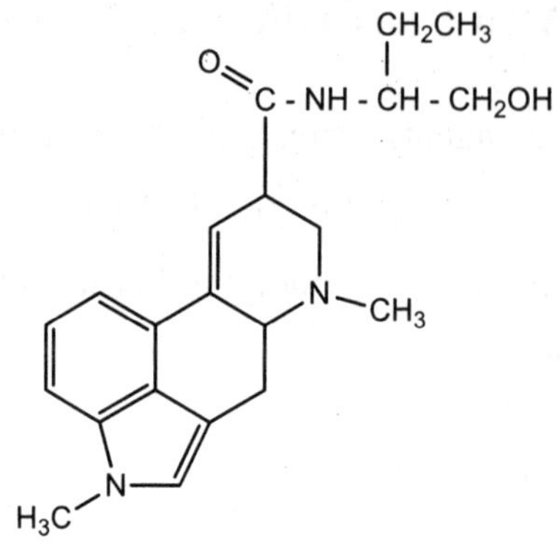

1-Methyl-D-lysergic acid butanolamide

It is a diethylamide lysergic acid derivative, a semi-synthetic ergot derivative

Mechanism of action: It antagonizes the effects of serotonin in blood vessels and gastrointestinal smooth muscle. It is a serotonin antagonistat 5-HT_1/5-HT_2act on central nervous system, which directly stimulates the smooth muscle leading to vasoconstriction.

Use: It is used for the treatment of migraine cluster and other vascular headache.

B. Dihydroergotamine

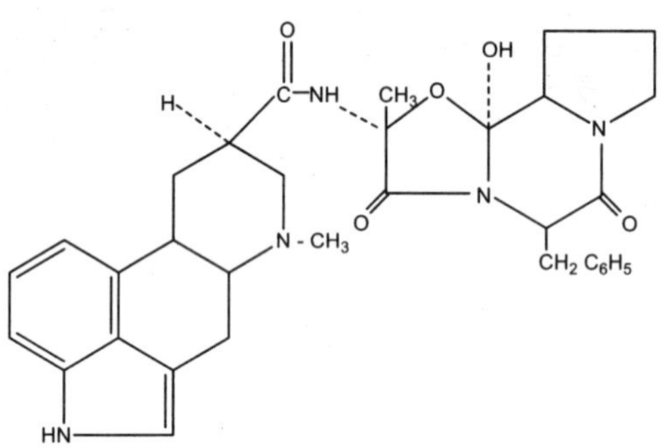

9, 10 - Dihydroergotamine

It is an ergot alkaloid and a semi synthetic derivative of ergotamine.

Mechanism of action: It binds to serotonin 5-HT_{1A}, 5-HT_{2A} and 5-HT_{2C} - receptors, α-adrenergic, serotonin and dopamine receptors. Vasoconstriction effect is by stimulating α-adrenergic and serotonin receptors. The anti-migraine activity is generally attributed to the agonist effect at 5-HT_1 receptors.

Use: It is used as a vasoconstrictor, specifically for the treatment of migraine.

3.1.2 Quinazolines

Prazosin, Tetrazosin and Doxozosin are selective α_1 antagonist contains 4-amino - 6, 7-dimethoxy quinazoline ring. These drugs possess quinazoline, piperazine and acyl moieties. The presence of 4th amino group and hetero moiety at 2nd position is essential for α_1-receptor antagonistic activity.The nature of acyl group has a significant effect on pharmacokinetic properties (Table 5.2).

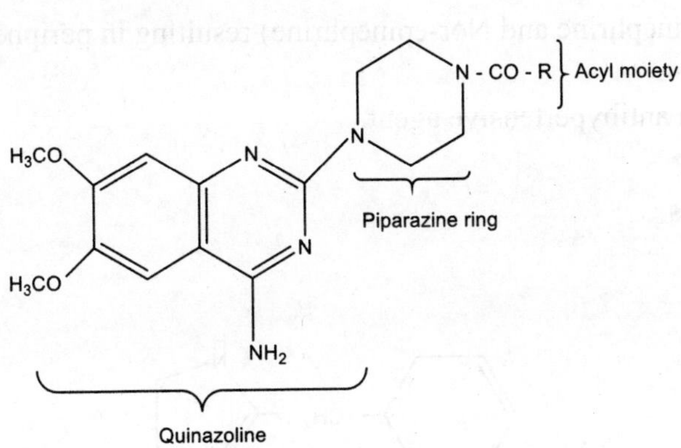

Table 5.2Structure of Quinazoline derivatives

S. No	Name	R
1.	Prazosin	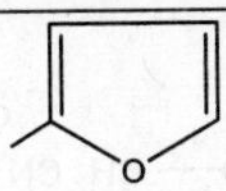
2.	Tetrazosin	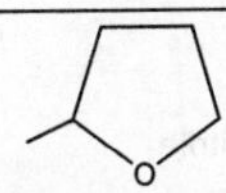
3.	Doxazosin	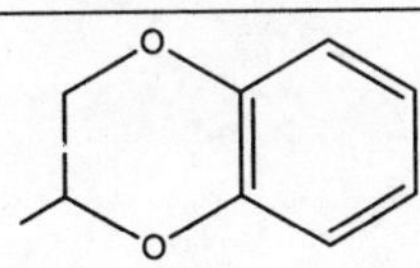

A. Prazosin (Minipress - XL)

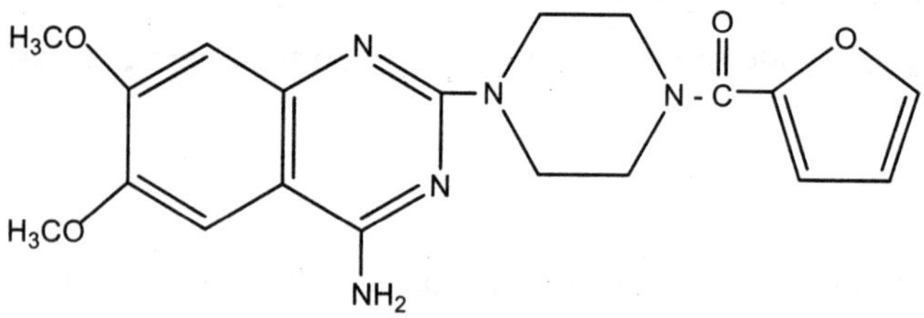

1- (4 - Amino - 6, 7 - dimethoxy - 2 - quinazolinyl)
- 4 - (2 - furanyl carbonyl) - piperazine

Mechanism of action: It acts by inhibiting the postsynaptic α1-adrenoceptors on vascular smooth muscle. It inhibits the vasoconstrictor effect of circulating and locally released catecholamines (Epinephrine and Nor-epinephrine) resulting in peripheral vasodilation.

Use: It is used as an antihypertensive agent.

3.1.3 Imidazolines

A. Tolazoline

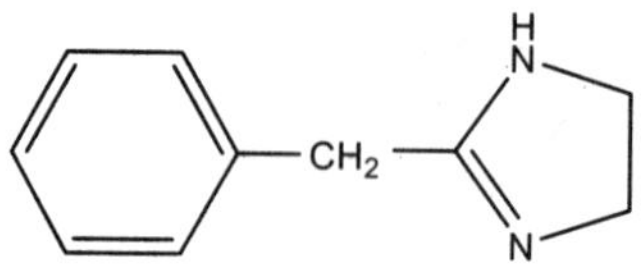

2 - Benzyl - 2 - imidazoline

Synthesis

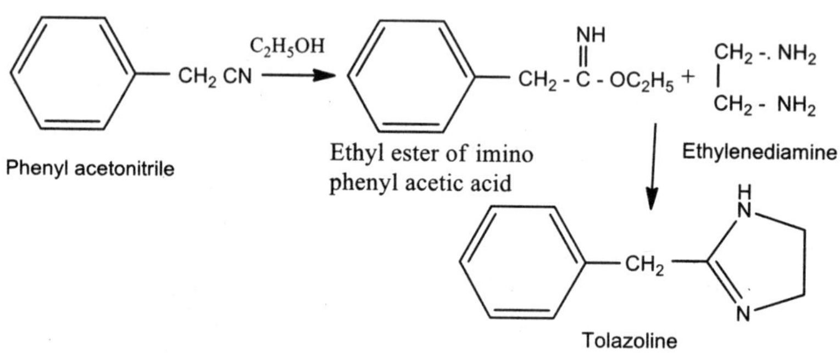

Mechanism of action: It is a non-selective α-receptor antagonist and a histamine agonist. By direct effect on vascular smooth muscle it acts as vasodilator.

Use: It is used as antihypertensive and vasodilatory agent. It is used in the treatment of persistent pulmonary hypertension of the new born. It is mainly used in Raynaud's disease.

B. Phentolamine (Regitine)

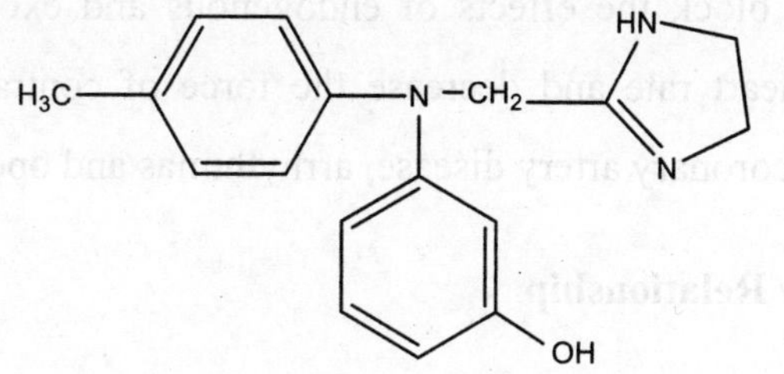

3 - {[(4, 5 - Dihydro - 1H - imidazol - 2 - yl) methyl] (4 - methyl phenyl) - amino} phenol

Mechanism of action: It is a non-selective α- adrenergic antagonist. It causes peripheral vasodilation through direct relaxation of vascular smooth muscle. Positive inotropic and chronotropic effects increase cardiac output.

Use: It is an antihypertensive and vasodilator.It is also used for the treatment of pheochromocytoma and Raynaud's syndrome.

3.1.4 β-Haloalkylamines

A. Phenoxybenzamine(Dibenzyline)

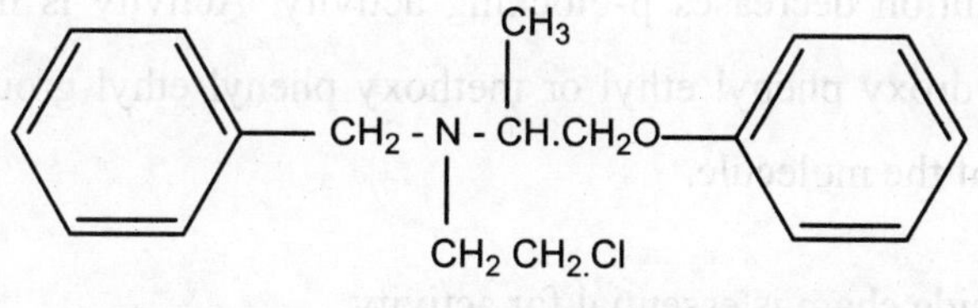

N - (2 - Chloro ethyl) - N - (1 - methyl - 2 - phenoxy ethyl) benzene methanamine

Mechanism of action: It is a non-selective α - adrenergic antagonist. It produces its therapeutic actions by blocking α- receptors, leading to a muscle relaxation and a dilatation of the blood vessels results in a lowering of blood pressure.

Use: It is used as an antihypertensive agent.

3.2 β - ADRENERGIC BLOCKING AGENTS

3.2.1 Introduction

All these agents block the effects of endogenous and exogenous catecholamine. These drugs slow the heart rate and decrease the force of contraction.It is used in the treatment hypertension, coronary artery disease, arrhythmias and open angle glaucoma.

3.2.2 Structure Activity Relationship

β - Blockers are structurally similar to β-agonist. The catechol ring can be replaced by a variety of ring system without loss of antagonistic activity. Aryl oxy propanol amines are more potent β-blockers than aryl ethanol amine. Most of the currently clinically used β-blockers are aryl oxy propanol amine derivatives.

$Ar - O - CH_2 - CH(OH) - CH_2 - NHR$

Aryloxy propanolamines

$Ar - O - CH(OH) - CH_2 - NHR$

Aryloxy ethanolamines

- Replacement of catechol hydroxyl group with chlorine or phenyl ring system retains β-blocking activity. eg. Pronethalol, Dichloroisoproterenol.
- N, N - disubstitution decreases β-blocking activity. Activity is maintained when phenyl ethyl, hydroxy phenyl ethyl or methoxy phenyl ethyl groups are added to amine as a part of the molecule.
- The two-carbonside chain is essential for activity.
- Introduction of $-OCH_2-$ group into the molecule between the aromatic ring and the ethylamine side chain provides β-blocking agents. eg. Propranolol.
- Nitrogen atom should be of 2 ° amine for optimum β-blocking activity.

- β-blockers exhibits a high degree of stereo selectivity in the production of their β-blocking effect. The carbon of side chain bearing hydroxyl group must be (S) configuration for optimal affinity to the β-receptor. eg. Levobunolol, Timolol.

- Replacement of ethereal oxygen in aryl oxy propanol amine with S, CH_2 or - N - CH_3 decreases the β-blocking activity.

- Most effective substitution at amino group of the aryl oxy propanol amine β-blocker is tert-butyl or isopropyl group.

- N-methyl group at side chain decreases the activity.

- The activity decreases if aromatic portion is converted to phenanthrene or anthracene ring.

3.2.3 Classification

β - Blockers are classified into two main types

I. Classificationbased on chemical structure

i. Aryloxy propyl amines: eg. Propranolol, Nadolol, Practolol, Metaprolol.

ii. Aryl ethanol amines: eg. Isoproterenol, Dichloroisoproterenol, Pronethalol.

II. Classification based on Generation

The first generation β-blockers are nonselective that they block both β_1 and β_2. The second generation β-blockers are cardio selective that they are selective for β_1-adreneo receptor. The third generation β-blockers are mixed α_1/β_1 blockers. They are used as vasodilators.

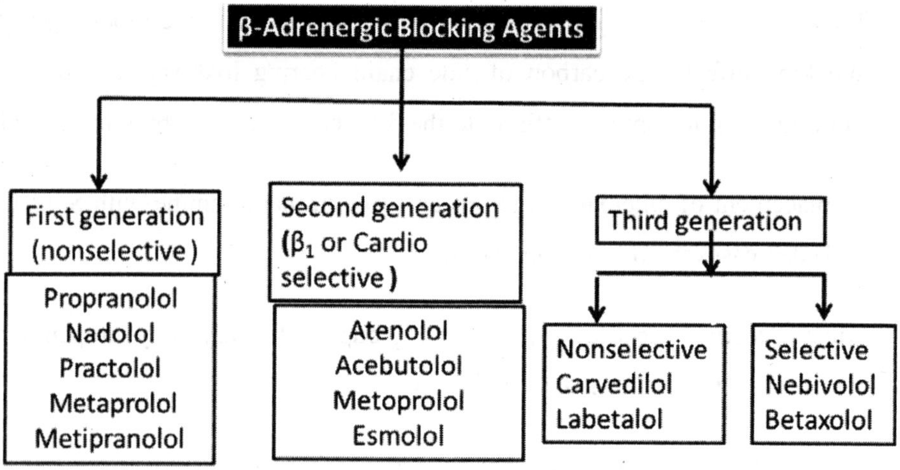

3.2.3.1 Aryloxy propyl amines

Aryloxy propylamines derivatives are given in Table 5.3

$$Ar - O - CH_2 - \underset{\substack{| \\ OH}}{CH} - CH_2\,NH\,.R$$

Table 5.3 General Structure ofβ-blockers

S. No	Name	Ar	R
1.	Metoprolol	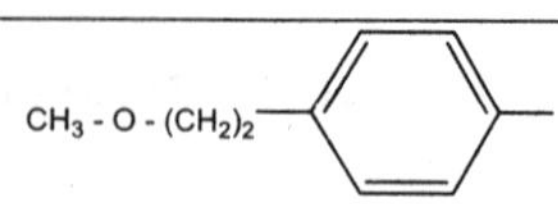	$-CH(CH_3)_2$
2.	Atenolol	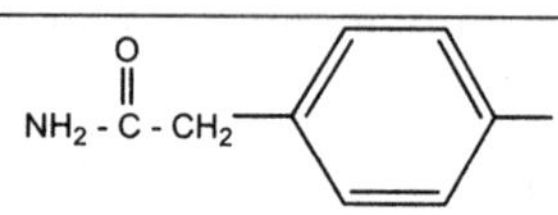	$-CH(CH_3)_2$
3.	Acebutolol	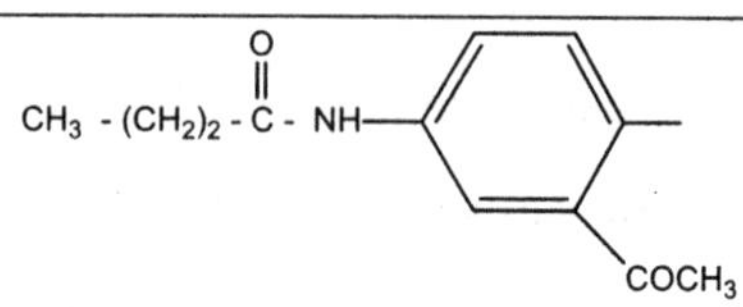	$-CH(CH_3)_2$
4.	Propranolol	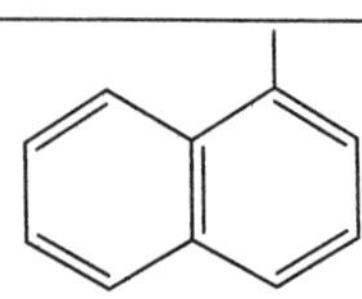	$-CH(CH_3)_2$

5.	Metipranolol	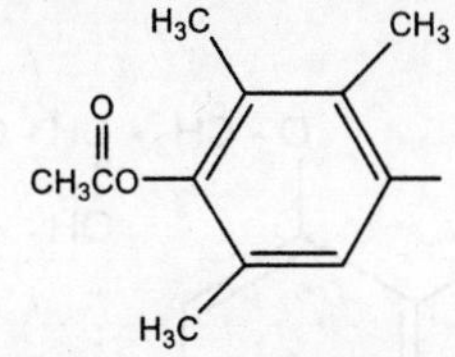	$-CH(CH_3)_2$
6.	Esmolol	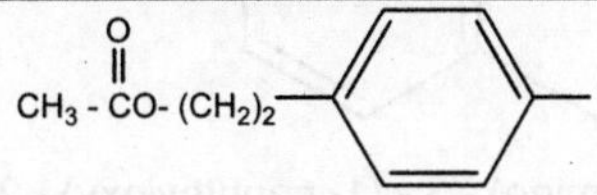	$-CH(CH_3)_2$
7.	Betaxolol	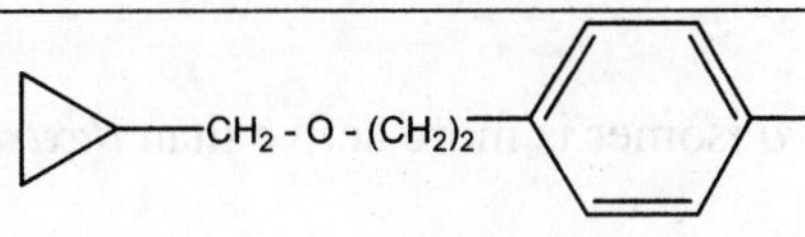	$-CH(CH_3)_2$
8.	Bisoprolol	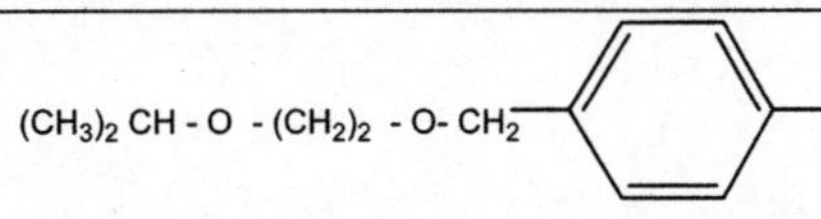	$-CH(CH_3)_2$

3.2.3.1.1 General Method of Preparation of Aryloxy Propyl Amine

The corresponding phenol reacts with epichlorohydrin and gives epoxide or chlorohydrin depending upon the reaction condition. The separation of both is not necessary because both can be converted into aryloxy propanolamine either through condensation or by aminolysis of the epoxy group with isopropyl amine or tert-butylamine.

A. Propranolol (Ciplar)

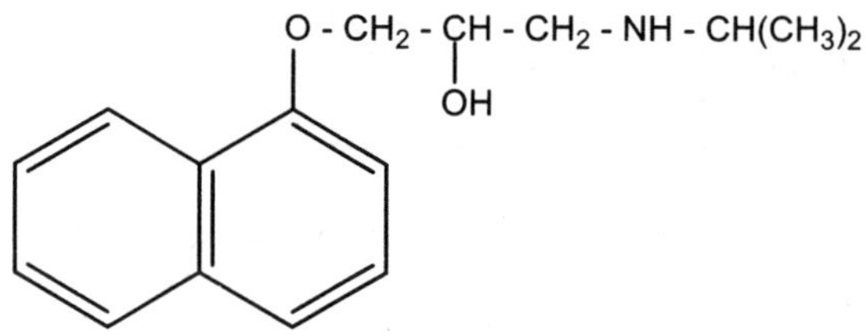

1- (Isopropyl amino) - 3 - (1- naphthyloxy) - 2 - propanol

The *levo* isomer is more active than *dextro* isomer

Synthesis

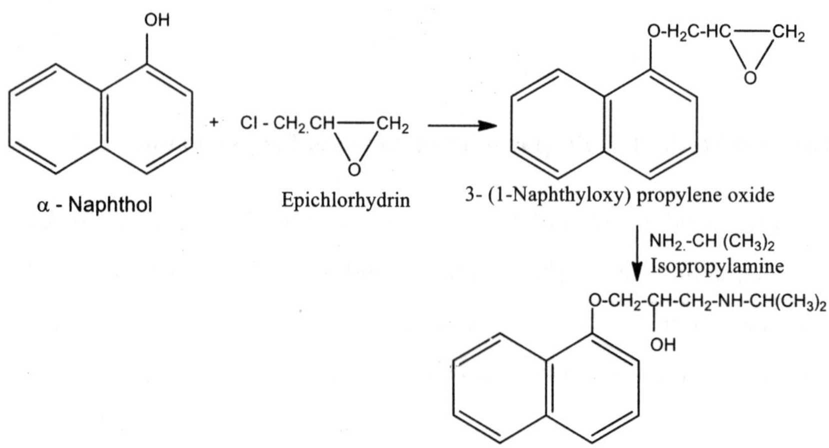

Propranolol

Mechanism of action: It competes with sympathomimetic neurotransmitters such as catecholamines for binding at β1-adrenergic receptors in the heart, inhibiting sympathetic stimulation. This results in a reduction in resting heart rate, cardiac output, systolic and diastolic blood pressure and reflex orthostatic hypotension.

Use: It is an effective antihypertensive agent. It is also used to treat arrhythmias, angina pectoris, post myocardial infarction, migraine prophylaxis and essential tremor.

B. Atenolol (Anol)

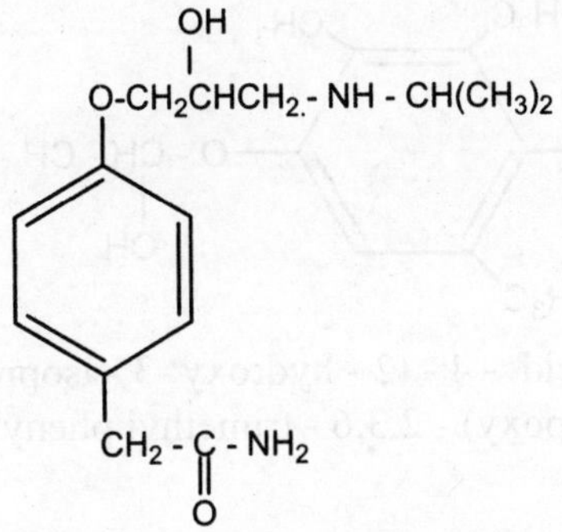

4 - {2 - Hydroxy - 3 - [(1 - methylethyl) amino] propoxy} benzeneacetamide

Mechanism of action: It inhibits stimulation of β1-receptor sites, located mainly in the heart, decreasing cardiac excitability, cardiac output and myocardial oxygen demand. It also acts to decrease the release of renin from the kidneys, aiding in reducing blood pressure.

Use: It is mainly used in the treatment of essential hypertension.

C. Metoprolol (Metomac)

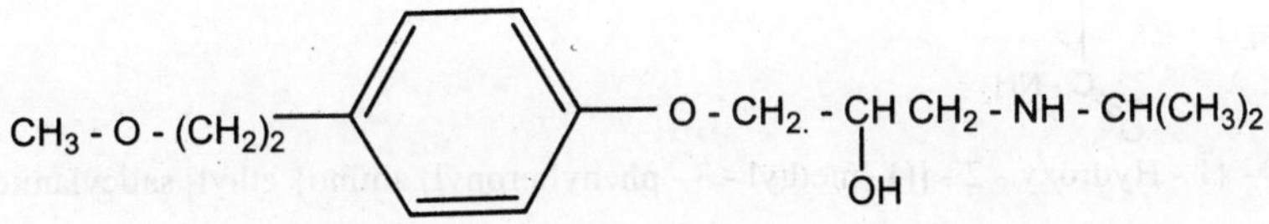

1 - [4 - (2 - Methoxy ethyl) phenoxy] - 3 - [(1- methyl ethyl) amino] - 2 - propanol

Mechanism of action: It acts by binding at β-adrenergic receptors in the heart it decreases the heart rate, cardiac output and blood pressure.

Use: It is used in the treatment of angina and hypertension.

D. Metipranolol (OptiPranolol)

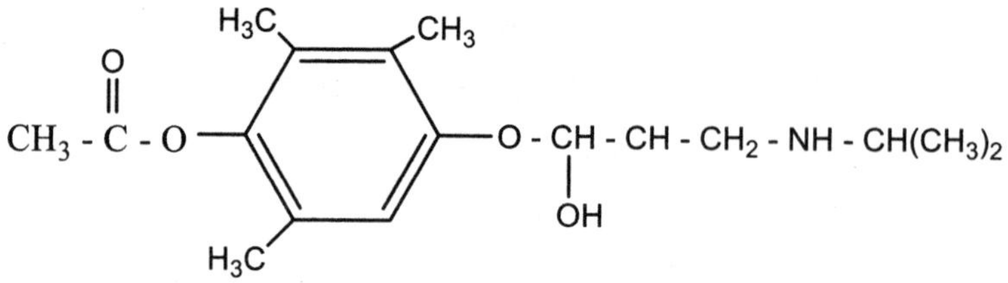

Acetic acid - 4 - (2 - hydroxy -3 - isopropylamino-
propoxy) - 2,3,6 - trimethyl phenyl ester

Mechanism of action: It binds toβ_1 and β_2 adrenergic receptors.It has only weak local anesthetic (membrane-stabilizing) and myocardial depressant activity. It appears that the ophthalmic β-adrenergic blocking agents reduce aqueous humor production.

Use: It is used as an anti-arrhythmic, antihypertensive and anti-glaucoma agent.

E. Labetalol (Labetamac)

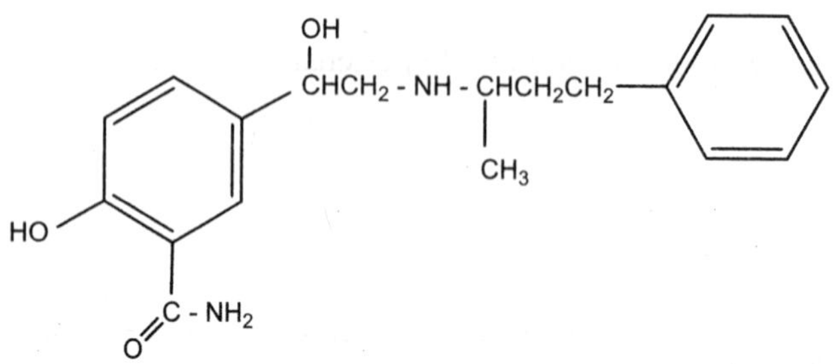

5 - {1 - Hydroxy - 2 - [(1- methyl - 3 - phenyl propyl) amino} ethyl] salicylamide

It is a competitive inhibitor of β_1, β_2 and α_1-adrenergic receptor. It is optically active because it has two optically active centers.1R, 1'R isomer possess β-antagonistic activity and 1S, 1 'R isomer possess α-antagonistic activity

Mechanism of action: It is a dual α_1 and β_1/β_2-adrenergic receptor blocker and competes with other catecholamines for binding to these sites. It is highly selective for postsynaptic α_1-adrenergic and non-selective for β-adrenergic receptors. It is about equipotent in blocking both β_1/β_2- receptors.

Use: It is a useful antihypertensive agent.

F. Carvedilol (Carloc)

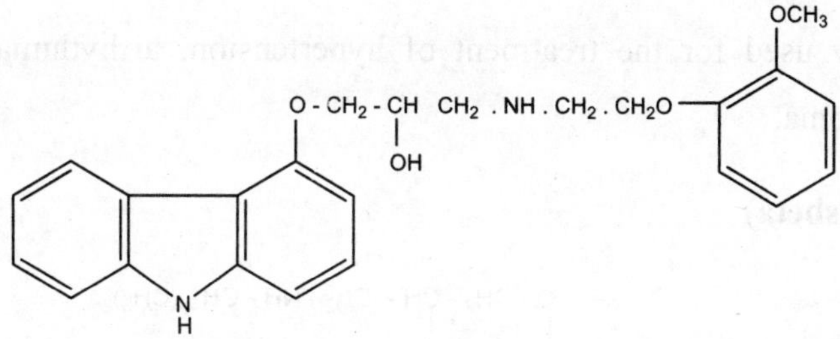

1- (9H - Carbazol - 4 - yloxy) - 3 - [2 - (2 - methoxy phenoxy) ethyl amino] - 2 - propanol

It acts as both α and β -adrenergic blocking agent. Only S- isomer is β-blocking and both enantiomers have α- blocking activity.

Mechanism of action: It is both a non-selective β-adrenergic receptor blocker (β_1, β_2) and α-adrenergic receptor blocker (α_1). It reversibly binds to β-adrenergic receptors on cardiac myocytes and prevents response to the sympathetic nervous system, leading to decreased heart rate and contractility.

Use: It is used in treating hypertension and congestive heart failure.

G. Betaxolol (Glocoptic)

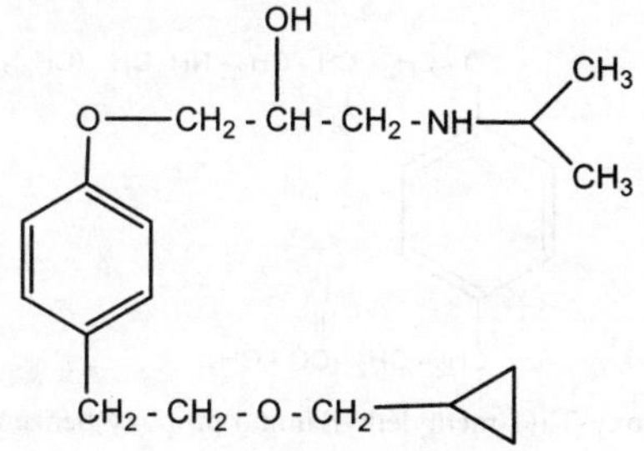

1-(Isopropylamino)-3-[P-(cyclopropylmethoxyethyl)phenoxy]-2-propanol

Mechanism of action: It acts by blocking the β_1-adrenergic receptors in the heart and bronchial and vascular smooth muscle. This causes bronchospasm and coronary vasodilatation.

Use: It is mainly used for the treatment of hypertension, arrhythmias, coronary heart disease and glaucoma.

H. Bisoprolol (Bisbeta)

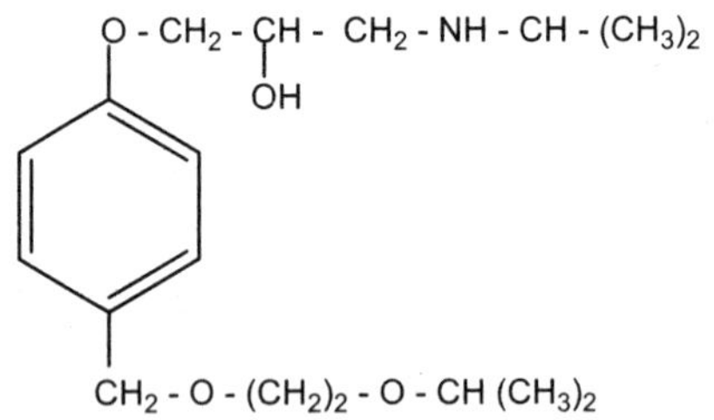

(RS)-1-(4-(2-isopropoxyethoxymethyl)phenoxy)-3-(ısopropylamino)-2-propanol

Mechanism of action: It selectively blocks β1-adrenergic receptors in the heart and vascular smooth muscle. This result in a reduction of heart rate, cardiac output, systolic and diastolic blood pressure and possibly reflex orthostatic hypotension.

Use: It is used for the management of heart failure, angina pectoris and mild to moderate hypertension and for secondary prevention of myocardial infarction.

I. Esmolol (Brevibloc)

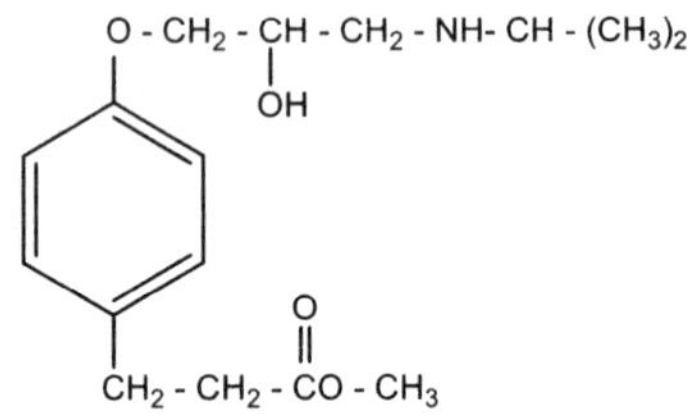

Methyl-4-(2-hydroxy-3-((1-methylethyl)amino)propoxy)benzene propanoate

Mechanism of action: It blocks β_1-receptor in cardiac tissue, it is said to be cardioselective.

Use: It is used as an antiarrhythmic agent.

Chapter 6

CHOLINERGIC AND ANTICHOLINERGIC DRUGS

I. INTRODUCTION

Motor nerves are divided into the somatic nervous system and autonomic nervous system. Somatic nervous system regulates the voluntary contraction of the skeletal muscles and autonomic nervous system (ANS) regulates the involuntary control of smooth, cardiac muscles and glands. The ANS composed of two divisions; Sympathetic and Parasympathetic generally serve the same visceral organs but cause essentially opposite effects. Sympathetic is responsible for the response commonly referred to as **"fight or flight"** while parasympathetic is referred to as **"rest and digest"**.

1.1 Neurotransmitter Acetylcholine

In the ANS, acetylcholine (ACh) is the neurotransmitter in the pre-ganglionic sympathetic and parasympathetic neurons. ACh is also the neurotransmitter at the adrenal medulla, all the parasympathetic innervated organs, the sweat glands and the piloerector muscle of the sympathetic ANS.

The preganglionic motor neurons of the sympathetic system arise in the spinal cord. They pass into sympathetic ganglia, which are organized into two chains that run parallel to either side of the spinal cord. The neurotransmitter of preganglionic neuron is ACh and postganglionic neuron is Noradrenaline. Parasympathetic stimulation causes slowing down the heartbeat, lowering of blood pressure, constriction of pupils, increased blood flow to the skin and viscera and increases peristalsis of the GI tract.

1.2 Biosynthesis and Catabolism of Acetylcholine

- Cholinergic neurons contain a large number of small membrane bound vesicle containing Ach near the synaptic portion of cell membrane.
- Ach is synthesized in the cytoplasm from acetyl-CoA and choline by the catalytic action of *choline acetyl transferase.*

- Acetyl-CoA is synthesized in mitochondria which is present in nerve endings.
- Free choline circulating in blood plasma readily crosses the blood-brain barrier and is taken up by cholinergic nerve terminals, for the most part, by a high- affinity choline uptake system that is temperature, energy and sodium-dependent.
- The rate-limiting steps in ACh synthesis are the availability of choline and acetyl-CoA.
- During increased neuronal activity the availability of acetyl-CoA from the mitochondria is upregulated as is the uptake of choline into the nerve ending from the synaptic cleft.
- Newly formed ACh is stored in synaptic vesicle.
- The release of ACh results from depolarization of the nerve terminal by the action potential, which alters membrane permeability to Ca^{2+}. Calcium enters the nerve terminal and causes the quantal release of ACh, which depolarizes the postsynaptic membrane.
- The released ACh combines with the receptor at target organ, remain bound for less than a milli second and is quickly hydrolyzed by *acetyl cholinesterase* into choline and acetate.

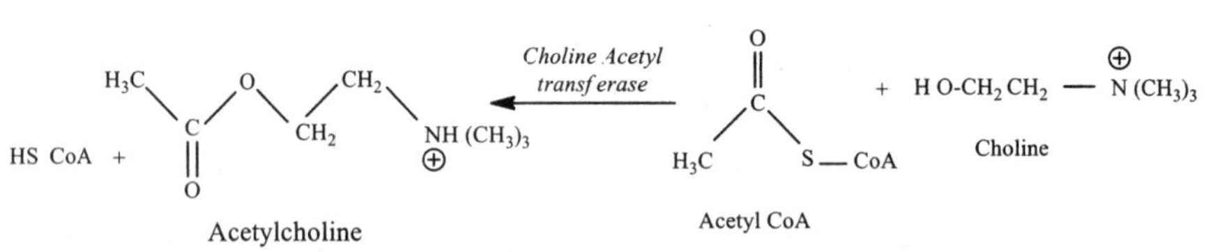

Fig.6.1 Biosynthesis of Acetylcholine

1.3 Cholinergic Receptors

There are two types of cholinergic receptors: **Nicotinic and Muscarinic receptor**

1.3.1 Nicotinic Receptor

Nicotinic receptors so named, because they are specifically stimulated by nicotine present in tobacco. They are ligand-gated ion channels receptor that form pores in cells plasma membrane, mediating fast signal transmission at synapse. Many types of neuronal nicotinic receptors are located at synapses between neurons, such as in the CNS where they are involved in cognitive function, learning and memory, arousal, reward, motor control and analgesia. Nicotinic receptors can be divided into following types depending upon their location as

Nicotinic receptor	N1 or NM receptors	N2 or NN receptors
Location	Neuromuscular junction	Autonomic ganglia.CNS and adrenal medulla
Function	Contraction of skeletal muscle	Transmission of cholinergic signals in the autonomic ganglia and secretion of Epinephrine and Nor-epinephrine from adrenal medulla.

1.3.2 Muscarinic Receptor

The prototype agonist for this receptor is muscarine, so named, they specifically stimulated by muscarinic. All muscarinic receptors are G-protein coupled receptors muscarinic being G-protein coupled receptors mediate a slow metabolic response. Binding of acetylcholine to a muscarinic AChR causes a conformational change in the receptor that is responsible for its association with and activation of an intracellular G protein, the latter converting GTP to GDP in order to become activated and dissociate from the receptor. Muscarinic receptors are involved in a large number of physiological functions including heart rate and force, contraction of smooth muscles and release of neurotransmitters. They are divided into following subclasses

Subclass	M_1	M_2	M_3	M_4	M_5
Location	CNS, gastric parietal cells and autonomic ganglia.	Heart (SA node, AV node, atria, Ventricle)	Smooth muscle, exocrine glands, iris, ciliary muscle	CNS	CNS

Function	Gastric acid secretion, GI motility, CNS response such as memory, arousal, attention and analgesia.	lowers conduction velocity at Sinoatrial and atrioventricular nodes, thus lowering heart rate	Increase exocrine secretion , Smooth muscle contraction, regulate pupil constriction, Promote eye, mouth, lung and skin lubrication

2. CHOLINOMIMETIC (or) PARASYMPATHOMIMETIC AGENTS

2.1 Introduction

Cholinergic drugs or Cholinomimetics or Parasympathomimetics are drugs producing action similar to acetylcholine by interacting with cholinergic receptor or increasing the availability of acetylcholine at these sites.

These agents mimic the action at parasympathetic system. Cholinomimetic drugs are either cholinergic agonist that are resistant to the hydrolytic action of *cholinesterase* or agents that inhibit *cholinesterase.*

2.2 Structure Activity Relationship

Structural features essential for activity are: the onium group, the ester function and the choline moiety.

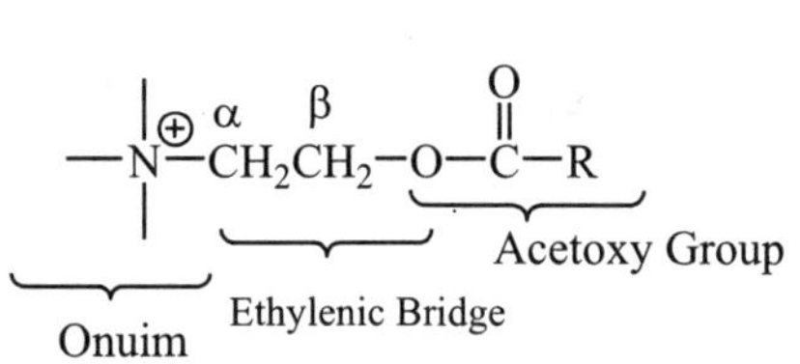

i) Modification of Onium

- The trimethyl ammonium group or onium group is essential for intrinsic activity.

- Even though trimethyl ammonium group is the optimal functional moiety, some exceptions are known. eg: Pilocarpine, Nicotine and Oxotremorine.
- Replacement with 1°, 2°and 3° amine for trimethyl ammonium group result in less activity.
- If one of the methyl group is replaced by ethyl or larger alkyl group the activity decreases.
- Replacement of all three methyl group in quaternary amine with ethyl or higher alkyl groups results in antagonist activity.
- The replacement of phosphonium, sulfonium or arsenonium isosteres for ammonium ion decreases the activity.

ii) Modification of Acetoxy Group

- Ester group is essential for affinity, binds with threonine and asparagine pockets at the receptor site. The ester group of ACh contributes to the binding of the compound to the muscarinic receptor.
- When acyl group is substituted by its higher homologues, less active compound is formed.
- Since ester group makes it liable to hydrolysis, alternate groups were included and found that replacing the ester with carbamate, ether or ketone function resists hydrolysis while maintaining activity.
- When methyl group is replaced by amine (replacing the ester with carbamate) cholinergic activity increases. Carbachol, has both muscarinic and nicotinic properties.
- The concept that the ester i.e. carbamic or other group is not essential for activity but may enhances the affinity of the molecule for the receptor.

- Studying a series of n-alkyl trimethyl ammonium salt revealed that for maximal muscarinic activity, the quaternary ammonium group should be followed by a chain of five atoms (five - atom rule). (A “rule of five” states that there should be no more than 5 atoms between the Nitrogen and the terminal Hydrogen). As the chain length increased from two, activity is rapidly lost.

iii) Modification of Ethylenic Bridge

- Shortening or lengthening the chain of atoms that separates the ester group from the onium moiety reduces muscarinic activity.

- Substitution of methyl group on α or β - carbon of ethylenic group result if equipotent or greater cholinergic activity. But larger than methyl group decreases the activity

  ✓ A methyl substitution in α-carbon, decreases both nicotinic and muscarinic activity, but muscarinic activity to greater extent

  ✓ Introduction of methyl group on the β carbon atom reduces the nicotinic activity but not muscarinic activity (e.g. Methacholine).

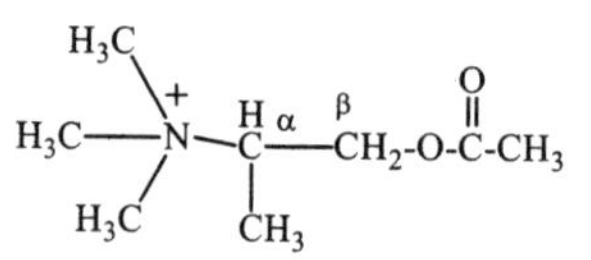

Methyl group in alpha carbon
Not As potent as Ach
Selective to Nicotinic receptor
Not Used clinically

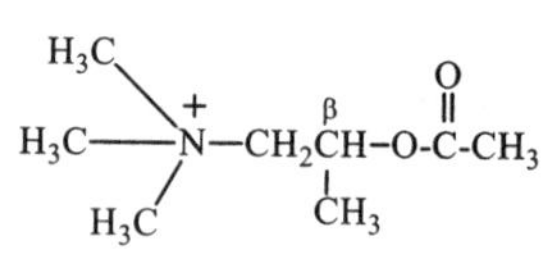

Methyl group in Beta carbon
As potent as Ach
Selective to Muscarinic receptor
Used clinically

- Due to the presence of methyl group on carbon atom, Methacholine (acetyl - β - methyl choline) is longer acting, since it is hydrolyzed by *acetyl cholinesterase* (AChE) enzyme at a much slower rate than acetyl choline and is almost totally resistant to hydrolysis by *butyryl cholinesterase* (pseudo cholinesterase).

- Hydrolysis by *acetyl cholinesterase* is more affected by β-substitution than α-carbon.

- Replacement of acyl group with aromatic or higher molecular weight ester produces cholinergic antagonist effect.

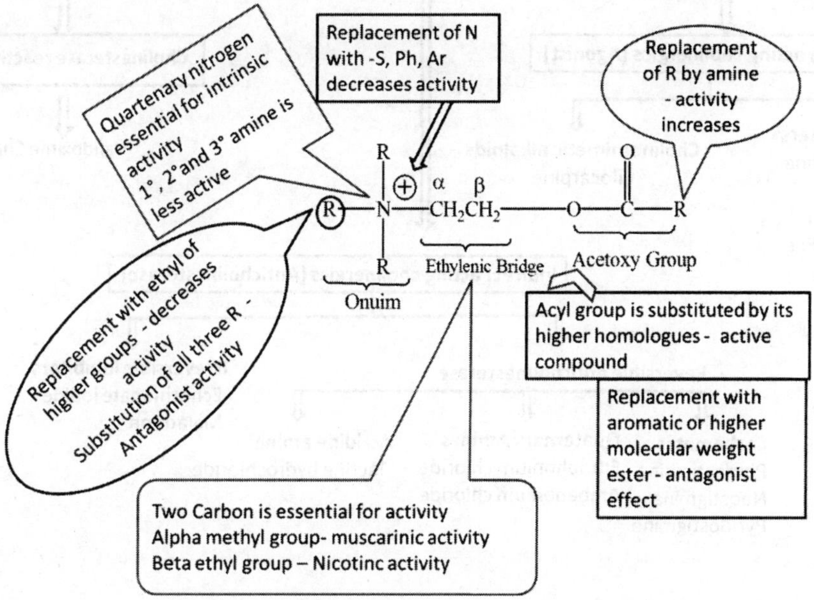

Fig. 6.2 SAR summary of Cholinomimetics

2.2.1 Therapeutic uses: These drugs are used commonly in ophthalmology, where they reduce elevated intraocular pressure in glaucoma and / or induce miosis. In GI disorders that involve, decreased smooth muscle contraction without obstruction. They may be used in the treatment of atonic constipation, congenital megacolon, postoperative intestinal ileus and post- vagotomy gastric atony. Vasospastic peripheral vascular disorders such as Raynaud's disease and dermatitis congelations, Sjogren's syndrome and Alzheimer's disease also been treated with these agents.

2.3 CLASSIFICATION

Based on the mechanism of action they are classified as

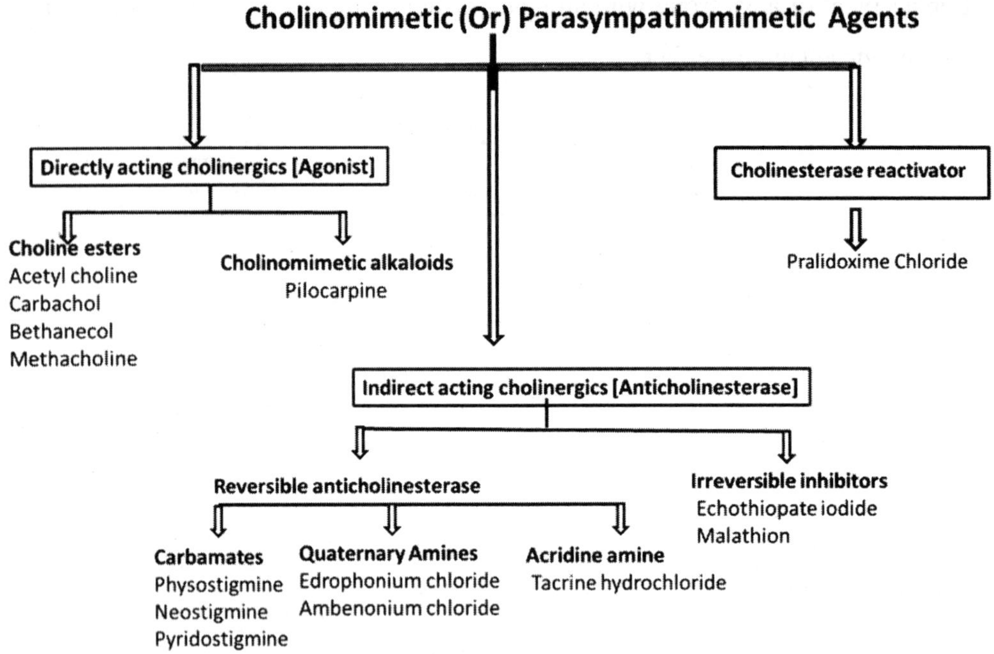

2.3.1 Direct Acting Cholinergic Drugs

The direct acting agents exert the effects by stimulating muscarinic and/or nicotinic receptor.

2.3.1.1 Choline Esters

Choline esters are synthetic derivatives of choline. The choline esters differ in relative sensitivity to hydrolysis and their relative nicotinic and muscarinic effect.

A. Acetylcholine (Miochox E)

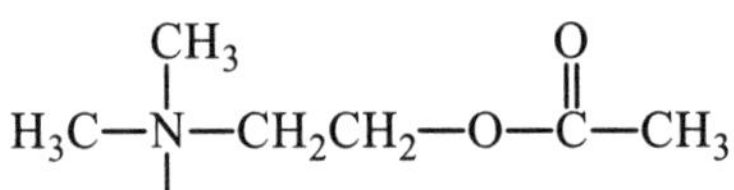

(2 - Acetyloxy ethyl) - trimethyl amide

Acetylcholine is a substance without which normal body function would not be possible. It does not penetrate into lipid membranes because of the presence of high polar ammonium group. So, when introduced externally it remains in the extracellular space and does not pass blood brain barrier. Therapeutically it has no importance because of its multiplicity of actions and its rapid inactivation by the *cholinesterases*. Acetylcholine has both muscarinic and nicotinic activity. All of the direct-acting cholinergic drugs have longer durations of action than acetylcholine.

Stereochemistry of Acetylcholine

Because of free rotation around most of the covalent bond, ACh can exist in number of conformations. Conformational isomers of ACh derived from rotation around -O-C-C-N- axis is shown in Fig. 6.3.

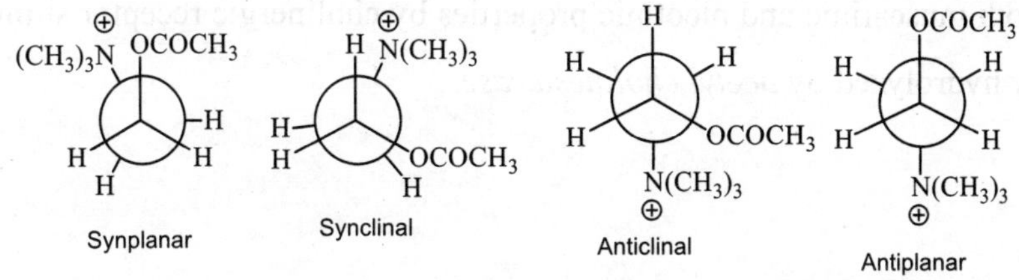

Fig. 6.3 Conformational Isomers of Aetylcholine

Acetylcholine probably interacts with muscarinic receptor by anticlinal conformation (dihedral angle between 110° to 117°) and nicotinic receptor by gauche conformation.

Mechanism of action: It is a central as well as peripheral neurotransmitter that transmits signals neurons to neurons or neurons to skeletal muscle. It produces myriads of action which depends on types of receptor on which it acts. Acetylcholine acts on muscarinic (M1, M2, M3) and nicotinic receptor (Nn Nm). Muscarinic receptors are GPCR in contrary nicotinic receptors are ionotropic receptor. Broadly action on muscarinic receptor produces relaxation of heart, contraction of GIT, pupil, increased gastric and salivary secretion whereas action on nicotinic receptor produces skeletal muscle contraction and involved in cognitive function.

Use: It is a topical ophthalmic drug to induce miosis, during certain intraocular surgical procedures, such as cataract surgery, iridectomy, penetrating keratoplasty and other anterior segment surgery. Systemically administered ACh is rapidly hydrolyzed by *acetyl cholinesterase* so it has no clinical use. It is a cardiac depressant and effective vasodilator.

B. Carbachol (Carbastat)

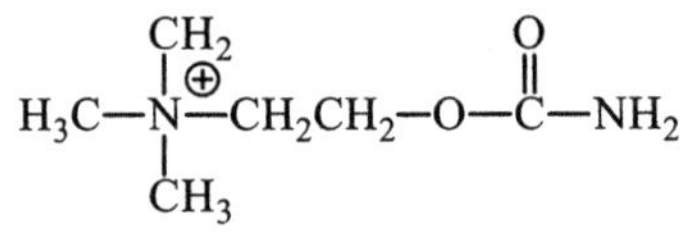

2- [(Amino carbanoyl) oxy]-N,N,N - trimethyl ethylamine

Carbachol is an ester of carbamic acid, the terminal methyl group of ACh is replaced by amino group, which is not responsive to hydrolysis by *cholinesterase*. It possesses both muscarinic and nicotinic properties by cholinergic receptor stimulation. It is more slowly hydrolyzed by *acetyl cholinesterase*.

Synthesis

Method - I

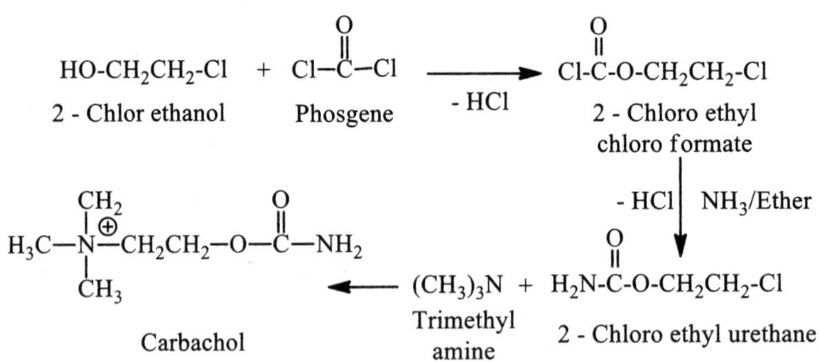

Method - II

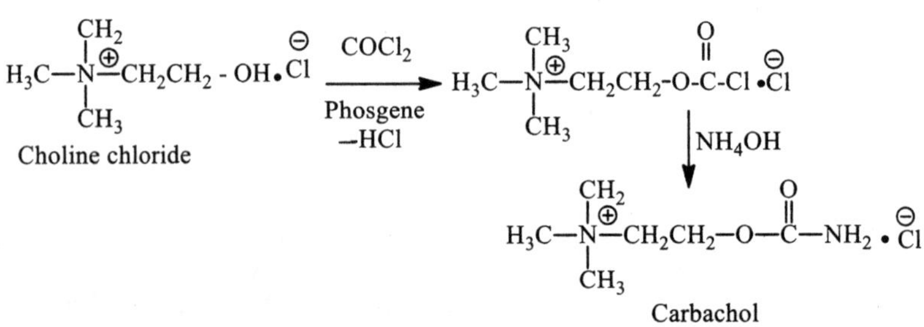

Mechanism of action: It is a parasympathomimetic drug stimulates both muscarinic and nicotinic receptors. In topical ocular and intraocular administration its principal effects are miosis and increased aqueous humour outflow.

Use: It is used for the treatment of glaucoma and ophthalmic surgery.

C. Bethanechol (Duvoid)

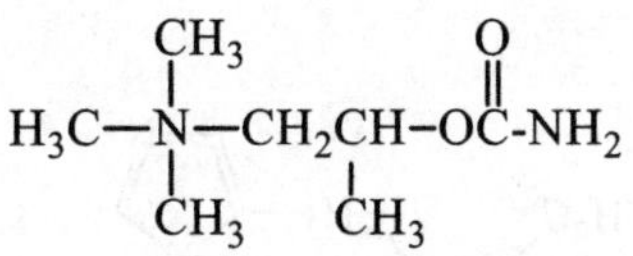

2 - [(Amino carbonyl) oxy] - N,N,N - trimethyl propyl amine

Bethanechol is a carbonic ester of β-methyl choline. It is not rapidly hydrolyzed by *acetyl cholinesterase* and has strong muscarinic action but little nicotinic action.

Mechanism of Action: It directly stimulates cholinergic receptors in the parasympathetic nervous system while stimulating the ganglia to a lesser extent. Its effects are predominantly muscarinic, inducing little effect on nicotinic receptors and negligible effects on the cardiovascular system.

Use: It produces smooth muscle contractions. It is not well absorbed from GI tract. It can be given subcutaneously but not by IM or IV because of its severe side effects. It is used to relieve urinary retention and abdominal distention after surgery.

d. Methacholine (Provocholine)

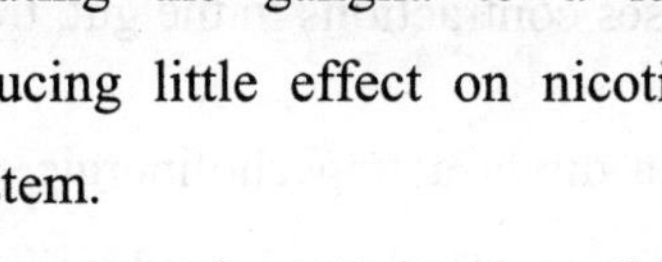

(2- Acetoxy) - trimethyl propyl amine

Methacholine exist in (S) and (R) - enantiomers. (S) - enantiomer has muscarinic activity. They are used as racemic mixture.

Mechanism of action: It induces bronchoconstriction by agonizing the muscarinic receptors used to test asthmatics and in bronchial hyperreactivity.

Use: It is used to treat Raynaud's syndrome and glaucoma.

2.3.1.2 Cholinomimetic Alkaloids

A. Pilocarpine (Miocarpine)

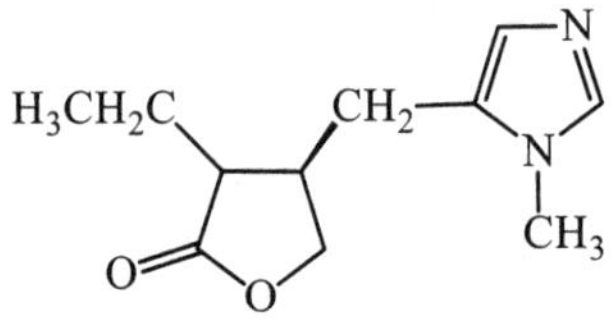

(3S - cis) - 3 - Ethyl dihydro - 4 - [(1- methyl -1H -imidazo l- 5yl) - methyl] - 2 - (3H) - furanone

Pilocarpine is an alkaloid obtained from the dried leaflets of *Pilocarpus jaborandi* (or) *Pilocarpus microphyllus* in which it occurs to the extent of about 0.5% together with other alkaloids. It is a non-selective agonist on the muscarinic receptors. It acts on M_3 receptor in smooth muscle causes contractions in the gut, trachea and eye.

Mechanism of action: It is a direct acting cholinergic parasympathomimetic agent. It increases secretion by the exocrine glands and produces contraction of the iris sphincter muscle and ciliary muscle by mainly stimulating muscarinic receptors.

Use: It is used for the treatment of symptoms of dry mouth caused by radiotherapy for cancer of head and neck and the symptoms associated with Sjogren's syndrome.

2.3.2 Indirect Acting Cholinergic Agonist

Cholinesterase inhibitors are very important class of compounds related to cholinomimetics. There are two types of cholinesterase,

i) *Acetyl cholinesterase*

ii) *Butyryl cholinesterase* (*Pseudo cholinesterase*)

They differ in their location in the body and their substrate specificity. *Acetyl cholinesterase* present in the surface of glial cell in synapse, catalyzes the hydrolysis of

Acetylcholine to choline and acetic acid. Inhibition of *Acetyl cholinesterase* prolongs the duration of the neurotransmitter in the junction and produces pharmacological effect similar to those of Acetylcholine. *Butyryl cholinesterase* is located in the human plasma and the properties are similar to *acetyl cholinesterase.*

Acetyl cholinesterase has two important sites namely anionic site and esteric site. The anionic site possesses a glutamate residue and in esteric site a histidine imidazole ring and a serine hydroxyl groups are present. The imidazole group of histidine accepts a proton from the serine hydroxyl group at the esteric site creating a strong nucleophilic area. The anionic site of enzyme binds with quaternary ammonium nitrogen of the Acetylcholine through ionic and hydrophobic forces. The activated serine attacks the carbonyl carbon of Acetylcholine resulting in tetrahedral intermediate. The tetrahedral intermediate is unstable and decomposes to acetylated enzyme and choline. The acetyl-enzyme is cleaved by general base catalyst to regenerate the free enzyme. By changing the acylating group on the substrate or on the enzyme inhibitor, the rate of regeneration of enzyme can be changed; hence the duration of inhibition can be controlled.

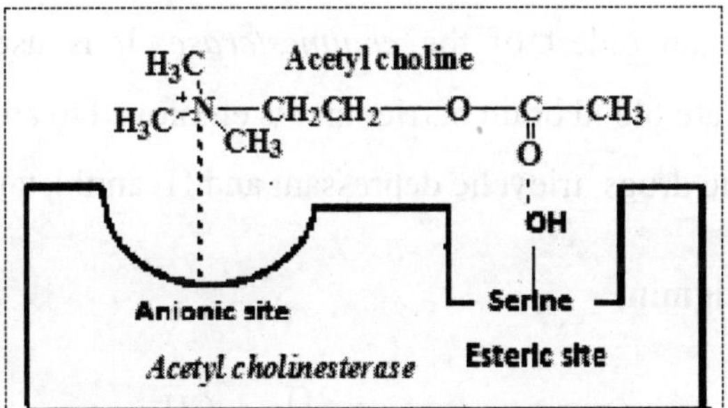

Fig. 6.4 Binding site of Acetyl Choline with *Acetylcholinesterase*

Based on the duration of inhibitory activity they are classified as reversible and irreversible inhibitors. Reversible inhibitors are used in the treatment of glaucoma, myasthenia gravis, stimulation of gastrointestinal and urinary tract motility, reversal of neuromuscular blockade and atropine poisoning. Irreversible *cholinesterase* inhibitors are organophosphates.

2.3.2.1 Reversible Inhibitors

2.3.2.1.1 Carbamates

A. Physostigmine (Antilirium)

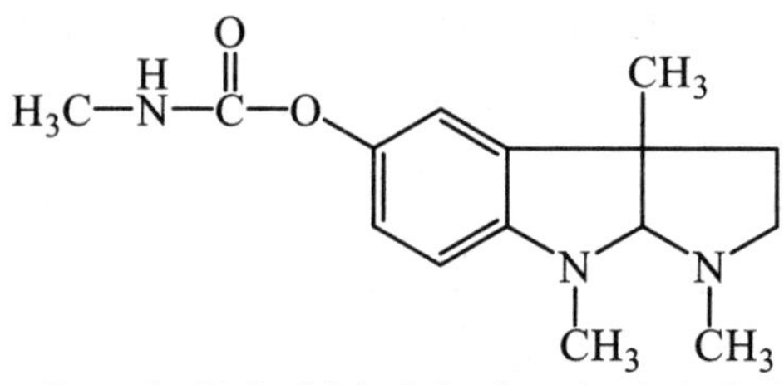

Pyrrolo [2,3 - b] indol - 5 - ol - 1, 2, 3, 3a, 8, 8a - hexahydro - 1,3a, 8 - trimethyl methyl carbamate

It is an alkaloid obtained from the dried ripe seed of *Physostigma venenosum*.

Mechanism of action: It inhibits destruction of acetylcholine by *acetylcholinesterase.* This action increases acetylcholine concentration at cholinergic transmission sites and prolongs and exaggerates effects of acetylcholine that are blocked by toxic doses of anticholinergics.

Use: Physostigmine is an oldest of the *cholinesterase.* It is used in the treatment of glaucoma. It can penetrate blood brain barrier and is employed to antagonize the toxic CNS effects of antimuscarinic drugs, tricyclic depressant and H_1 antihistamines.

B. Neostigmine (Prostigmin)

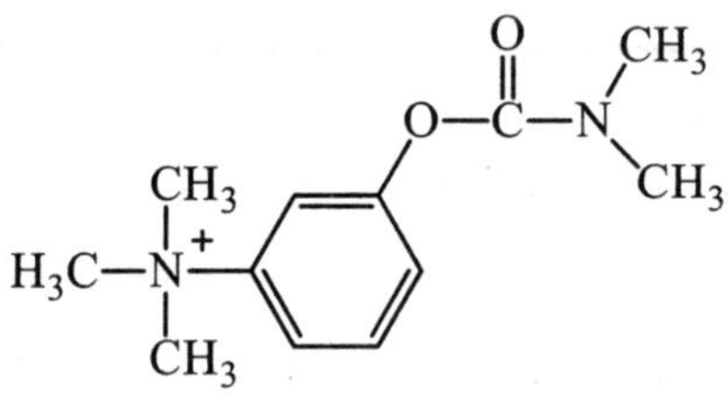

3 - [(Dimethyl carbamoyloxy) phenyl] - trimethylazanium

Synthesis

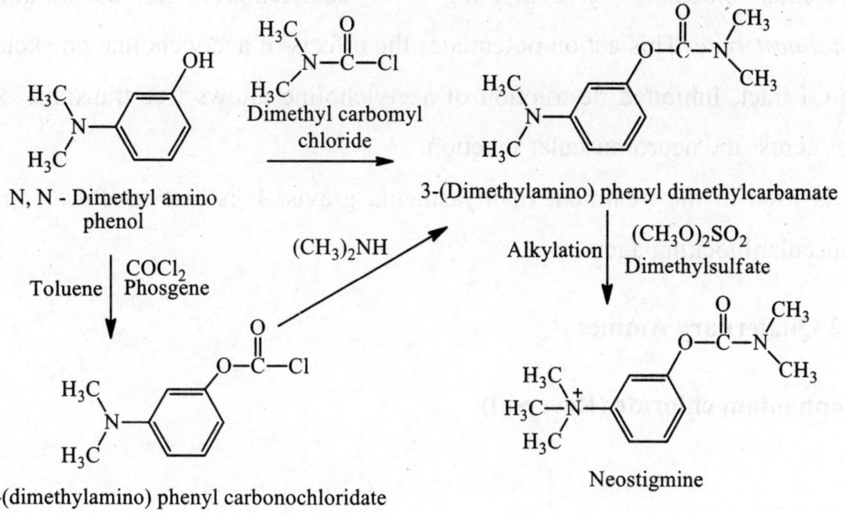

Mechanism of action: It is a parasympathomimetic, specifically, a reversible *cholinesterase* inhibitor. It inhibits *acetylcholinesterase* which is responsible for the degradation of acetylcholine. So, with *acetylcholinesterase* inhibited, more acetylcholine is present thereby increasing acetylcholine accumulation at myoneural junction and facilitating nerve impulse transmission across the junctions. It does not cross the blood-brain barrier.

Use: It is used in the treatment of myasthenia gravis.

C. Pyridostigmine (Mestinon)

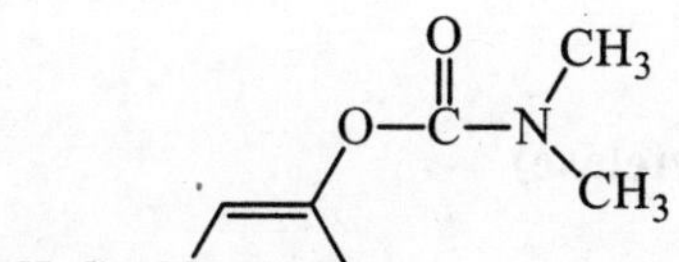

3-{(Dimethylamino) - carbonyl] - oxy}-1-methyl pyridine

Mechanism of action: It improves muscle strength compromised by myasthenia gravis or neuromuscular blockade by competing with acetylcholine for its binding site on *acetylcholinesterase.* This action potentiates the effects of acetylcholine on skeletal muscle and the GI tract. Inhibited destruction of acetylcholine allows free transmission of nerve impulses across the neuromuscular junction.

Use: It is used in the treatment of myasthenia gravis. It is also useful as antagonist of neuromuscular blocking agent.

2.3.2.1.2 Quaternary Amines

A. Edrophonium chloride (Reversol)

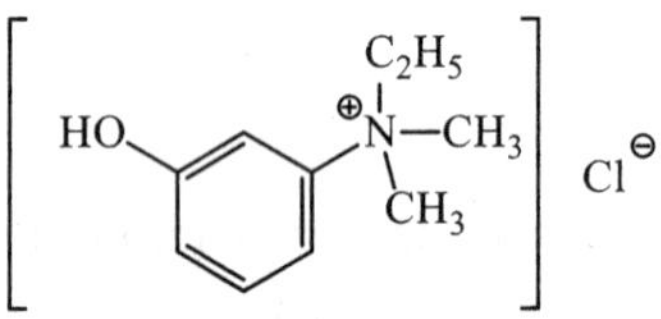

Ethyl (m-hydroxy phenyl) dimethyl ammonium chloride

Mechanism of action: It improves muscle strength compromised by myasthenia gravis or neuromuscular blockade by competing with acetylcholine for its binding site on *acetylcholinesterase.* This action potentiates the effects of acetylcholine on skeletal muscle and the GI tract. Inhibited destruction of acetylcholine allows free transmission of nerve impulses across the neuromuscular junction.

Use: It is used in the diagnosis of myasthenia gravis. It is also used in myasthenia and cholinergic crisis.

B. Ambenonium chloride (Mytelase)

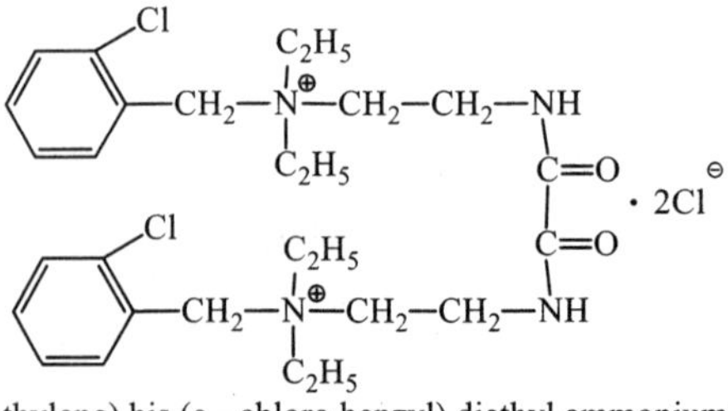

[Oxalyl bis (imino ethylene) bis (o - chloro benzyl) diethyl ammonium] dichloride

Mechanism of action: It attaches to *acetylcholinesterase* and blocks its breakdown. This action prolongs and exaggerates acetylcholine's effects, producing cholinergic responses, such as miosis, increased intestinal and skeletal muscle tone, bronchoconstriction, bradycardia and increased salivary and sweat gland secretion.

Use: It is used in the treatment of myasthenia gravis in patient who do not respond to Neostigmine or Pyridostigmine.

2.3.2.1.3 Acridine Amine

A. Tacrine hydrochloride (Cognex)

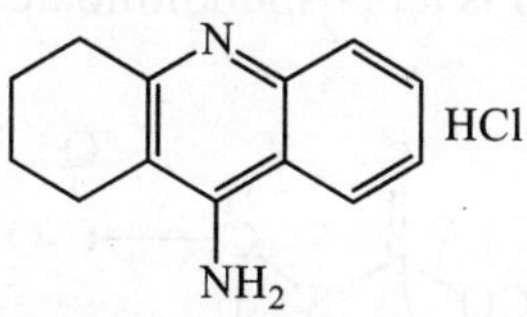

5,6,7,8 - tetrahydroacridin - 9 - amine

Mechanism of action: It is an *anticholinesterase* agent which reversibly binds with and inactivates *cholinesterases*. This inhibits the hydrolysis of acetylcholine released from functioning cholinergic neurons, thus leading to an accumulation of acetylcholine at cholinergic synapses. The result is a prolonged effect of acetylcholine.

Use: It is used in the treatment of Alzheimer's diseases.

2.3.2.2 Irreversible Inhibitors

They belong to a class of organophosphorus esters and both AChE and BuChE are inhibited irreversibly. These agents are nerve poisons and have been used in warfare, in bio-terrorism and as agricultural pesticides.

A. Echothiophate iodide (Phospholine iodide)

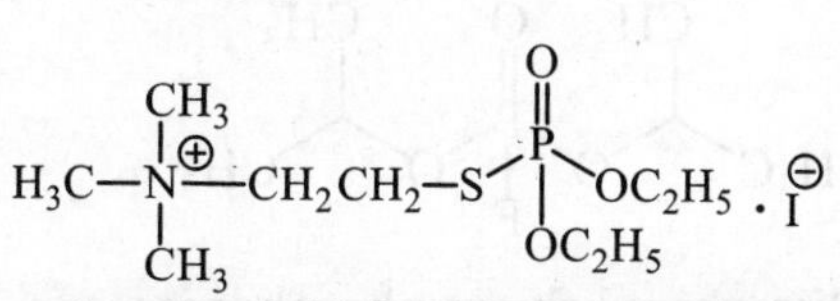

2 - [(Diethoxy phosphinyl) thio] - N,N,N - trimethyl ethyl ammonium iodide

Mechanism of action: It is a long-acting *cholinesterase* inhibitor for topical use which enhances the effect of endogenously liberated acetylcholine in iris, ciliary muscle and other parasympathetically innervated structures of the eye. It binds irreversibly to *cholinesterase* and is long acting due to the slow rate of hydrolysis by *cholinesterase.*

Use: It is a long acting irreversible anti-AChE drug, used in the treatment of glaucoma.

B. Malathion (Ouide)

Malathion is an effective pesticide, which is more effective on insects than on humans because it requires biotransformation to the phosphate form, which can only be carried out by insects. Malathion is a phosphodithioate ester.

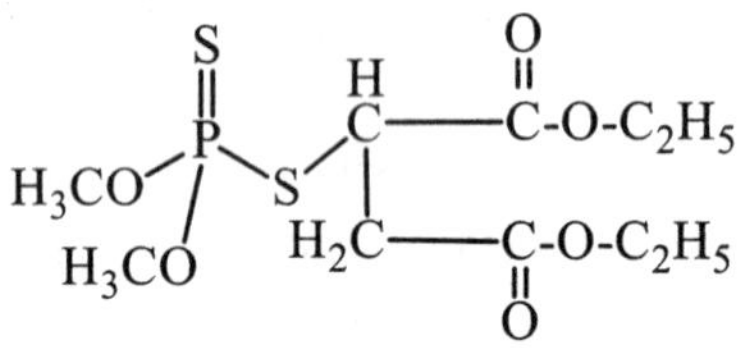

2 - [(Dimethoxy phosphino thioyl)thiol]butanoicacid diethyl ester

Mechanism of action: It is a parasympathomimetic organophosphate compound that is used as an insecticide for the treatment of head lice. Malathion is an irreversible cholinesterase inhibitor and has low human toxicity.

Use: It is used extensively for controlling insects on vegetables, fruits and cereal crops. It is also used for controlling insects affecting man and animals.

C. Isoflurophate (Dyflos)

Isoflurophate is an organophosphate. It covalently binds to acetyl *cholinesterase* and inhibits acetyl *cholinesterase* irreversibly.

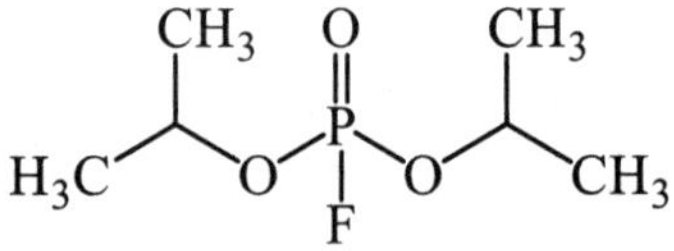

Diisopropyl fluoro phosphonate

Mechanism of action: It is an irreversible cholinesterase inhibitor with actions similar to that of Echothiophate.

Use: It is used to treat glaucoma.

D. Parathion (Folidol)

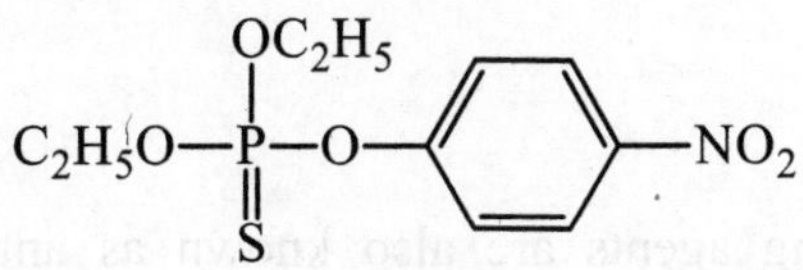

O,O - Diethyl - *O* - *p* - nitrophenyl phosphoro thioate

Parathion is a weak *cholinesterase* inhibitor

Mechanism of action: It is a *cholinesterase* inhibitor. It generally disrupts the nervous system by inhibiting *acetylcholinesterase.*

Use: It is used as an agricultural insecticide. It is especially used for controlling aphids, spider mites and scale insects.

2.3.2.3 *Cholinesterase* Reactivator

A. Pralidoxime chloride (Protopam chloride)

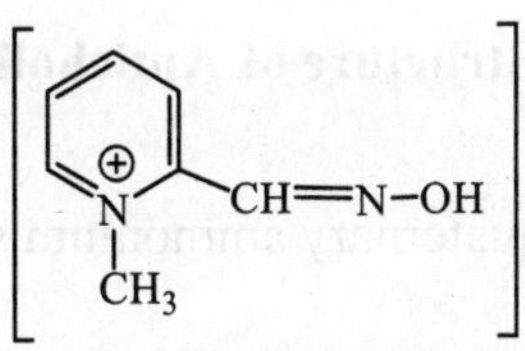

2 - Formyl - 1 - methyl pyridinium chloride oxime

Mechanism of action: It is an antidote to organophosphate pesticides and chemicals. Organophosphates bind to the esteratic site of *acetylcholinesterase,* which results initially in reversible inactivation of the enzyme. *Acetylcholinesterase* inhibition causes acetylcholine to accumulate in synapses, producing continuous stimulation of cholinergic fibers throughout the nervous systems. If given within 24 hours after organophosphate exposure, pralidoxime reactivates the *acetylcholinesterase* by cleaving the phosphate-ester bond formed between the organophosphate and *acetylcholinesterase.*

Use: It is used as an antidote for poisoning by Parathion and related pesticides.

3. CHOLINERGIC BLOCKING AGENTS (or) ANTISPASMODICS

3.1 Introduction

Cholinergic blocking agents are also known as antimuscarinic, anticholinergic, parasympatholytic or cholinolytic drugs. Antimuscarinic drug are those which antagonizes the effect of Acetylcholine by binding to muscarinic receptors. Because of the ability to relax smooth muscle, they are also referred as antispasmodics. Nicotinic antagonists which block certain action of Acetylcholine are referred as Ganglionic blockers and neuromuscular blockers.

3.2 Structure Activity Relationship

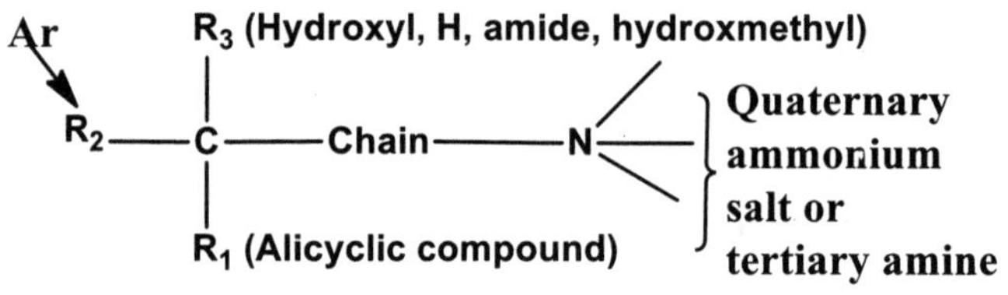

Fig. 6.5 General Structure of Anticholinergic Agent

- Nitrogen substituent may be quaternary ammonium salt or a tertiary amine with different alkyl groups.
- Most potent derivatives have Quaternary ammonium salt.
- Tertiary amine protonated at physiological P_H also possess antagonist activity.
- Alkyl group can be methyl, ethyl, propyl or isopropyl group.

- The nitrogen atom (cationic site) and pivotal carbon are separated by a chain may be ester, ether or hydrocarbon. Effective binding occurs with anticholinergic agents with ester group since it is similar to acetyl choline.

- R_1 or R_2 could be aromatic, carbocyclic or heterocyclic, but if both of cyclic it results in more antagonist activity. The rings may be same or different ring. One aromatic moiety is essential for Vander Waals interaction with the receptor in pivotal carbon. One cycloaliphatic or other hydrocarbon (olefinic group) required for hydrophobic interaction with the receptor.

- The R_3 group can be hydrogen, hydroxyl, hydroxymethyl, amide or component of the R_1 and R_2 group. Antagonist with hydroxyl or hydroxymethyl show more potency.

3.3 Therapeutic Uses

Anticholinergic drugs of non-quaternary amine derivative will cross the blood brain barrier (BBB) and have therapeutic actions or side effects, involving the central nervous system; if anticholinergic drugs are quaternary amines, they will not cross the blood brain barrier, thus they are devoid of CNS activity.

Therapeutic uses following inhibition of parasympathetic transmission are

1) Peripheral

i) Mydriasis: dilatation of pupil of the eye.

ii) Cycloplegia: a paralysis of the ciliary structure of the eye.

iii) Antisialagogue: decrease saliva production.

iv) Antispasmodic: decrease motility of smooth muscle and urinary incontinence.

v) Anhidrotic: reduces perspiration.

2) Central: Antiparkinson and anti-motion sickness.

3.4 Classification

Cholinergic blockers are classified chemically as

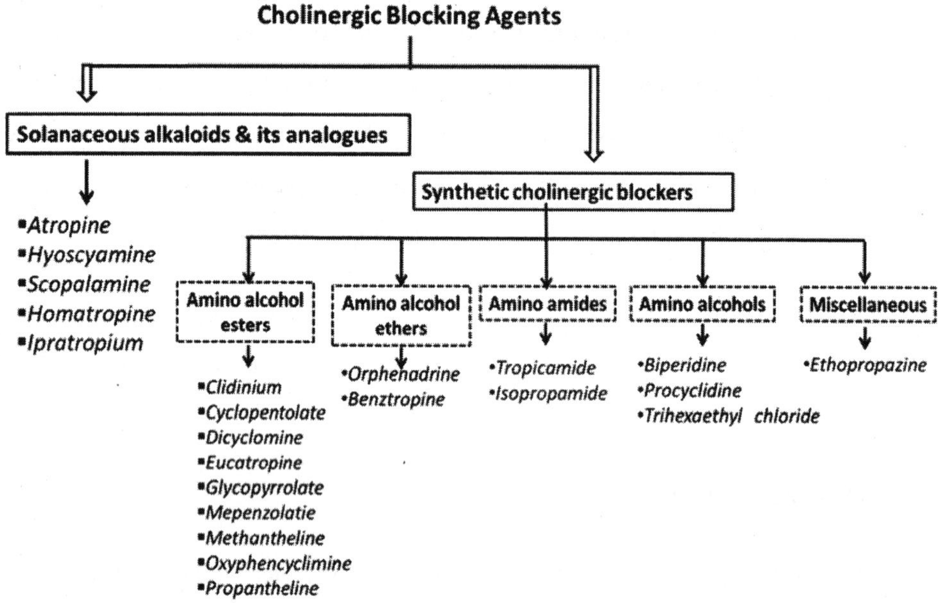

3.4.1 Solanaceous Alkaloids

This group includes Atropine, Hyoscyamine and Scopolamine. These alkaloids are found in *Atropa belladonna* and *Datura stramonium*. Atropine occurs along with Hyoscyamine. Hyoscyamine is optically active. $[\alpha]_D - 22^0$, but readily racemises to Atropine, when warmed with ethanolic solution.

A. Atropine sulphate (Atreza)

Atropine is a tropine ester of racemic tropic acid and is optically inactive. Atropine is isolated from natural sources, results from racemization of (-) Hyoscyamine, during the isolation process.

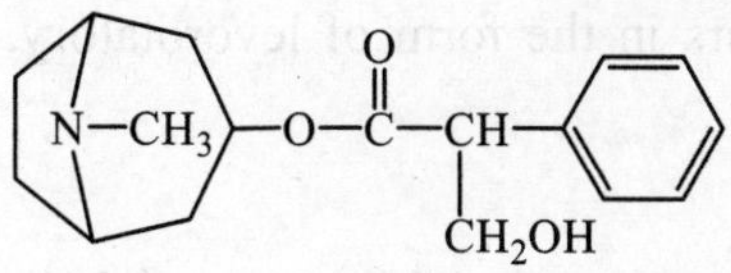

(8 - methyl -8-aza bicyclo [3.2.1] oct -3-yl) -3-hydroxyl -2- phenyl proponoate

Mechanism of action: It inhibits acetylcholine's muscarinic action at the neuro effector junctions of smooth muscles, cardiac muscles, exocrine glands, SA and AV nodes and the urinary bladder. In small doses, Atropine inhibits salivary and bronchial secretions and diaphoresis. In moderate doses, it increases impulse conduction through the AV node and increases heart rate. In large doses, it decreases GI and urinary tract motility and gastric acid secretion.

Use: It produces a mydriatic effect. It is used as an antidote to prevent the muscarinic effect of ACh accumulation due to organophosphate poison. It is used in rhinitis for symptomatic relief in cold. In cathartic preparation it is also used as antispasmodic.

B. Hyoscyamine sulphate (Anaspaz)

It is a levorotatory isomer of Atropine also known as *levo* atropine. The *dextro* form does not exist in nature.

Mechanism of action: It competitively inhibits acetylcholine at autonomic postganglionic cholinergic receptors. It acts mainly to reduce salivary, bronchial gastric secretion and sweat gland secretions.

Use: It is used as antispasmodic.

C. Scopolamine hydrobromide or Hyoscine (Biospan)

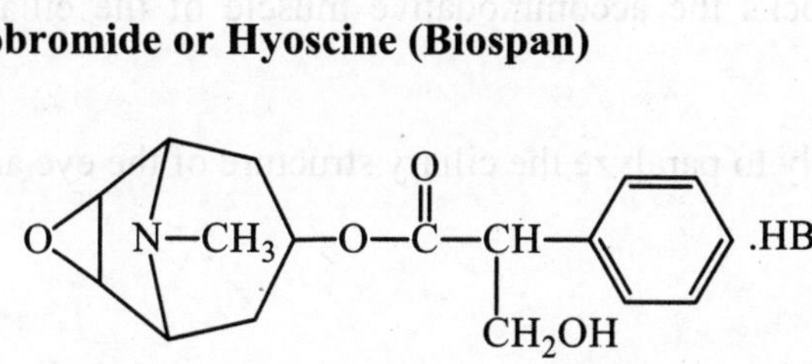

(-) (S) - 3 - Hydroxy - 2 - phenyl propionic acid - (1R, 2R,4S,7S,9S) - 9 - methyl - 3 - oxa - 8 - aza bicyclo (3.3.1.$0^{2,4}$) non - 7 - yl ester

It is an alkaloid occurs in the form of levorotatory, found in various members of solanaceae.

Mechanism of action: It competitively inhibits acetylcholine at autonomic postganglionic cholinergic receptors. It reduces GI smooth-muscle tone; decreases gastric secretions and GI motility; reduces bladder detrusor muscle tone; reduces nasal, oropharyngeal and bronchial secretions; and decreases airway resistance by relaxing smooth muscles in the bronchi and bronchioles. It also blocks neural pathways in the inner ear to relieve motion sickness and depresses the cerebral cortex to produce sedation and hypnotic effects.

Use: It is effective in preventing motion sickness. It is a competitive blocking agent of the parasympathetic nervous system, but it differs markedly from Atropine in its action on the higher nerve centre.

D. Homatropine hydrobromide (Hydromet)

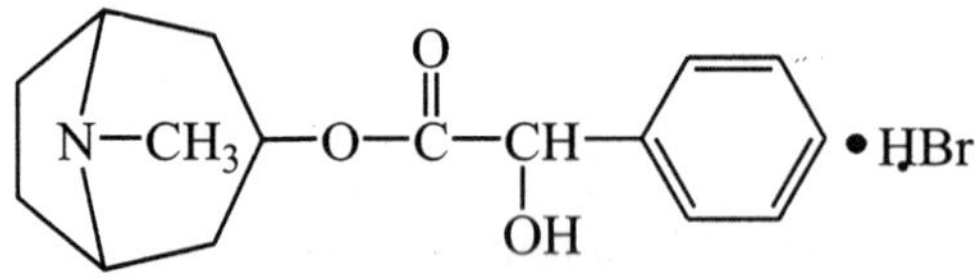

1αH, 5αH - Tropan -3α - ol hydrobromide

Mechanism of action: It is a competitive muscarinic receptor antagonist. It act in similar manner as atropine, producing similar parasympatholytic effects. By blocking muscarinic receptors and cholinergic signaling pathways, homatropine blocks the response of the iris sphincter muscle and cause the pupil to become unresponsive to light upon dilation or mydriasis. It also blocks the accommodative muscle of the ciliary body to cholinergic stimulation.

Use: It is used topically to paralyze the ciliary structure of the eye and to effect mydriasis.

E. Ipratropium bromide (Atrovent)

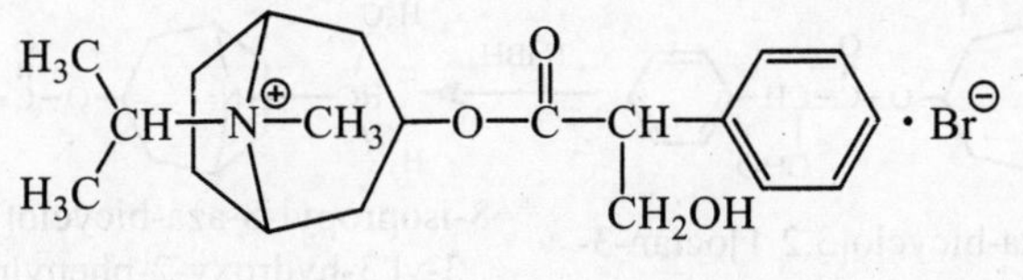

(+) - Endo -3- (3 - hydro -1- oxo - 2 - phenylpropoxy) - 8-methyl - 8 - (1-methylethyl) - 8 - azoniabicyclo (3.2.1) octane bromide

Ipratropium is a quaternary ammonium derivative of Atropine

Synthesis

Method – I: From Atropine: Atropine is quaternized with isopropyl bromide give Ipratropium bromide.

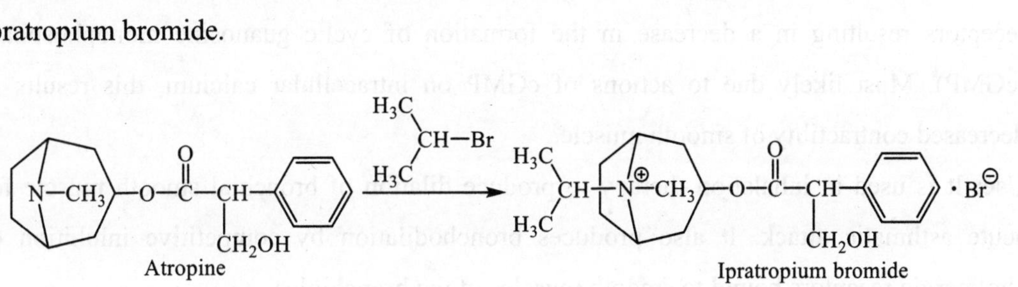

Method - II: From Succinaldehyde

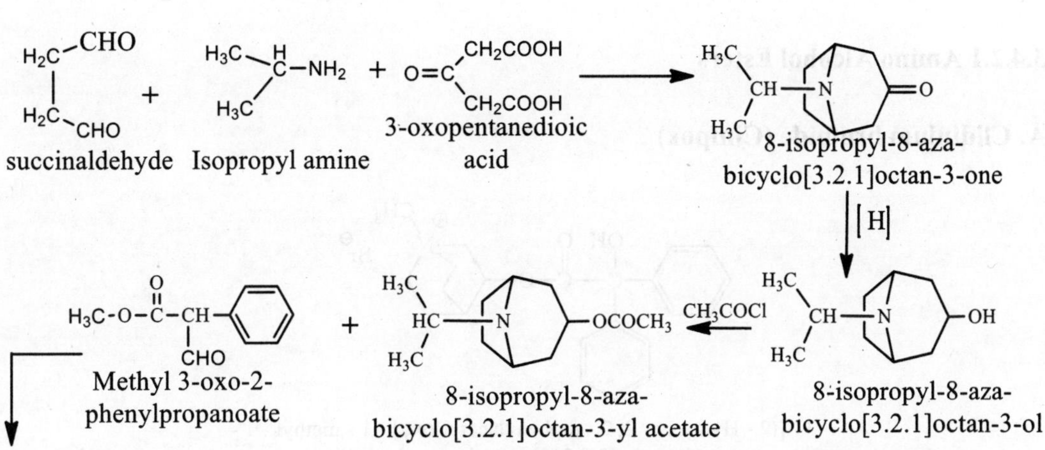

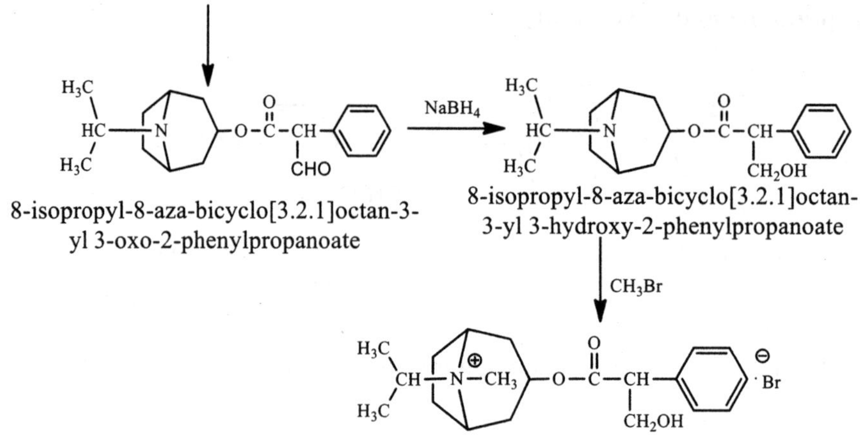

8-isopropyl-8-aza-bicyclo[3.2.1]octan-3-yl 3-oxo-2-phenylpropanoate

8-isopropyl-8-aza-bicyclo[3.2.1]octan-3-yl 3-hydroxy-2-phenylpropanoate

Ipratropium bromide

Mechanism of action: It is an anticholinergic agent blocks muscarinic cholinergic receptors resulting in a decrease in the formation of cyclic guanosine monophosphate (cGMP). Most likely due to actions of cGMP on intracellular calcium, this results in decreased contractility of smooth muscle.

Use: It is used in inhalation therapy to produce dilation of bronchial smooth muscle for acute asthmatic attack. It also produces bronchodilation by competitive inhibition of cholinergic receptors bound to smooth muscles of the bronchioles.

3.4.2 Synthetic Cholinergic Blocking Agents

3.4.2.1 Amino Alcohol Esters

A. Clidinium bromide (Cinipox)

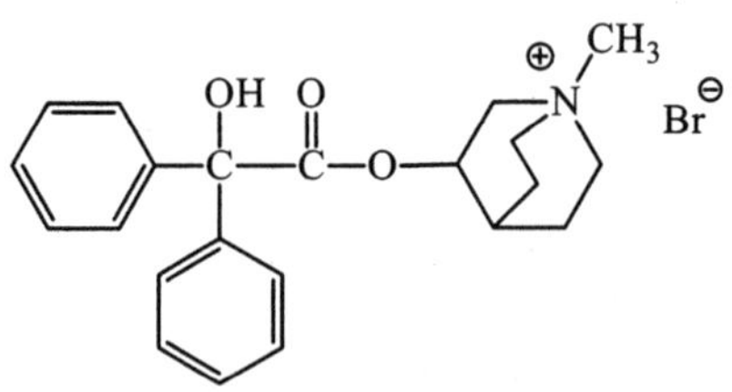

3 - [(2 - Hydroxy - 2, 2 - diphenylacetyl)oxy] - 1 - methyl - 1 - azabicyclo [2.2.2] octan - 1 - ium bromide

Mechanism of Action: It inhibits muscarinic actions of acetylcholine at postganglionic parasympathetic neuro effector sites primarily by inhibiting the M1 muscarinic receptors.

Use: It is used as anticholinergic agent, in combination with minor tranquillizer Chlordiazepoxide. It is used for peptic ulcer, hyperchlorhydria and ulcerative or spastic colon.

B. Cyclopentolate hydrochloride (Cyclogik)

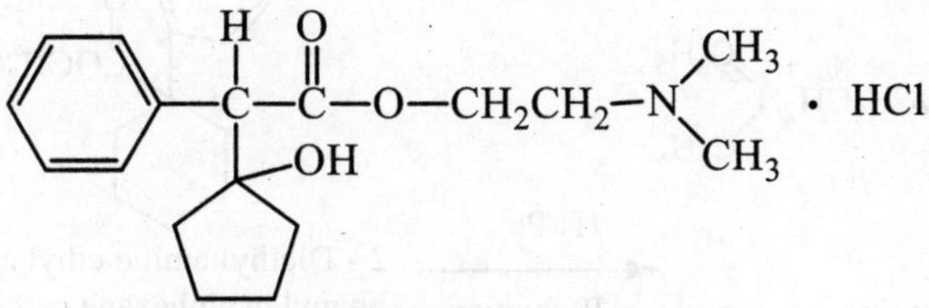

2 - (Dimethylamino) ethyl (1 - hydroxy cyclopentyl) (phenyl) acetate

Mechanism of action: It blocks muscarinic receptors and produces dilatation of the pupil (mydriasis) and prevents the eye from accommodating for near vision (cycloplegia).

Use: It is used as mydriatic agent.

C. Dicyclomine hydrochloride (Colimex)

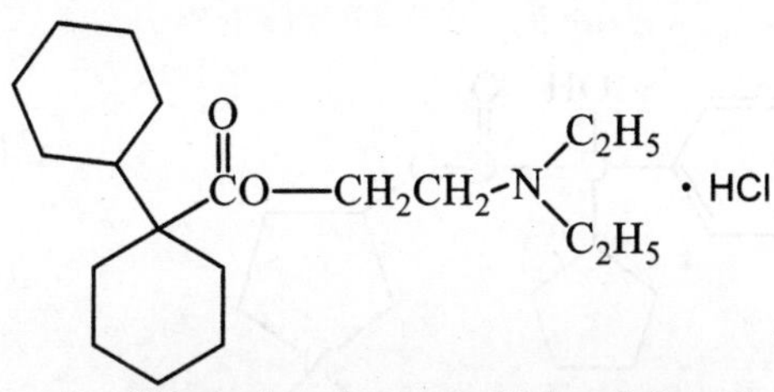

2 - (Diethyl amino) ethyl bicyclohexyl - 1 - carboxylate hydrochloride

Synthesis

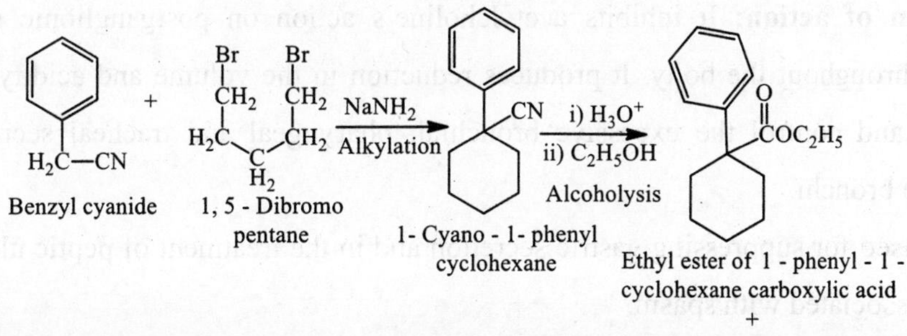

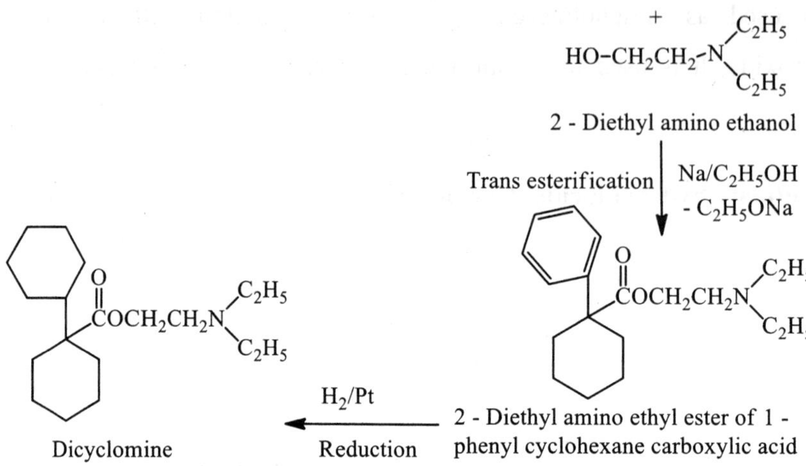

Mechanism of action: It inhibits acetylcholine's muscarinic actions at postganglionic parasympathetic receptors in smooth muscles, secretory glands and the CNS. These actions relax smooth muscles.

Use: It is also used in dysmenorrhea, pylorospasm and biliary dysfunction.

D. Glycopyrrolate (Cuvposa)

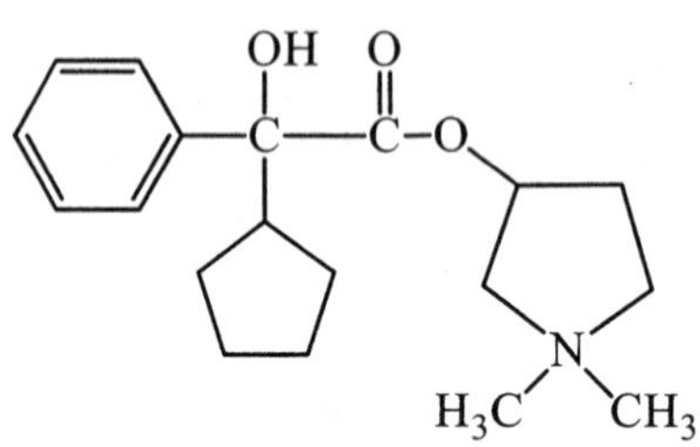

3 - Hydroxy - 1,1- dimethyl pyrrolidium - α - cyclopentyl mandelate

Mechanism of action: It inhibits acetylcholine's action on postganglionic muscarinic receptors throughout the body. It produces reduction in the volume and acidity of gastric secretions and control the excessive bronchial, pharyngeal and tracheal secretions and dilating the bronchi.

Use: It is used for suppressing gastric secretion and in the treatment of peptic ulcer and GI disorders associated with spasm.

E. Methantheline bromide (Hiprex)

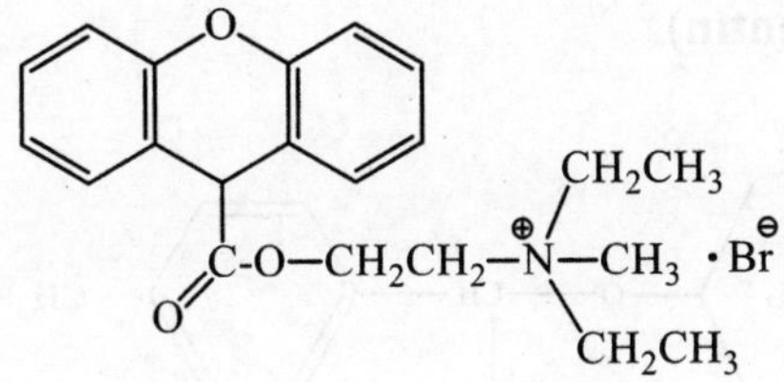

N - Methyl - N - ethyl - N - {2 - [(9H - xanthene - 9 - yl carbonyl) oxy] ethyl} - 2 - ethyl ammonium bromide

Mechanism of action: It inhibits the muscarinic actions of acetylcholine. Depending on the dose, anticholinergics may reduce the motility and secretory activity of the gastrointestinal system and the tone of the ureter and urinary bladder and may have a slight relaxant action on the bile ducts and gallbladder.

Use: It is a potent anticholinergic agent and acts on nicotinic cholinergic receptor.

F. Propantheline bromide (Spastheline)

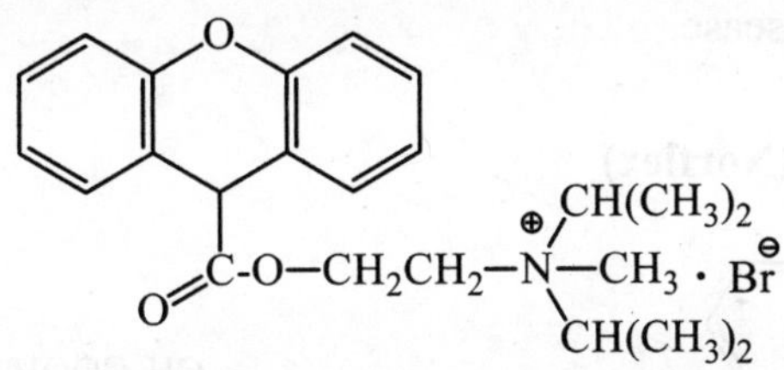

N - Methyl - N - (1 - methyl ethyl) - N - {2 - [(9H - xanthene - 9 - yl carbonyl) oxy] ethyl} - 2 - proponyl ammonium bromide

Mechanism of action: It is an anticholinergic drug that reduces the effect of acetylcholine, a chemical released from nerves that stimulates muscles, by blocking the receptors for acetylcholine on smooth muscle (a type of muscle). It also has a direct relaxing effect on smooth muscle.

Use: It is used as antispasmodic and in the treatment of peptic ulcer.

3.4.2.2 Amino Alcohol Ethers

A. Benztropine mesylate (Cogentin)

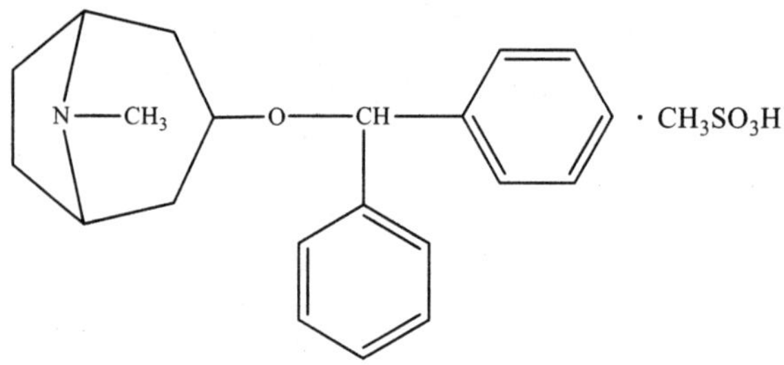

3-Benzhydryloxy-8-methyl-8-azabicyclo[3.2.1]octane;methanesulfonic acid

Mechanism of action: It blocks acetylcholine's action at cholinergic receptor sites. This restores the brain's normal dopamine and acetylcholine balance, which relaxes muscle movement and decreases drooling, rigidity and tremor. It also inhibit dopamine reuptake and storage, which prolongs dopamine's action.

Use: It has anticholinergic, antihistaminic and local anaesthetic activities. It is used in the treatment of Parkinson's disease.

B. Orphenadrine citrate (Norflex)

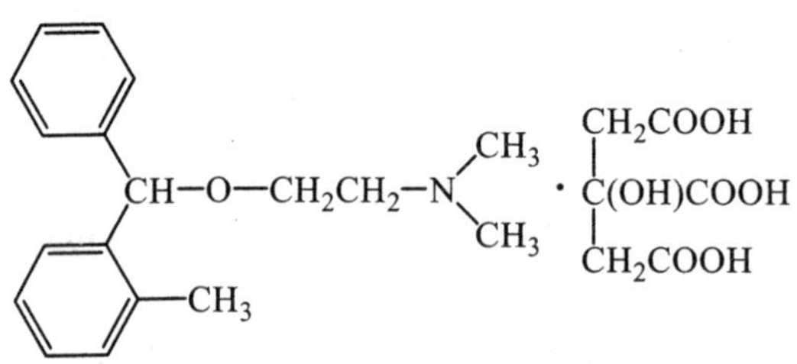

N, N - Dimethyl - 2 - (o - methyl - α -phenyl benzyloxy) ethylamine citrate

Mechanism of action: It reduces muscle spasms by acting on cerebral motor centers or medulla. Postganglionic anticholinergic effects and some antihistaminic and local anesthetic action contribute to skeletal muscle relaxation.

Use: It is used for the symptomatic treatment of Parkinson's disease. It is also used as skeletal muscle relaxant.

3.4.2.3 Amino Alcohols

A. Biperiden hydrochloride (Akineton)

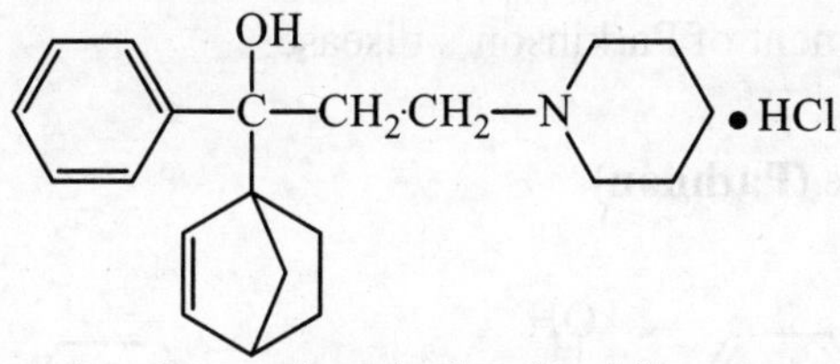

5α - Norbornen - 2 - yl - α - phenyl - 1 - piperidine propanol hydrochloride

Mechanism of action: It blocks acetylcholine's action at cholinergic receptor sites. This action restores the brain's normal dopamine and acetylcholine balance, which relaxes muscle movement and decreases rigidity and tremors. It also inhibits dopamine reuptake and storage, which prolongs dopamine's action.

Use: It is used in all types of Parkinson's disease.

B. Procyclidine hydrochloride (Kemadrin)

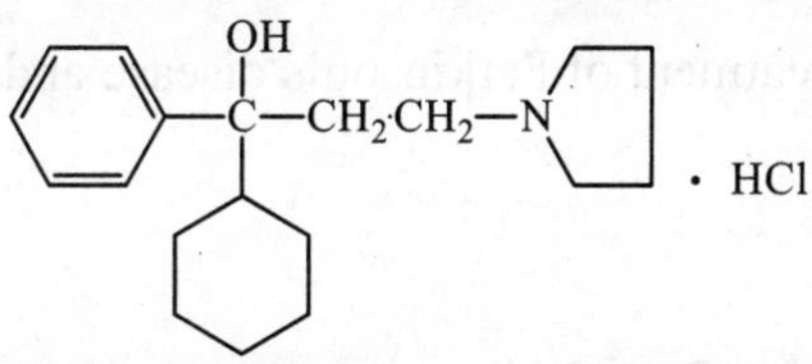

1- Cyclohexy - 1- phenyl - 3 - pyrrolidin - 1 - yl -1- propanol hydrochloride

Synthesis

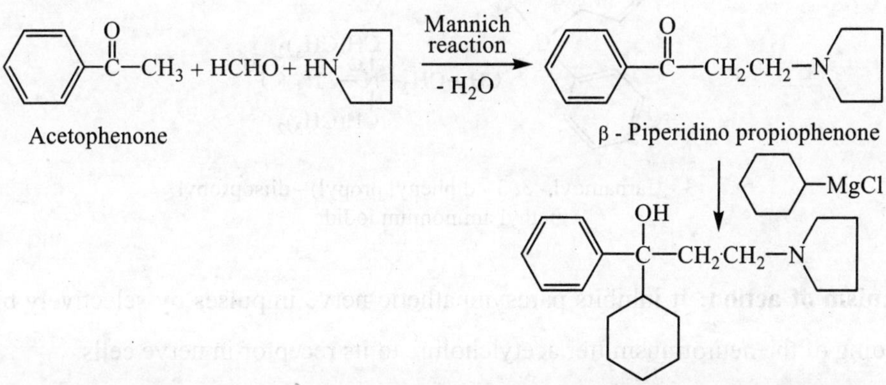

Procyclidine hydrochloride

Mechanism of action: It acts by blocking central cholinergic receptors and thus balancing cholinergic and dopaminergic activity in the basal ganglia. Its antispasmodic effects are thought to be related to the blockage of central cholinergic receptors M1, M2 and M4.

Use: It is used in the treatment of Parkinson's disease.

C. Tridihexethyl chloride (Pathilon)

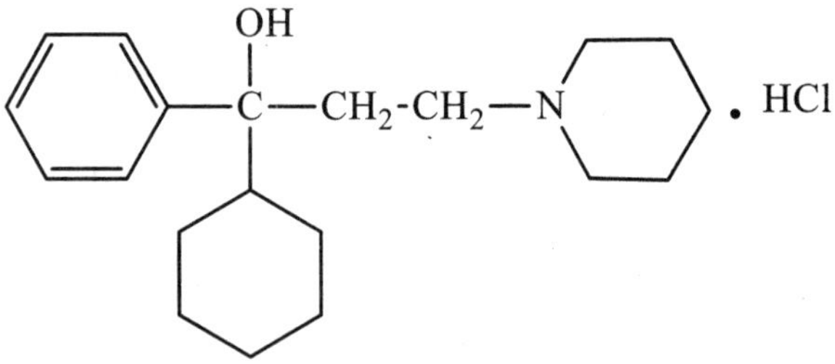

(*R*) - 1 - cyclohexyl - 1 - phenyl - 3 - (piperidin - 1 -yl) propan - 1 - ol hydrochloride

Mechanism of action: It binds to muscarinic acetylcholine receptor. It may block all three types of muscarinic receptors including M-1 M-2 and M-3 receptors.

Use: It is used in the treatment of Parkinson's disease and also used as an antispasmodic.

3.4.2.4 Amino Amides

A. Isopropamide iodide (Gastabid)

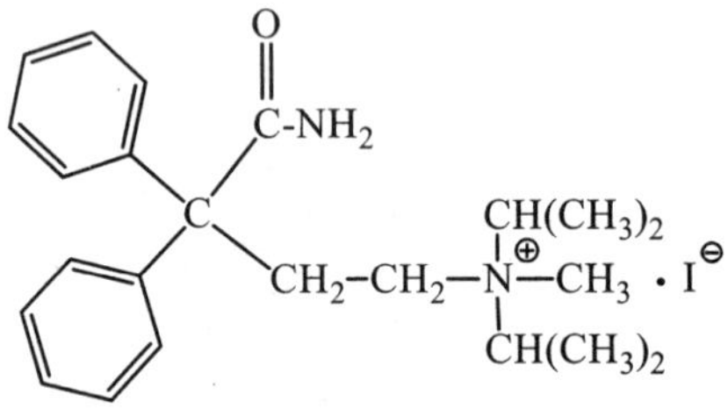

(3 - Carbamoyl - 3, 3 - diphenyl propyl) - diisopropyl methyl ammonium iodide

Mechanism of action: It inhibits parasympathetic nerve impulses by selectively blocking the binding of the neurotransmitter acetylcholine to its receptor in nerve cells.

Use: It is a potent anticholinergic drug. It has antispasmodic and antisecretory effects. It is used in the treatment of peptic ulcer. It is given along with Trifluperazine.

B. Tropicamide (Mydriacyl)

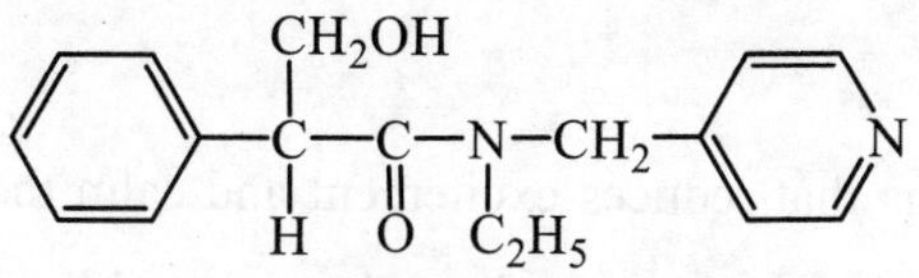

N - Ethyl - 3 - hydroxy - 2 - phenyl - N - (pyridin - 4 - yl methyl) propanamide

Mechanism of action: It blocks the receptors in the muscles of the eye (muscarinic receptor M4). It also acts by blocking the responses of the iris sphincter muscle to the iris and ciliary muscles to cholinergic stimulation, producing dilation of the pupil and paralysis of the ciliary muscle.

Use: It is used to dilate pupil for an eye examination and other ophthalmologic practices.

3.4.2.5 Miscellaneous

A. Ethopropazine hydrochloride (Parsidol)

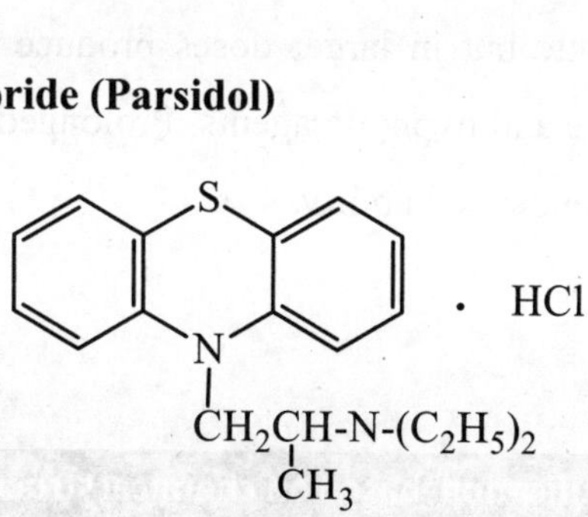

10 - [2 - (Diethyl amino) propyl] phenothiazine hydrochloride

Mechanism of action: It partially blocks central cholinergic receptors, thereby helping to balance cholinergic and dopaminergic activity in the basal ganglia; salivation may be decreased and smooth muscle may be relaxed. Its local anesthetic effect is due to its antagonism of the NMDA glutamate receptor.

Use: It is useful in the symptomatic treatment of Parkinsonism.

SEDATIVE AND HYPNOTICS

Chapter 7

1. INTRODUCTION

Sedatives are the drugs that reduces excitement and calm the patients without producing sleep. Hypnotics are drugs which produce sleep resembling normal sleep. Both sedative and hypnotics are CNS depressant but those with quick onset, shorter duration and steeper dose respond curve are preferred as hypnotics while more slowly acting drugs with flatter dose respond curves are employed as sedatives. Hypnotic drugs are used to induce sleep when sleeplessness is not due to a definite stimulus such as pain, itching which prevents sleep or awake the patient.

Sedative and hypnotic drugs are clinically used as anti-anxiety, anti-epileptics, muscle relaxants pre-anaesthetic medication and as an adjunctive therapy in psychiatry. Sedatives at therapeutic dose are anxiolytic but in larger doses produce hypnosis. Drowsiness is a side effect common to all sedative and hypnotic agents. Prolonged over dosage of these drugs can result in habituation and dependence liability.

2. CLASSIFICATION

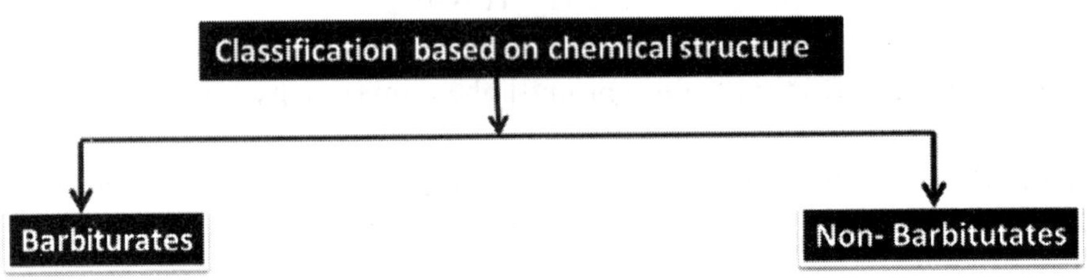

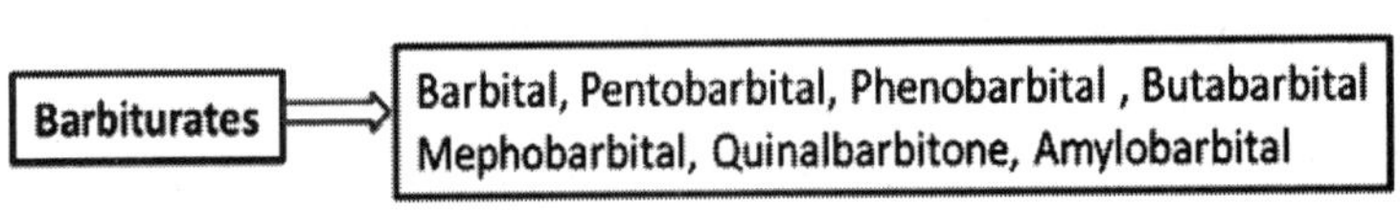

Non - Barbitutates

- **Benzodiazepine and related compounds :** Chlordiazepoxide , Clonazepam, Diazepam, Prazepam, Nitrazepam, Flurazepam, Halazepam, Lorazepam, Oxazepam , Temazepam , Chlorazepate
- **Triazolo - 1, 4- benzodiazepines:** Triazolam, Alprazolam, Estazolam
- **Imidazo pyridine:** Zolpidem
- **Cyclo pyrrolone:** Zopiclone
- **Pyrazolo pyrimidine:** Zaleplon
- **Piperidindione derivatives:** Methyprylone, Glutethimide
- **Carbamic acid ester:** Meprobamate. Ethinamate
- **Piperazine derivative :** Hydroxyzine hydrochloride
- **Disubstituted quinazolinone derivative:** Methaqualone
- **Chloral derivative:** Chloral hydrate
- **Acetylenic alcohol :** Ethchlorvynol
- **Cyclic ether:** Paraldehyde
- **Parasympatholytic :**Scopolamine
- **Inorganic salts:** Potassium bromide, Magnesium sulfate
- **Aromatic tertiary alkylamine:** Diphenhydramine
- **Precursors of serotonin :** L - tryptophan, 5- Hydroxy tryptophan

2.1 Barbiturates

Barbiturates are derived from barbituric acid or 2, 4, 6 – trioxo hexahydro pyrimidine. In general, the barbiturates exert a significant depressant action on the cerebrospinal axis. The relative degree of depression, sedation, hypnosis, antiepileptics or anaesthesia depends on the nature of the barbiturates, its dose and route of administration. Barbituric acid was first synthesized by combining urea from animal and malonic acid from apple.

2.1.1 Classification

Barbiturates are further classified based on their duration of action as follows.

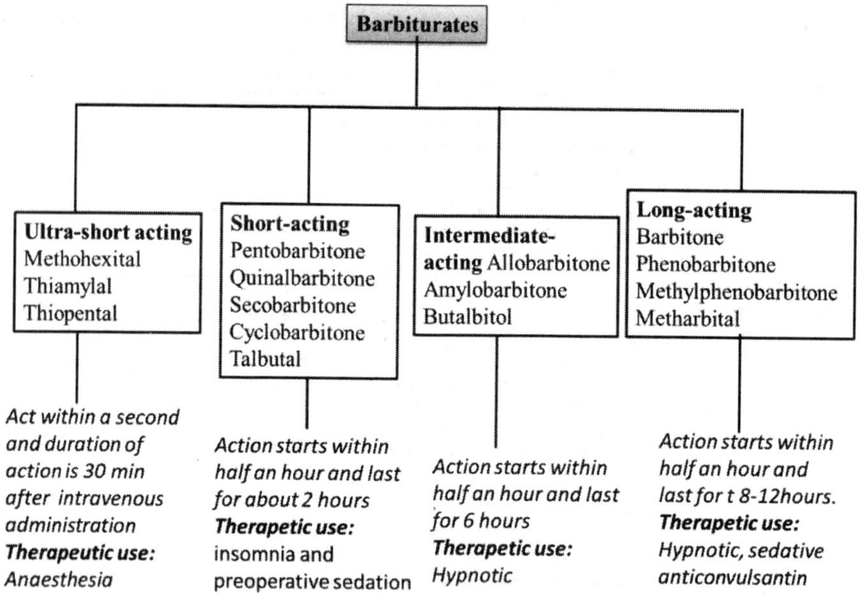

2.1.2 Mechanism of Action

The mechanism of action of barbiturate is inhibition of CNS by stimulating the inhibitory neurotransmitter system in the brain called Gamma amino butyric acid (GABA) system. Barbiturates as well as Benzodiazepines produce its desired pharmacological effect by allosterically binding to $GABA_A$ receptor complex by enhancing the GABA inhibitory response. GABA is the main inhibitory neurotransmitter for this receptor. When GABA binds the receptor, it triggers a conformational change in the pore, allowing more Cl^- to enter into the cell. This results in a hyperpolarization of the cell membrane, consequently increasing the firing threshold and producing an inhibition of action potential firing.

Upon binding, barbiturates/benzodiazepines lock the $GABA_A$ receptor into a conformation that increases the binding of GABA. This lead to prolonged opening of the channel. This influx of chloride creates a negative effect on neurotransmission. Therefore, an increase in the effect of GABA results in general suppression of the CNS. The $GABA_A$ receptor is composed of five protein subunits that ring a central chlorine ion channel. The majority of $GABA_A$ receptor subunits are α, β and γ.

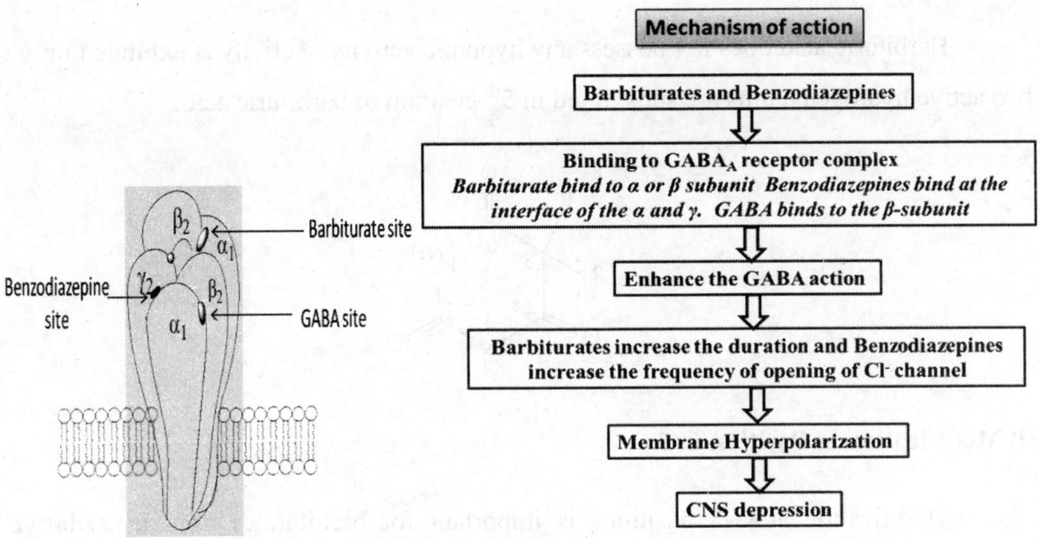

Fig. 7.1 Mechanism of action of Barbiturates and Benzodiazepine

- Barbiturate bind to α or β subunit of $GABA_A$ receptor and enhance the GABA action and prolong the inhibitory effects. Benzodiazepine bind to α and γ - subunits of $GABA_A$.
- Barbiturates increases the duration of opening of Cl^- channel, whereas Benzodiazepines increases the frequency of the opening.
- At higher doses, barbiturates may act as direct agonists at $GABA_A$ receptors and mimic the action of GABA which is responsible for barbiturate anaesthesia.
- Barbiturates also block the AMPA (α-Amino-3-hydroxy-5-methyl-4-isoxazole propionic acid) receptor a subtype of glutamate receptor, which is sensitive to an excitatory neurotransmitter glutamate. Glutamate restricts ion flow and increase the *trans* membrane action potential of the neuron.
- At very high concentration (anesthetic dose) it also depresses the voltages sensitive Na+ and K+ channel.

2.1.3 Structure Activity Relationship

Barbituric acid does not possess any hypnotic activity. Activity is exhibited only when two active hydrogen atoms are substituted in 5th position of barbituric acid.

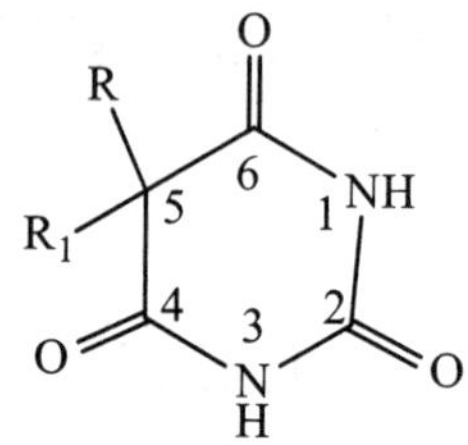

(i) Modification at Position C-5

Modification at C-5 positions is important for barbiturates used **as sedative** and **hypnotics**.

- Mono substitution at 5th carbon decreases the activity, because of the presence of one available proton at that site increases the acidity due to *tautomerism.* The proper acidity ratio of ionized and unionized form is important to cross the blood brain barrier **(BBB).**

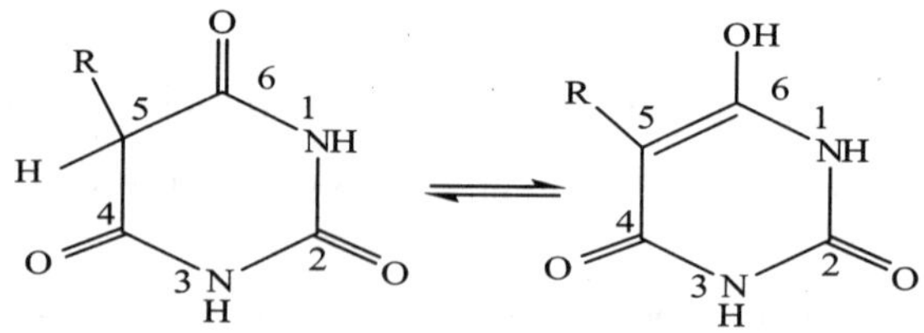

- The 5, 5'- disubstituted barbituric acid contains three lactam group that can undergo lactam-lactim *tautomerism.* The acidity of barbituric acid depends upon the number of substituent present in the position 5.

- Both the hydrogen at position 5 should be replaced, but the sum of the carbon of both substituents should be between 6 and 10 for optimal hypnotic activity. This sum is also indexed for duration of action.

- As the sum of alkyl group increases the lipid solubility of the compound also increases, it leads to increased onset of action and decreased duration of action.

- Greater the branching, more potent is the drug due to high lipid solubility and also have shorter duration of action. eg. Pentobarbital is more potent than Amobarbital.

- Branched cyclic or unsaturated chain reduces the duration of action due to its metabolic conversion to more polar inactive metabolites.

- Double bonds in the alkyl substituent group produces compound more readily vulnerable to oxidation. They have shorter duration of action. eg. Pentobarbitone.

- Shorter chain at C-5 resists oxidation and they are long acting barbiturates and long chain at that position is short acting.

- Stereo isomers have same potencies.

- Alicyclic or aromatic substituted analogues are more potent than aliphatic substituent. Only one of the substituents in position 5 may be closed chain.

- The presence of halogen in the 5 - alkyl group increases the potency.

- The polar substituent (OH, NH_2, COOH, CO, RNH) in the aromatic group at C-5 decreases the lipid solubility and potency.

(ii) Modification at Position 1 and 3

Modifications at nitrogen 1 or 3 position are important for barbiturates used as **anaesthetics** and **anticonvulsant.**

- Alkylation at position C-1 or C-3 may result in shorter onset and duration of action because N-methylation reduces the acidity value.

- Attachment of larger alkyl group to the nitrogen imparts anticonvulsant property to barbiturates.

- Attachment in both the nitrogen at N-1 and N-3 render the drug non-acidic making them inactive.

(iii) Modification at Position 2, 4 and 6

Modification at oxygen is important for barbiturates used as **anaesthetics.**

- The replacement of oxygen by sulphur at C-2 increases the lipid solubility hence shortens the duration and onset of action.
- Introduction of more sulphur at position C-4 and C-6 decreases the hypnotic activity.
- These drugs are used as intravenous anaesthetics.eg. Thiopental

The structure of barbiturates with duration of action is represented in Table 9.1

Table 7.1 Barbiturates used as Sedative and Hypnotics

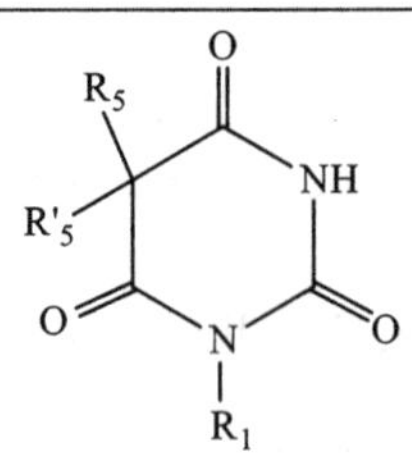

	Generic Name	Substituent's		
		R_1	R_5	R'_5
A	**Long duration of Action: (< 6 hrs)**			
1	Phenobarbital	- H	- C_2H_5	- C_6H_5
2	Mephobarbital	- CH_3	- C_2H_5	- C_6H_5
3	Barbital	-H	- C_2H_5	- C_2H_5
B	**Intermediate duration of Action:(3 to 6 hrs)**			
1	Amobarbital	- H	- C_2H_5	- $CH_2CH_2CH(CH_3)_2$

2	Butabarbital	- H	- C_2H_5	$CH_3CH_2CH(CH_3)$—
C	**Short Duration of Action: (> 3 hrs)**			
1	Pentobarbital	- H	- C_2H_5	$CH_3CH_2CH_2CH(CH_3)$—
2	Secobarbital	- H	- CH_2-CH=CH_2	$CH_3CH_2CH_2CH(CH_3)$—
3	Talbutal	H	- CH_2-CH=CH_2	$CH_3CH_2CH(CH_3)$—

2.1.4 General Synthesis of Barbiturates

The barbiturates are 5, 5'- dialkyl barbituric acid. The following scheme shows the synthesis of 5, 5' - dialkyl compounds condensing appropriate dialkyl malonate with urea makes all the barbiturates.

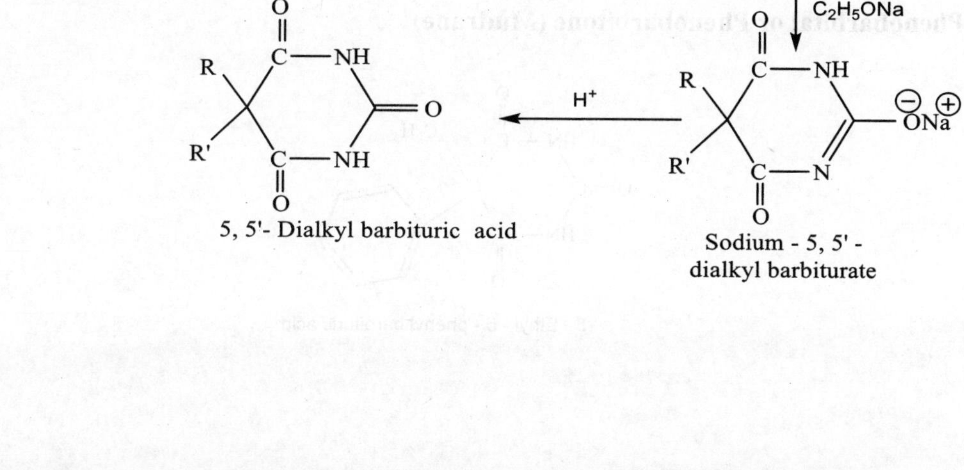

Substitution of thiourea for urea in the reaction produces 2- thio barbiturates

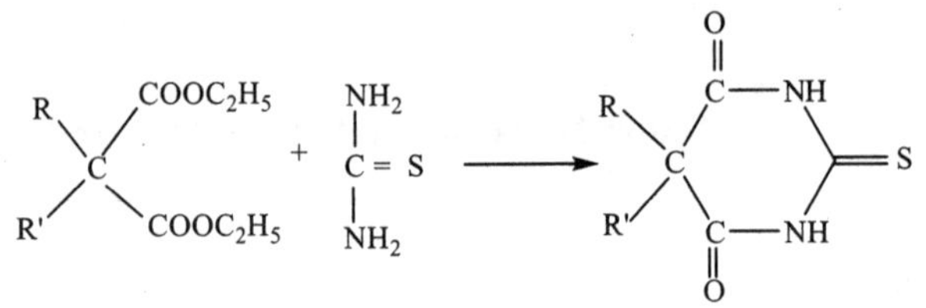

A. Barbital or Barbitone (Veronal)

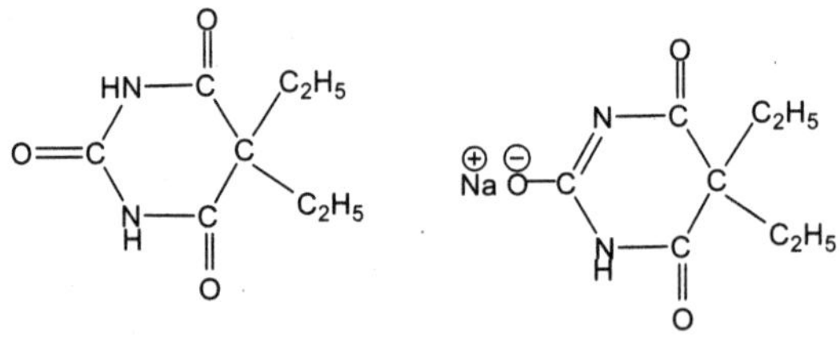

5,5' - Diethyl barbituric acid

Sodium - 5,5' - diethyl barbiturate

Synthesis

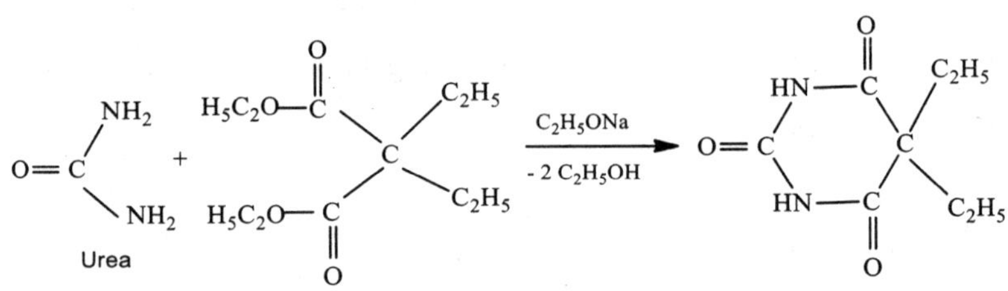

Urea

Diethyl malonic ester

Barbital

Use: It is a powerful hypnotic drug and generally used in the treatment of seizures.

B. Phenobarbital or Phenobarbitone (Mudrane)

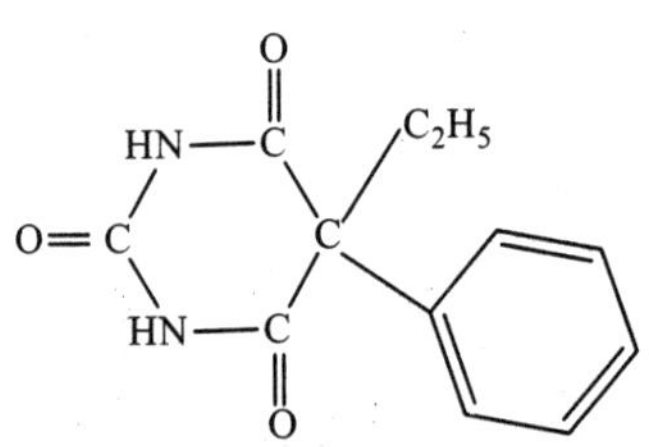

5 - Ethyl - 5 - phenvl barbituric acid

Use: It is used as sedative and hypnotic. It is a drug of choice for the treatment of grand mal and petit mal epilepsy.

C. Mephobarbital or Methylphenobarbitone (Prominal)

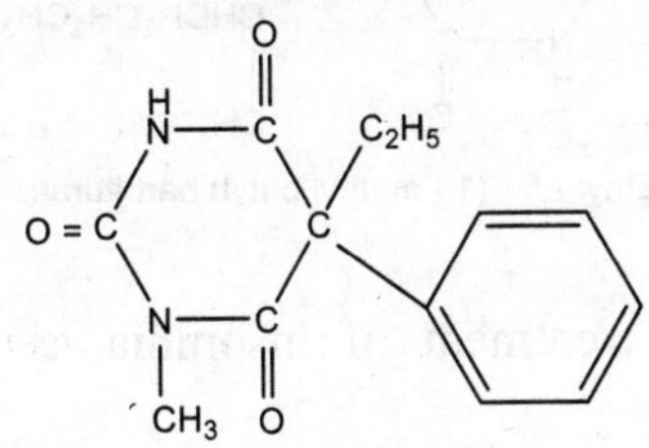

5 - Ethyl - 1- methyl - 5 - phenyl barbituric acid

Use: It is used as anticonvulsant with strong hypnotic activity.

D. Butabarbital (Butisol)

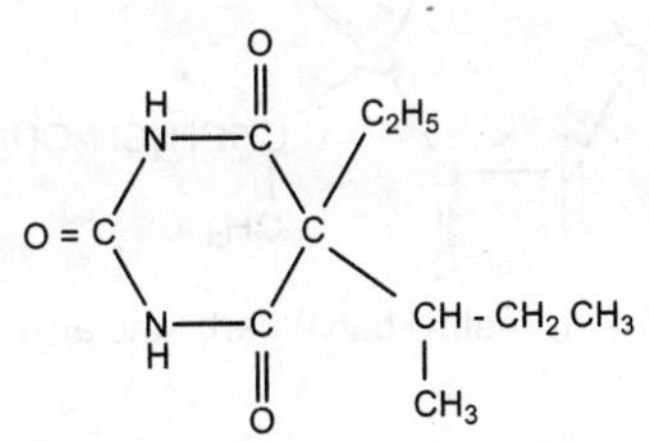

5 - Ethyl - 5 - (1- Methyl propyl) barbituric acid.

Use: It is used as sedative and hypnotic at different dose intervals.

E. Amobarbital or Amylobarbitone (Amytal)

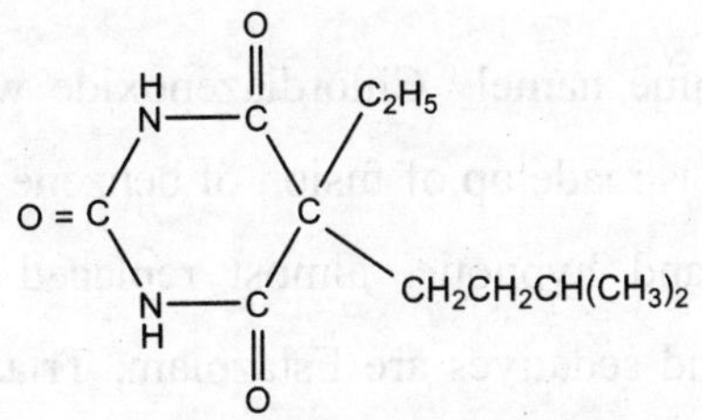

5 - Ethyl - 5 - isopentyl barbituric acid

Use: It is used in the treatment of insomnia and pre-operative medication.

F. Pentobarbital or Pentobarbitone (Barbinol)

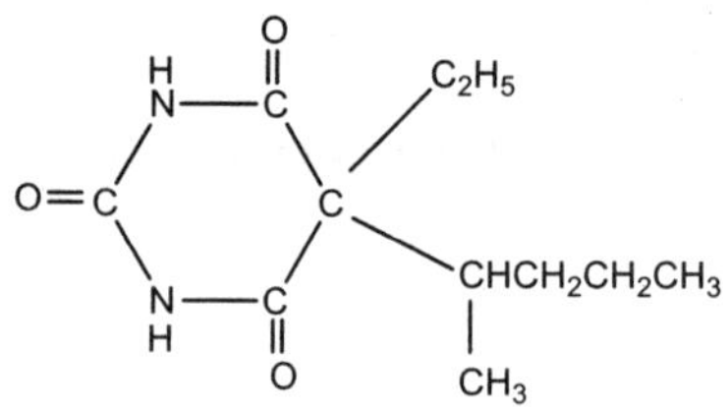

5 - Ethyl - 5 - (1 - methyl butyl) barbituratic acid

Use: It is used mostly in the treatment of insomnia, as basal anaesthetics and also in Strychnine poisoning.

G. Secobarbital or Quinalbarbitone (Seconal)

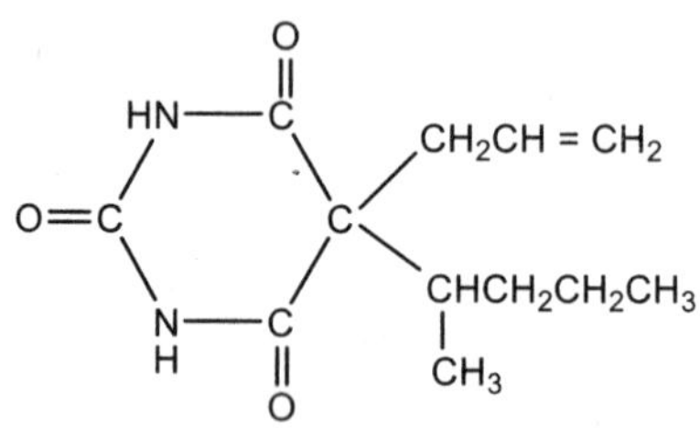

5 - Allyl - 5 - (1- methyl butyl) barbituric acid

Use: It is widely used as sedative and hypnotics. It is also used in status epileptics and toxic reactions to Strychnine and local anaesthetics.

2.2 Nonbarbiturates

2.2.1 Benzodiazepines

The first benzodiazepine namely Chlordiazepoxide was synthesized by accident in 1955. The chemical structure is made up of fusion of benzene ring with diazepine ring. It is a second-generation sedative and hypnotic, almost replaced barbiturates. Benzodiazepines normally used as hypnotic and sedatives are Estazolam, Triazolam, Quazepam, Flurazepam and Temazepam. Benzodiazepines also have uses in epilepsy (Diazepam, Clonazepam, Clobazam) anaesthesia (Midazolam), some motor disorders and occasionally in acute psychoses. The major clinical advantages of benzodiazepines are high efficacy, rapid onset of action and low toxicity.

2.2.1.1 Mechanism of Action

- ❖ The mechanism of action for the benzodiazepine is nearly the same as that of barbiturates. Like barbiturates, benzodiazepines bind at a unique site on the $GABA_A$ receptor. (Fig. 7.1).
- ❖ Benzodiazepine binds to the interface of γ and α subunit of $GABA_A$ receptor and enhance the GABA action that increase the frequency of chloride channel and results in general suppression of the CNS.
- ❖ Benzodiazepines bind at the interface of the γ subunit and any of the α_1, α_2, α_3, or α_5-subunits. Benzodiazepines with high affinity for the α_1 subunit are associated with sedatives and those with affinity for α_2 or α_3 subunits demonstrate anti-anxiety activity. Receptors containing the α_5 subunits may play a role in memory processes.
- ❖ Barbiturates increases duration and benzodiazepines increases frequency of opening of Cl^- channel.

2.2.1.2 Structure Activity Relationship

The basic structure of 1, 4 - benzodiazepine is shown below

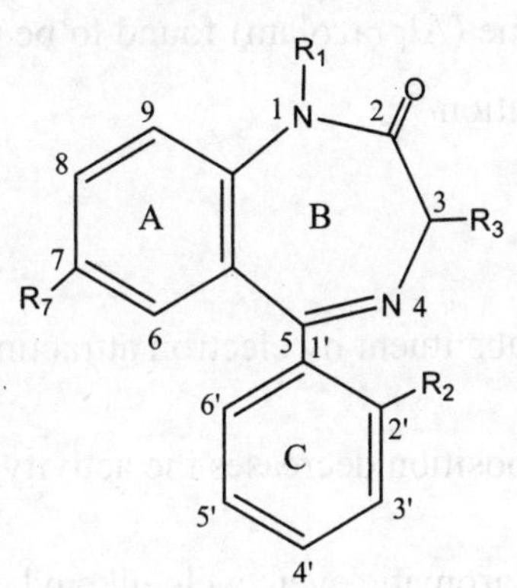

(i) Ring A substitution

- An electronegative substituent at position 7 is required for activity. As more the electro negativity the activity also increases.
- Position 6, 8 and 9 should not be substituted.

(ii) Ring B substitution

- Substitution at N^1 by alkyl, haloalkyl, alkynyl and amino alkyl group increases the activity.
- The 2- carbonyl function is optimal for activity.
- Alkyl substitution at position 3 decreases the activity, but the presence or absence of hydroxyl group is essential pharmacokinetically. Compound without 3-hydroxy group are non-polar and usually have long half-life. Compounds with the 3-hydroxy group have short half-life because of rapid conjugation with glucuronic acid.
- Saturation of 4, 5 double bond or a shift of this double bond to 3, 4 positions decrease the activity.
- A phenyl ring at position 5 promotes the activity.
- Triazolo benzodiazepine (Alprazolam) found to be more potent. They do not require any substitution at position 7.

(iii) Ring C Substitution

- The ortho or diortho substituent by electron attracting group increases the activity.
- Any substitution at 4' position decreases the activity dramatically.
- C-ring can be a hetero aromatic even cyclo alkenyl.

Benzodiazepine derivatives are given in Table 9.2

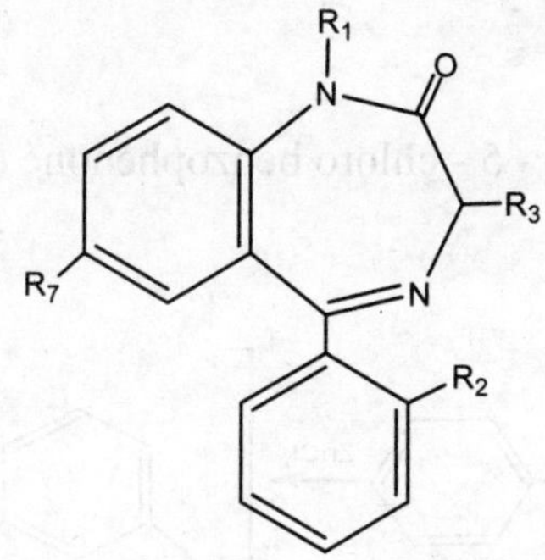

Table 7.1 Benzodiazepine Derivatives

S. No	Generic name	R_1	R_2	R_3	R_7
1.	Diazepam	$-CH_3$	- H	- H	- Cl
2.	Oxazepam	- H	- H	- OH	- Cl
3.	Lorazepam	- H	- Cl	- OH	- Cl
4.	Clorazepate	- H	- H	- COOH	- Cl

A. Diazepam (Alzepam)

Diazepam is the most successful sedative from benzodiazepine group. It is discovered by Strenhack and Hoffmann.

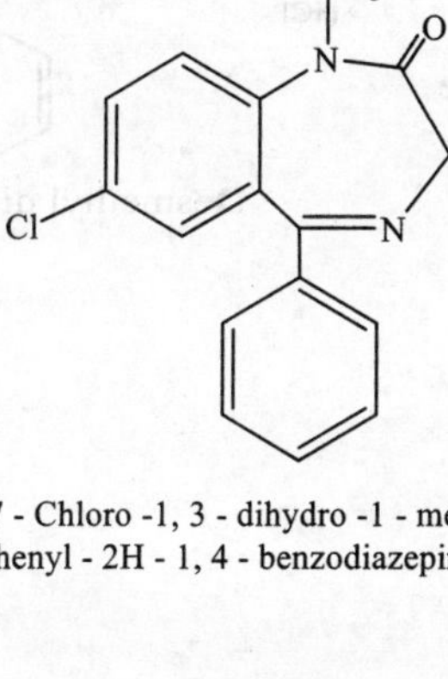

7 - Chloro -1, 3 - dihydro -1 - methyl - 5 - phenyl - 2H - 1, 4 - benzodiazepin - 2 - one

Synthesis

Method - I

Step - 1: Synthesis of 2 - Amino - 5 - chloro benzophenone (Intermediate)

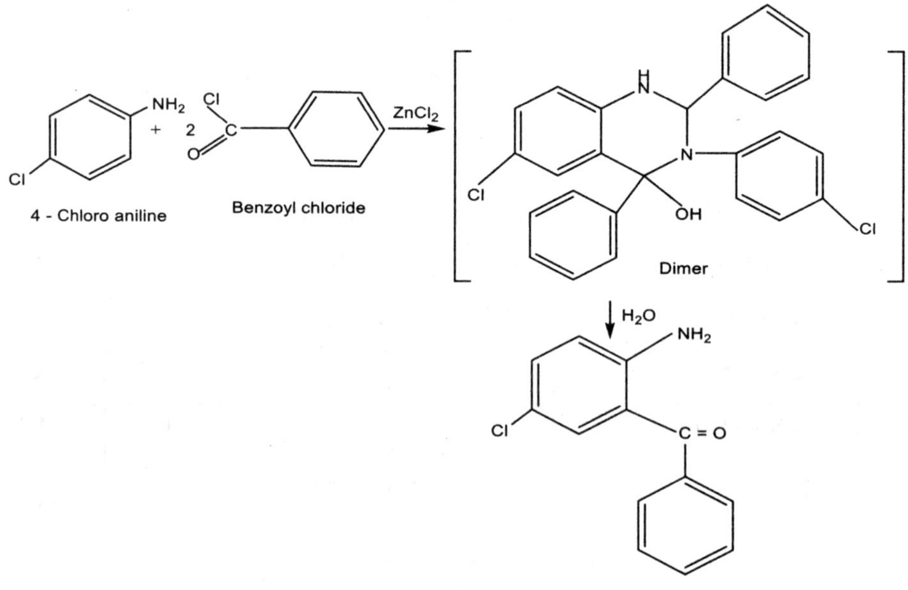

2 - Amino - 5 - chloro benzophenone

Step - 2: Synthesis of Diazepam

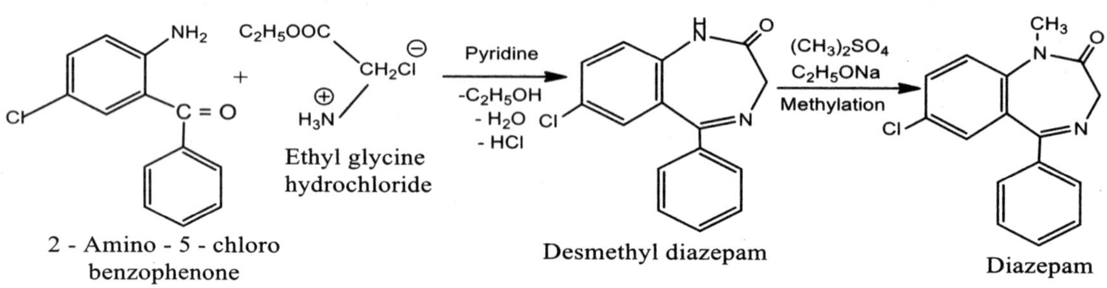

Method - II

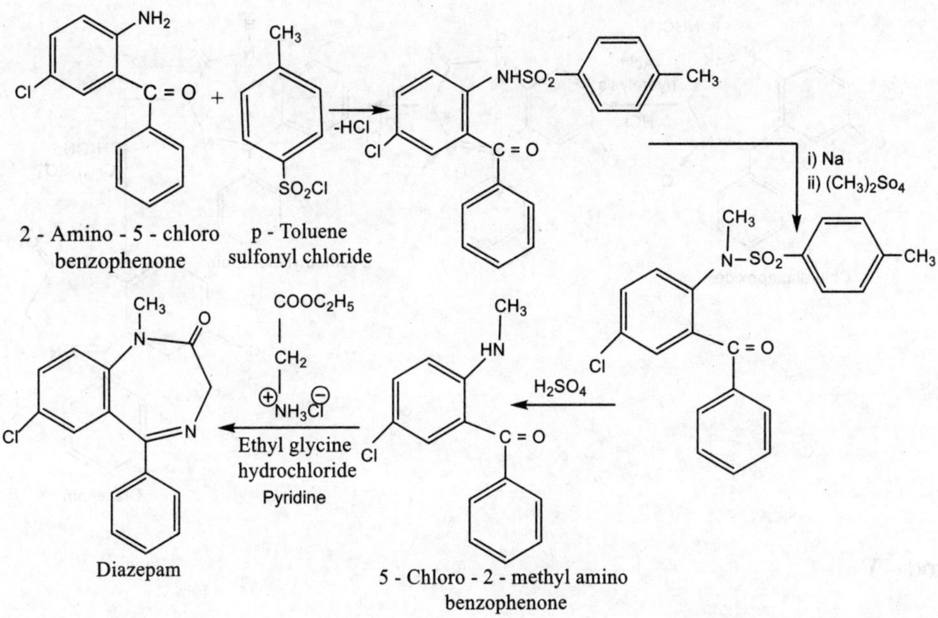

Method - III

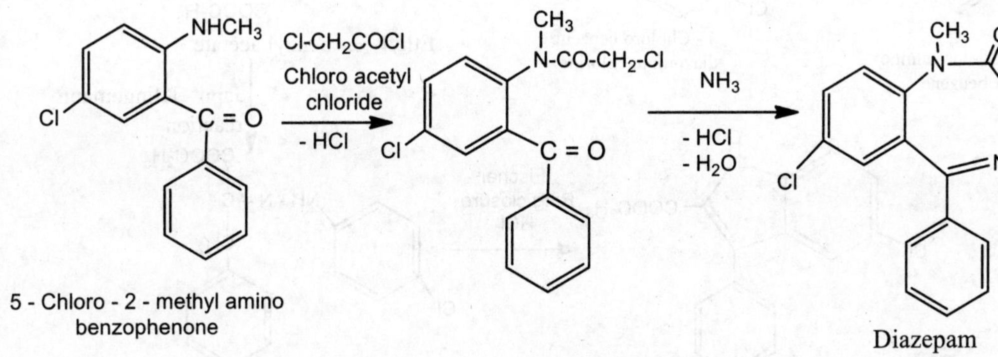

Method – IV: Diazepam can also be obtained by acid hydrolysis is of Chlordiazepoxide.

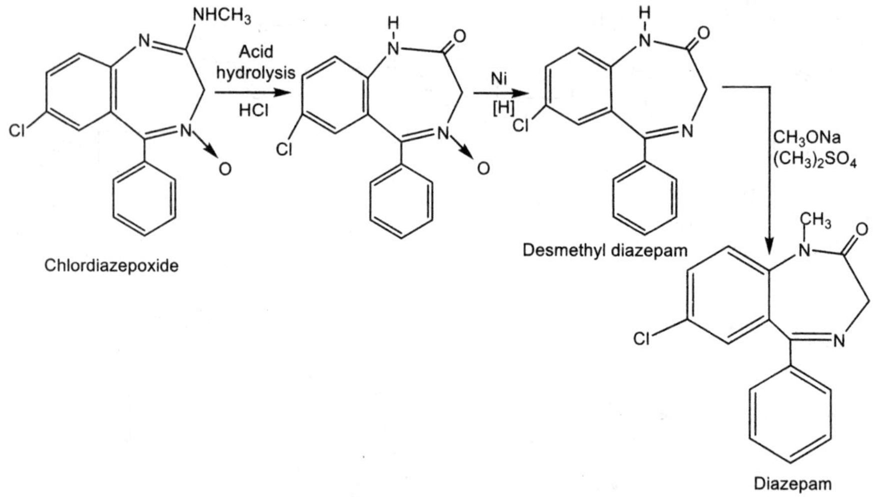

Method – V

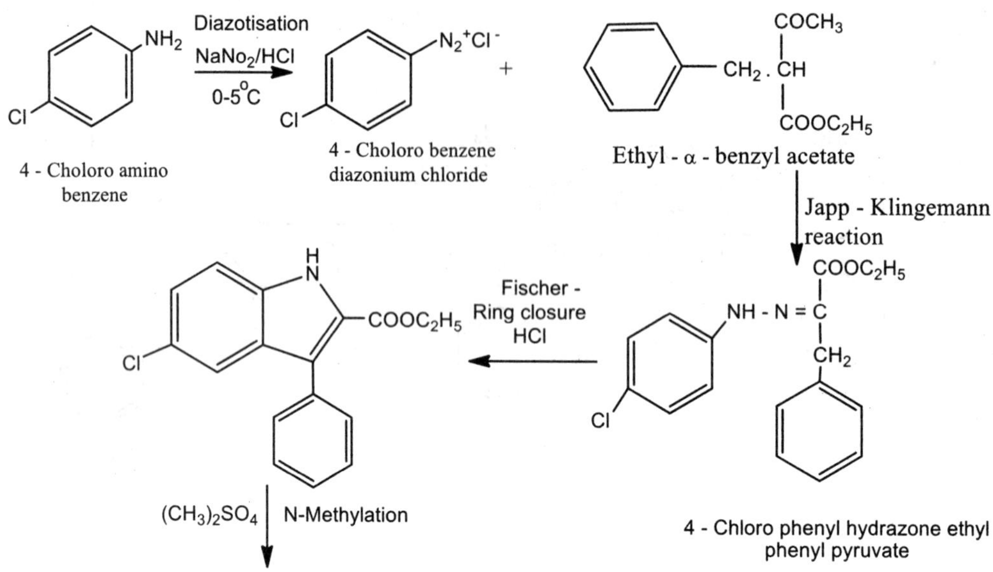

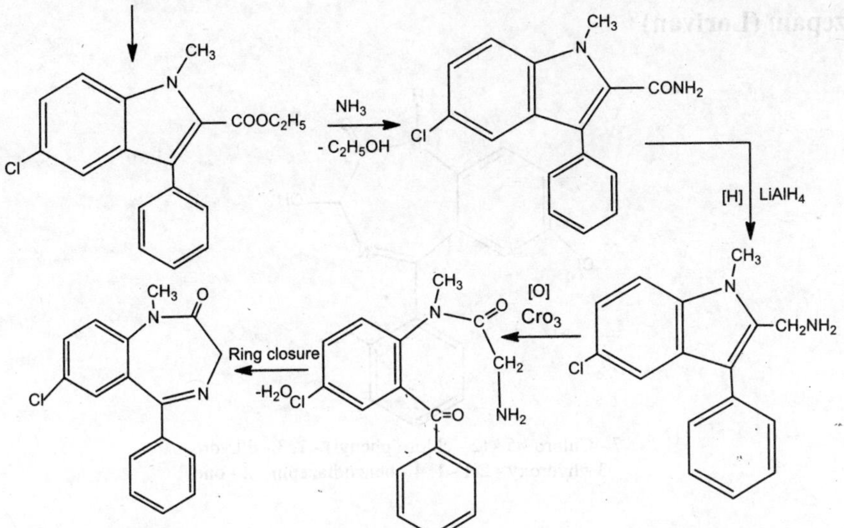

Use: It is used as skeletal muscle relaxant, anticonvulsant and antianxiety agent.

B. Oxazepam (Serepax)

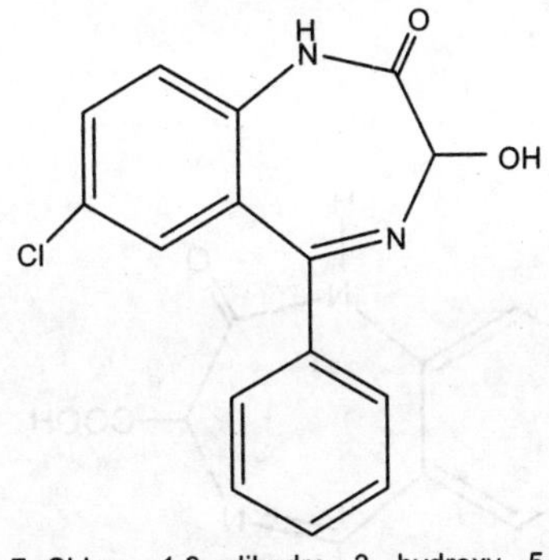

7- Chloro - 1,3 - dihydro - 3 - hydroxy - 5 - phenyl - 2H - 1,4 - benzodiazepin - 2 -one

Use: It is a mild sedative useful in the management and control of anxiety, tension, agitation, irritability and related symptoms. It is also useful for the control of acute tremulousness inebriation or anxiety associated with alcohol withdrawal.

C. Lorazepam (Lorivan)

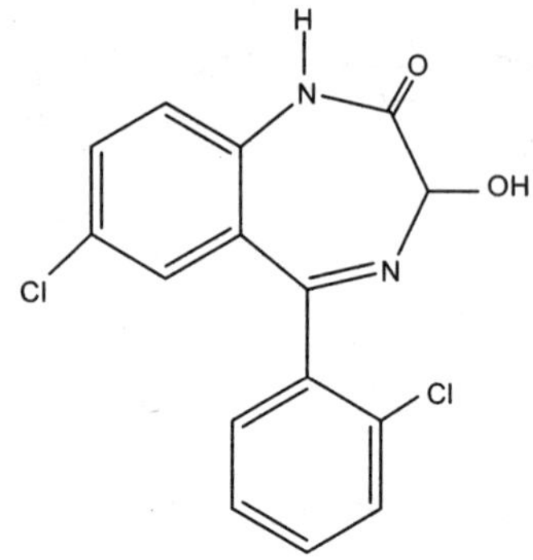

7 - Chloro - 5 - (2 - chloro phenyl) - 1, 3 - dihydro - 3 - hydroxy - 2H - 1, 4 - benzodiazepin - 2 - one

Lorazepam is 2'- Chloro substituted analogue of Oxazepam. The presence of 2' Chloro group increases the activity.

Use: It is used to treat anxiety disorders. It is used for the short term treatment of insomnia acute seizure and sedation.

D. Clorazepate (Tranxene)

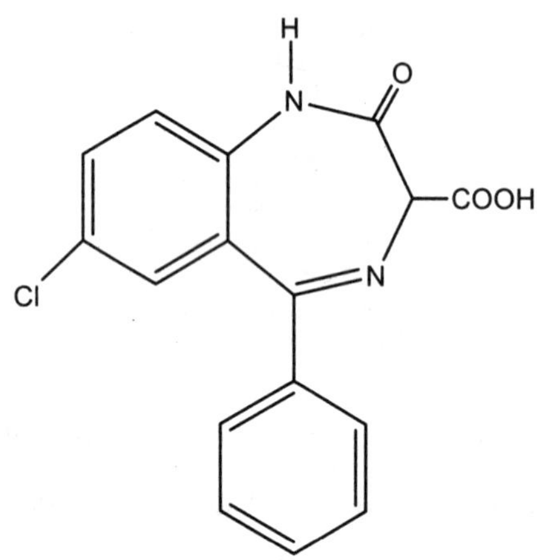

7 - Chloro - 2 - oxo - 5 - phenyl - 1, 3 - dihydro - 2H - 1, 4 - benzodiazepin - 3 - carboxylic acid

Use: It is used to treat anxiety disorders. It is also used as muscle relaxant and anticonvulsant.

E. Chlordiazepoxide (Librium/Depoxil)

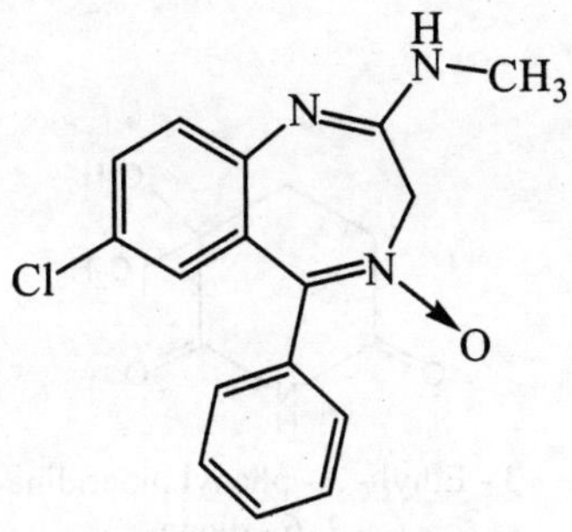

7 - Chloro - 2 - (methyl amino) - 5 - phenyl - 3H - 1, 4 - benzodiazepin - 4 - oxide

Use: It is used as antipsychotic, sedative and muscle relaxant.

2.2.2 Triazolo-1, 4-benzodiazepines

A. Alprazolam (Aleez/Aldep)

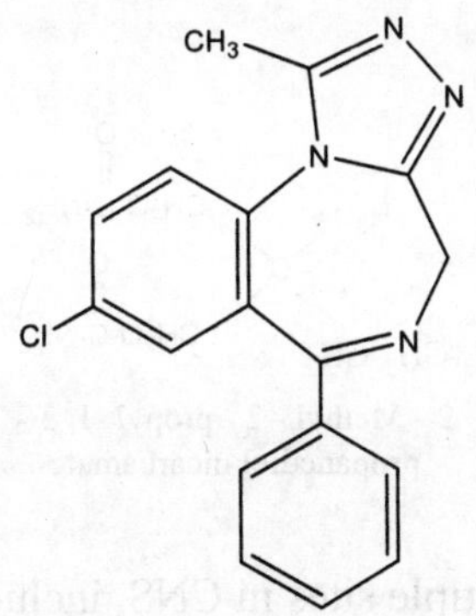

8 - Chloro - 1 - methyl - 6 - phenyl - 4H - S - triazolo - [4, 3-a] - [1,4] - benzodiazepine

Mechanism of action: It acts on benzodiazepine receptors BNZ-1 and BNZ- 2.It couple with GABA-A receptors to enhance GABA binding to its receptor.

Use: It is a highly potent anxiolytic. It also possesses sedative, hypnotic, skeletal muscle relaxant and anticonvulsant properties.

2.2.3 Piperidinedione Derivatives

A. Glutethimide (Glimid)

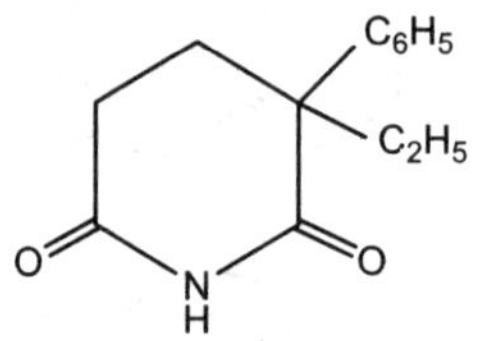

3 - Ethyl - 3 - phenyl piperidine - 2, 6 - dione

Mechanism of action: It is a GABA agonist which helps induced sedation.

Use: It is a hypnotic drug useful for inducing sleep in all types of insomnia. It induces sleep without depressing respiration.

2.2.4 Carbamic acid Ester

A. Meprobamate (Equanil)

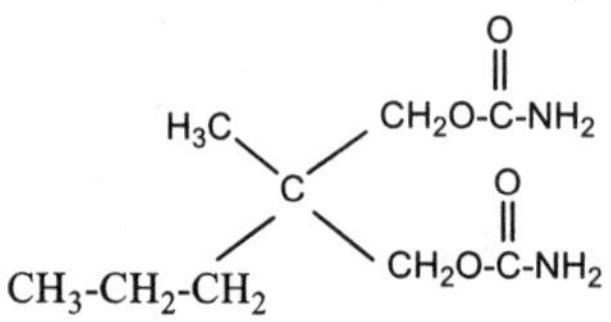

2 - Methyl - 2 - propyl -1, 3 - propanediol dicarbamate

Mechanism of action: It acts at multiple sites in CNS, including thalamus and limbic system. It inhibits spinal reflexes, causing CNS relaxation; its sedative effects may account for its anticonvulsant action. It also has muscle relaxant properties.

Use: It is used for the management of anxiety disorders or for short term relief of the symptoms of anxiety.

2.2.5 Acetylenic Alcohol

A. Ethchlorvynol (Placidyl)

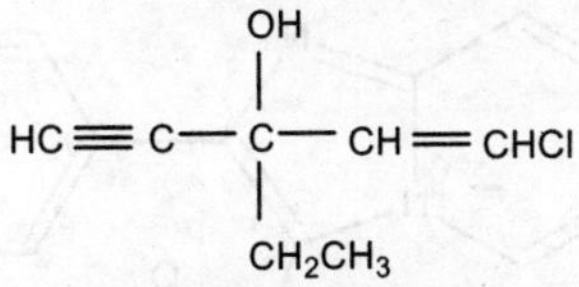

1 - Chloro - 3 - ethyl - 1 - penten - 4 - yn - 3 - ol

Mechanism of action: It depresses the central nervous system in a manner similar to that of barbiturates. Barbiturates bind at distinct binding sites associated with a Cl^- ionophore at the GABA receptor, increasing the duration of time for which the Cl^- ionophore is open. The post-synaptic inhibitory effect of GABA in the thalamus is, therefore, prolonged.

Use: It is a mild hypnotic that induce sleep within 15 minutes to 1 hour and has duration of action of approximately 5 hours.

2.2.6 Cyclic Ether

A. Paraldehyde (Paral)

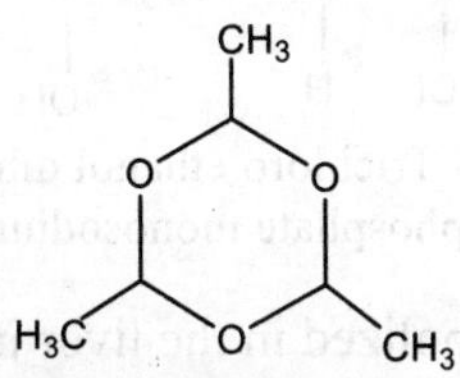

2, 4, 6 -Trimethyl - 1, 3, 5 - trioxane

It is a polymer of acetaldehyde of a type similar to trioxy methylene

Mechanism of action: It acts by reducing the release of acetylcholine in response to neuronal depolarization.

Use: It is one of the oldest sedative and hypnotics.

2.2.7 Imidazo pyridine

A. Zolpidem (Ambien/Lipiden)

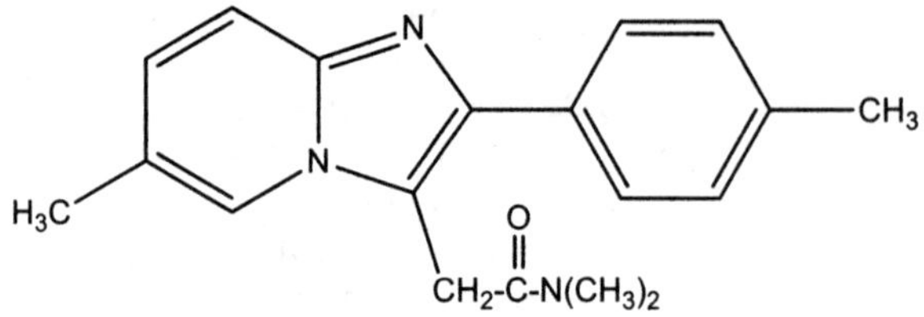

N, N - dimethyl - 2 - (6 - methyl - 2 - p - tolyl imidazo - [1, 2-a] - pyridin - 3 - yl) acetamide

Mechanism of action: It is a γ-Aminobutyric acid agonist. It act by binding to $GABA_A$ receptors at the same location as benzodiazepines and increase GABA effects in the central nervous system

Use: It is used to treat insomnia.

2.2.8 Miscellaneous

A. Triclofos sodium (Silence)

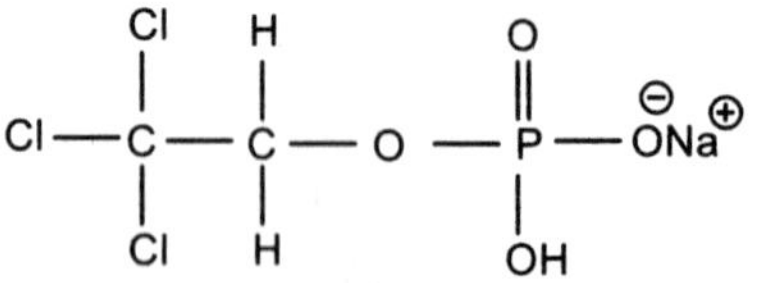

2, 2, 2 - Trichloro ethanol dihydrogen phosphate monosodium

Triclofos is a prodrug which is metabolized in the liver into the active drug trichloro ethanol.

Synthesis

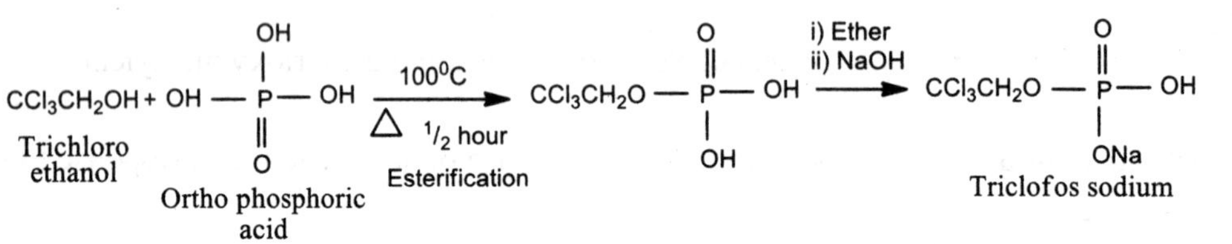

Mechanism of action: It is converted to Trichloro ethanol in the body. It act on brain and produces sleep. Trichloro ethanol decreases time taken to fall asleep and lengthen the sleep.

Use: It is a hypnotic drug suggested for insomnia, characterized by difficulty in falling sleep, nocturnal awakening and early morning awakening.

Chapter 8

ANTIPSYCHOTICS

1. INTRODUCTION

Antipsychotics are drugs, used to manage psychosis such as delusions, hallucinations, paranoia or disordered thought, mostly in schizophrenia and bipolar disorder. They are also known as neuroleptics or major tranquilizers. They act mainly on the lower brain area to produce emotional calmness and relaxation without significant sedation, hypnosis, motor impairment or euphoria. In addition, many of these drugs also act as skeletal muscle relaxants, antihypertensive, antiemetic and antiepileptic. The mechanism of action of antipsychotic agent is complex. It acts by blocking postsynaptic dopaminergic receptor and act as competitive antagonists of dopamine both centrally and peripherally.

2. CLASSIFICATION

This class of drugs fall into two categories:

(i) Typical Antipsychotics or First-Generation Antipsychotic Drugs. The typical or conventional, antipsychotics were first developed in the 1950s and used to treat schizophrenia. Typical antipsychotics may also be used for the treatment of acute mania, agitation and other conditions.

(ii) Atypical Antipsychotics or Second-Generation Antipsychotic Drugs. These new medications were approved for use in 1990s and used to treat schizophrenia, bipolar disorder, autism and as an adjunct in major depressive disorder.

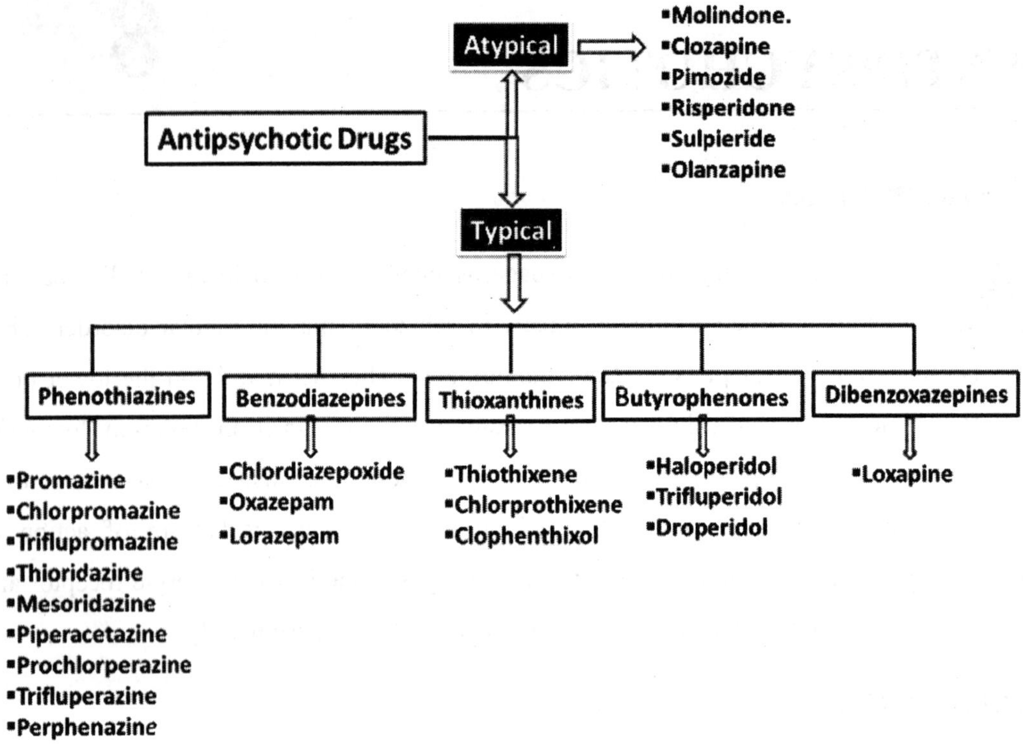

2.1 Typical Antipsychotics

2.1.1 Phenothiazines

Phenothiazine is a tricyclic ring of thiazine type, was first synthesized in the year 1883. Many drugs containing phenothiazine rings are clinically used as antihistaminic and antipsychotics. Phenothiazine act on specific post-synaptic receptor and block the post-synaptic dopamine receptor. They work on positive symptoms on psychosis such as hallucination, delusion, loss of association and bizarre behavior. The binding of sites of dopamine towards dopamine receptors are (Fig. 8.1)

- a flat hydrophobic area interacts with the phenyl ring and hydrogen bonding around the phenyl ring to accommodate the ring hydroxyl group.
- two carbon distance is essential between anionic and the ring site.

- protonated anionic site.

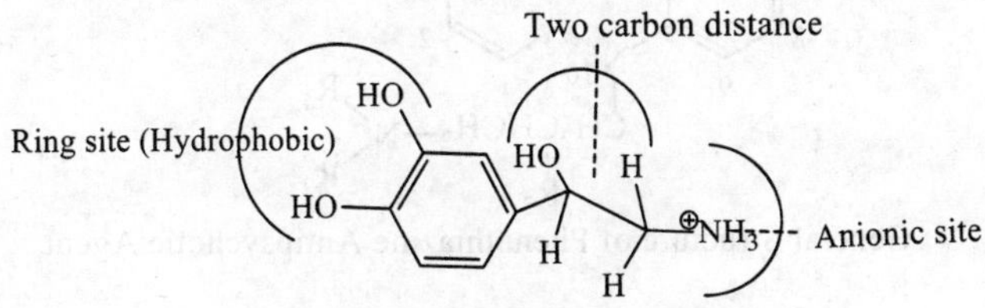

Fig. 8.1 Binding of Dopamine Receptor

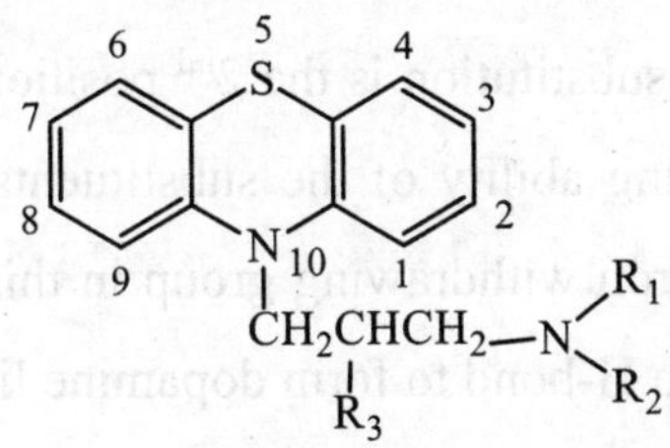

Phenothiazine shows neuroleptics effect mainly through interaction at D_2 type of dopamine receptor. The presence of electron withdrawing group (chloro) in the 2nd position of the ring is an important structural feature for neuroleptic property. The chloro group in the 2nd position tilts the protonated side chain towards the ring. This allows the favorable Vander Waal's forces of attraction of side chain with chloro substituent. The resulting conformation permits the superimposition of dopamine. Even though phenothiazine contains 3 carbon chain, two carbon distances is attained through the molecular bonding of the side chain towards ring. Phenyl ring interact with flat hydrophobic area of the receptor.

The protonated basic amino group form hydrogen bond with substituent at C_2 (unshared pair of electrons) which resembles Dopamine. The sulfur at C_5 is analogous to the p-hydroxyl group of Dopamine and it is also assigned as receptor binding function.

2.1.1.1 Structure Activity Relationship

Phenothiazines are chemically constituted by lipophilic linearly fused tricyclic system and hydrophilic basic amino alkyl side chain.

The structure activity relationship activities of these compounds are determined by:

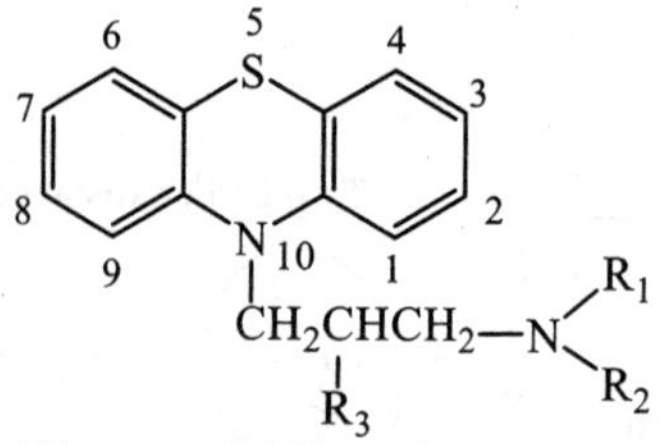

General Structure of Phenothiazine Antipsychotic Agent

(i) Phenothiazine Ring Substitution

- The best position for substitution is the 2nd position. Neuroleptic activity increases as electron withdrawing ability of the substituents increases. eg. Chlorpromazine The presence of electron withdrawing group in this position help bending the side chain nitrogen through H-bond to form dopamine like conformation.
- The presence of chlorine in 2nd position is essential for neuroleptic drugs.
- Presence of unshared election pair of an atom or atoms of the 2nd substituent increases the potency of the compound.
- Substituent at 3rd position shows significant activity when compared to unsubstituted compound but not as significant as substituent at 2nd position.
- Substitution at 1st and 4th position has a deleterious effect on antipsychotic activity.
- Oxidation of the ring sulphur to sulfoxide or sulfone decreases neuroleptic activity.

(ii) Modifications of alkyl side chain

- Three carbon atom chains between position 10 and the amino nitrogen is required. Two carbon side chain increases H_1 antagonism.
- Shortening or lengthening of the chain, at this position decreases the activity.

- The three- carbon atom side chain may be necessary for neuroleptic activity because it permits the maximum resemblance of most preferred conformational form of Dopamine.

- Substitution on the propylene chain of 10 - (3 - amino propyl) phenothiazine may also influence antipsychotic potency. For example.

    (a) Introduction of methyl group at C_1 decreases antipsychotic activity and may result in Imipramine like activity.

    (b) If oxygen is introduced at C_1 of the 3 - amino propyl side chain, it results into anti-depressant like action. eg. Chlorazine.

    (c) Introduction of methyl group at C_2 or C_3 of the side chain has little influence on activity.

    (d) Bridging of position 3 of the side chain to position 1 of the phenothiazine ring reduce neuroleptic activity.

(iii) Modification of basic amino group

- Maximum neuroleptic potency is retained in compound having 3 ° amino groups. Activity is reduced with 2° and 1° amino groups.

- Alkylation of amino group with large amino groups decreases neuroleptic activity.

- Activity is retained or increased if the amino group is incorporated in cyclic systems like piperidyl or piperazine eg. Mesoridazine.

- Potency of the compound increases with substitution of hydroxy, methyl, hydroxy ethyl group at C_4 of piperidine or piperazine.

- Piperazine phenothiazines may be esterified with long chain fatty acids to produce slowly absorbed long acting, lipophilic prodrug. eg. Fluphenazine decanoate.

The general structure of Phenothiazine drugs are given in Table 8.1.

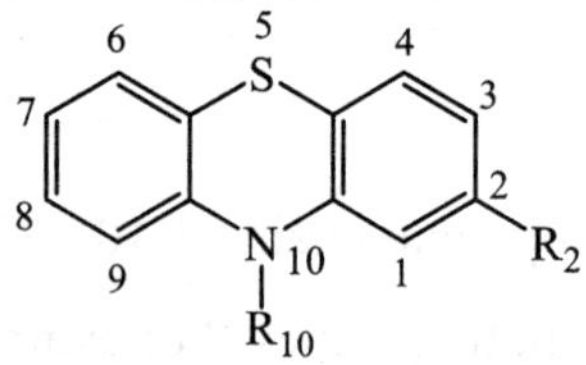

Table 8.1 Phenothiazine Derivatives

Generic Name	R_2	R_{10}
Promazine	- H	$-(CH_2)_3N(CH_3)_2$
Chlorpromazine	- Cl	$-(CH_2)_3N(CH_3)_2$
Triflupromazine	$-CF_3$	$-(CH_2)_3N(CH_3)_2$
Thioridazine	$-SCH_3$	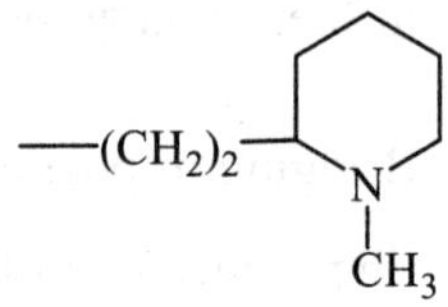
Prochlorperazine	- Cl	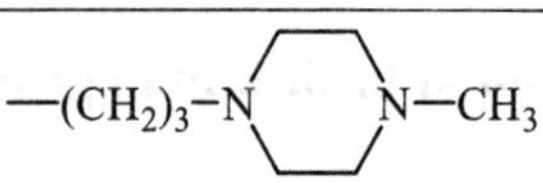
Trifluperazine	$-CF_3$	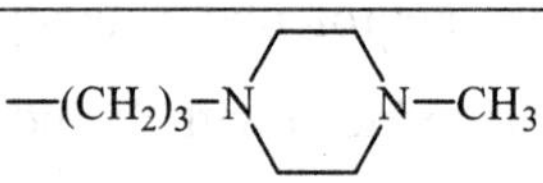

A. Promazine hydrochloride (Sparine)

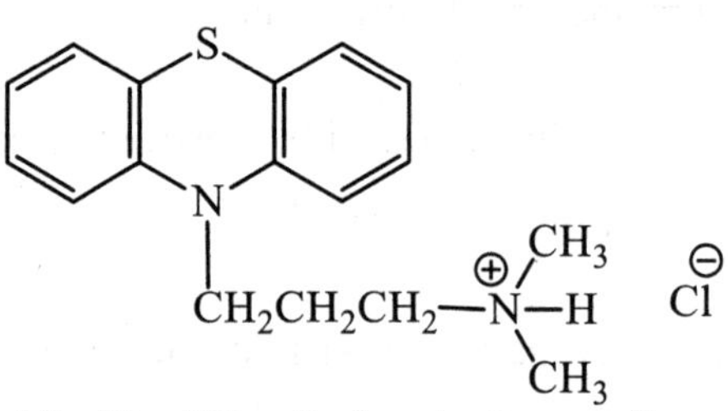

10 - [3 - (Dimethyl amino) propyl] phenothiazine hydrochloride

Mechanism of action: It is dopamine, muscarinic and histamine receptor antagonists. It shows antipsychotic effect by antagonizing D_2 dopamine and serotonin receptor.

Use: It is used to treat schizophrenia.

B. Chlorpromazine hydrochloride (Megatil)

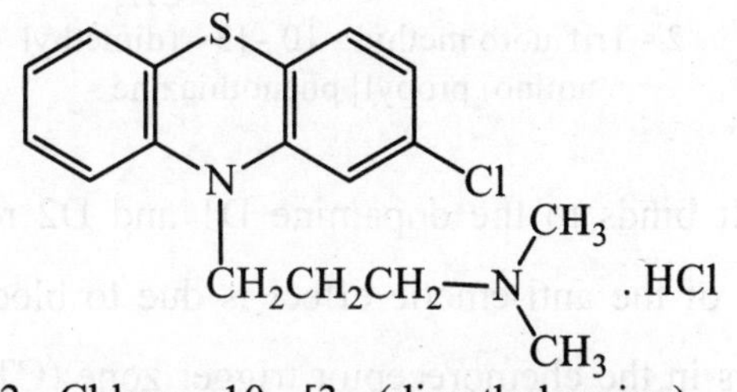

2 - Chloro - 10 - [3 - (dimethyl amino) propyl] phenothiazine hydrochloride

Synthesis

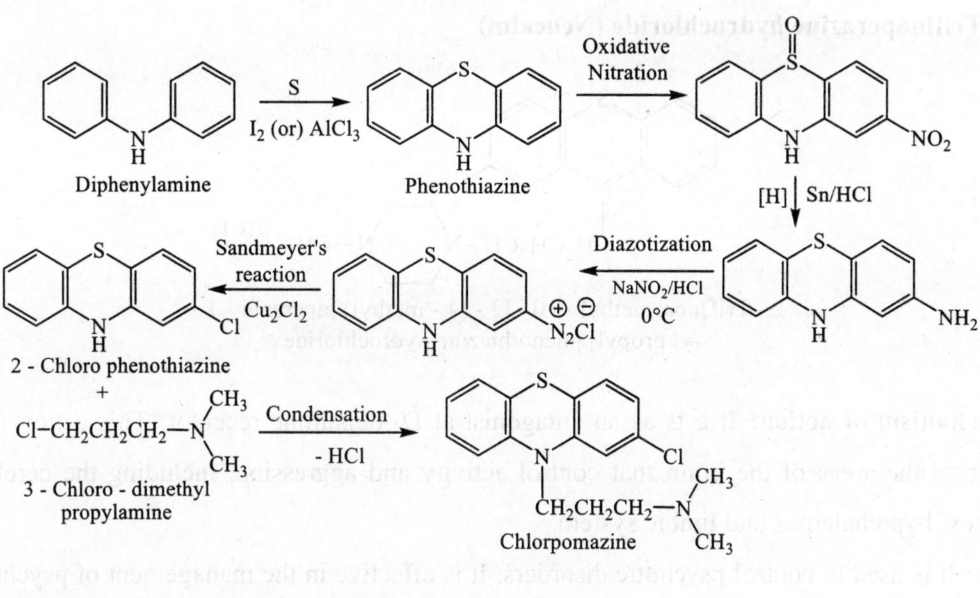

Mechanism of action: Same as Promazine hydrochloride.

Use: It is effective in the management of psychotic disorders, nausea and vomiting as well as much depressive illness.

C. Triflupromazine (Triazine)

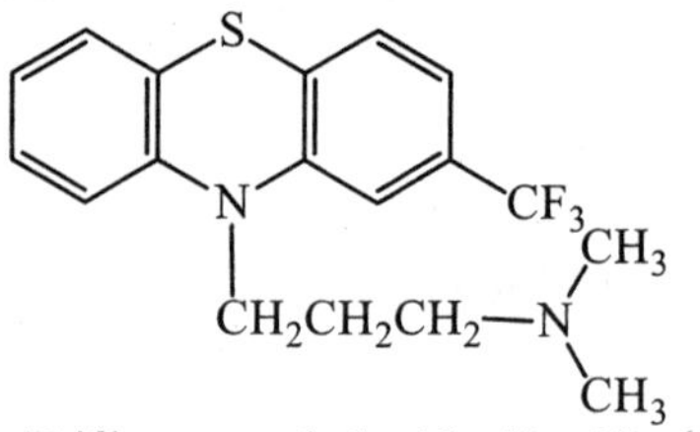

2 - Trifluoro methyl - 10 - [3 - (dimethyl amino) propyl] phenothiazine

Mechanism of action: It binds to the dopamine D1 and D2 receptors and inhibits their activity. The mechanism of the anti-emetic effect is due to blockage of the dopamine D2 neurotransmitter receptors in the chemoreceptor trigger zone (CTZ) and vomiting centre. It blocks the neurotransmitter dopamine and the vagus nerve in the gastrointestinal tract.

Use: It is used in the treatment of pain, nausea, vomiting and psychotic disorders.

D. Trifluoperazine hydrochloride (Neocalm)

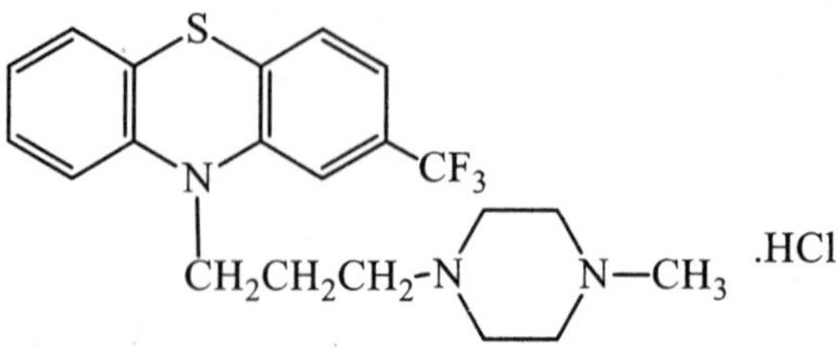

2 - Trifluoromethyl - 10 - [3 - (4 - methyl) piperazin - 1 - yl propyl] phenothiazine hydrochloride

Mechanism of action: It acts as an antagonist at D_2 dopamine receptor. This action may depress the areas of the brain that control activity and aggression, including the cerebral cortex, hypothalamus and limbic system.

Use: It is used to control psychotic disorders. It is effective in the management of psychotic disorders. It is also effective for the control of excessive anxiety, tension and agitation.

E. Thioridazine hydrochloride (Iorid)

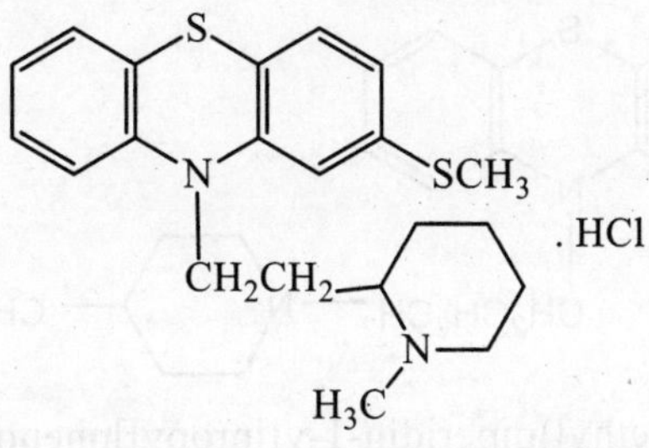

2 - Methyl thio - 10 - [2 - (1 - methyl piperidyl) ethyl] phenothiazine

Mechanism of action: It blocks dopaminergic D_1 and D_2 receptors in the brain; blocks α-adrenergic effect, depresses the release of hypothalamic and hypophyseal hormones and is believed to depress the reticular activating system thus affecting basal metabolism, body temperature, wakefulness, vasomotor tone and emesis.

Use: It is used to treat certain mental and mood disorders eg. Schizophrenia.

F. Prochlorperazine maleate (Novapar)

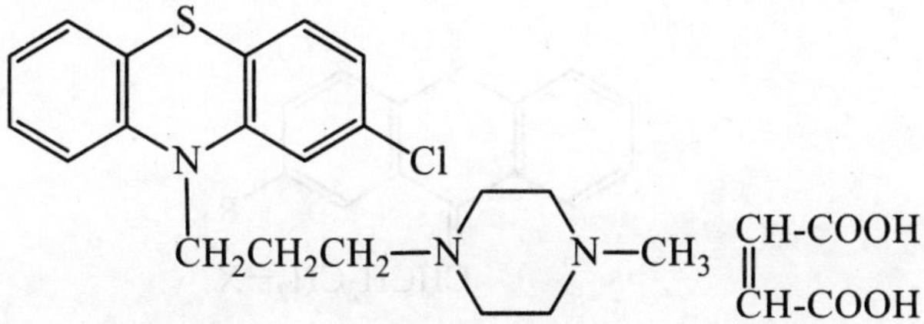

2 - Chloro - 10 - [3 - (4 - methyl - 1 - piperazinyl) propyl] phenothiazine maleate

Mechanism of action: It alleviates psychotic symptoms by blocking dopamine receptors, depressing release of selected hormones and producing α-adrenergic blocking effect in the brain.

Use: It is used as an antiemetic and antipsychotic.

G. Piperacetazine hydrochloride (Quide)

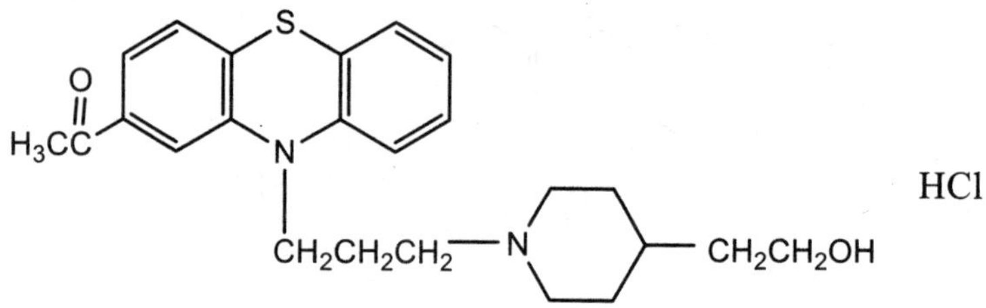

1-[10-[3-[4-(2-hydroxyethyl)piperidin-1-yl]propyl]phenothiazin-2-yl]ethanone

Mechanism of action: It acts depressing the chemoreceptor trigger zone and blocking D2 dopamine receptors in the brain. It also blocks histaminergic, cholinergic and noradrenergic receptors.

Use: It is used for schizophrenia.

2.1.2 **Thioxanthenes**

Thioxanthene is the parent system for the following neuroleptics and drug of this classification is represented in table 8.2

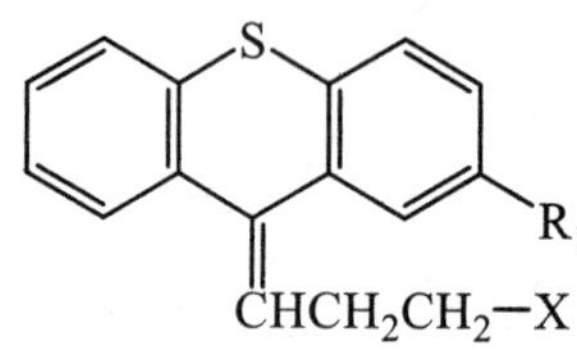

Table 8.2 Thioxanthene Derivatives

S. No	Compounds	R_1	X
1.	Chlorprothixene	- Cl	$-N(CH_3)_2$
2.	Thiothixene	$-SO_2-N(CH_3)_2$	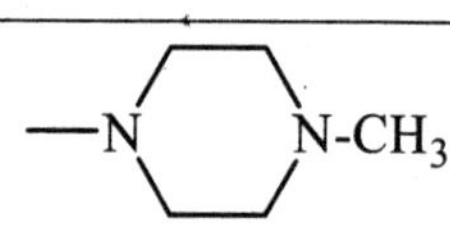

A. Chlorprothixene (Truxal)

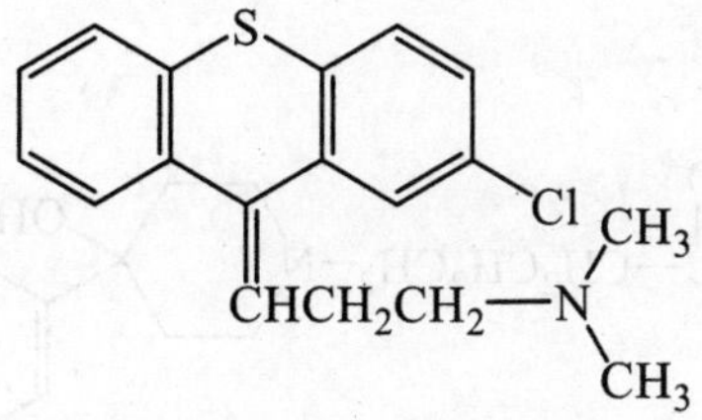

3 - (2 - Chloro - 9H - thioxanthen - 9 - ylidene) - N,N' - dimethyl - 1 - propan amine

Mechanism of action: It blocks dopaminergic D1 and D2 receptors in the brain; depresses the release of hypothalamic and hypophyseal hormones and also depress the reticular activating system thus affecting basal metabolism, body temperature, wakefulness, vasomotor tone and emesis.

Use: It is used in the treatment of acute and chronic schizophrenia and in psychotic and other conditions in which anxiety, agitation and tension predominate.

B. **Thiothixene (Navane)**

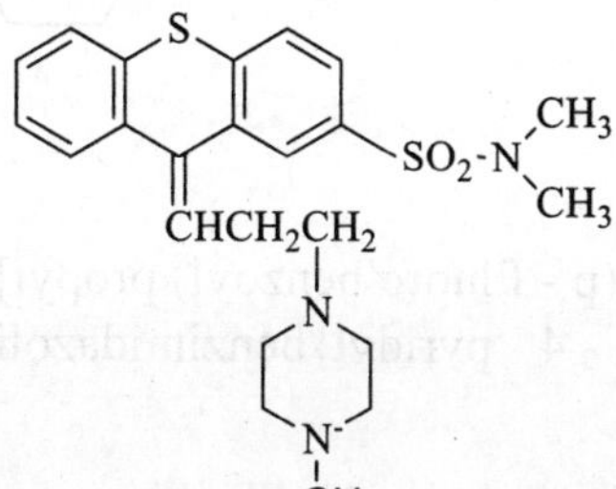

(9Z)-N,N-dimethyl-9-[3-(4-methylpiperazin-1-yl)propylidene]-9H-thioxanthene-2-sulfonamide

It is a typical antipsychotic of the thioxanthene class which is related to Chlorprothixene

Mechanism of action: It acts as an antagonist on different postsynaptic receptors like dopaminergic receptors, serotonergic receptors, histaminergic receptors and muscarinic receptors

Use: It is used in the treatment of psychoses like schizophrenia and bipolar mania.

2.1.3 Butyrophenones

A. Haloperidol (Agitol)

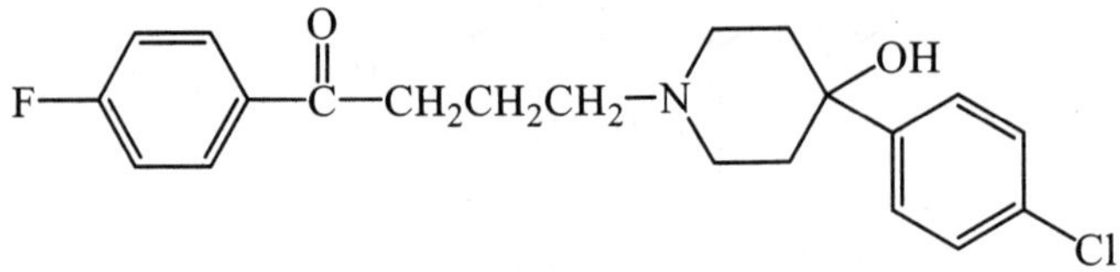

4 - [4 - (p - Chloro phenyl) - 4 - hydroxy - 1 - piperidinyl] - 4 - fluoro phenyl) - 1 - butanone

Mechanism of action: It blocks postsynaptic dopamine receptors in the limbic system and increase brain turnover of dopamine, producing an antipsychotic effect.

Use: It is used in the treatment of schizophrenia, acute psychosis and delirium.

B. Droperidol (Droperol)

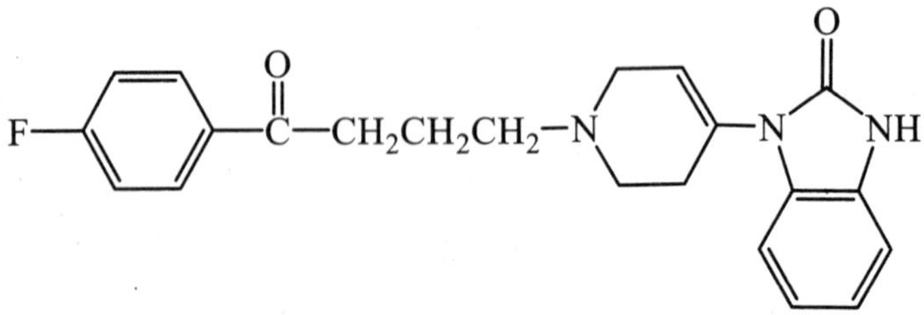

1 - {1 - [3 - (p - Fluoro benzoyl) propyl] - 1, 2, 3, 6 - tetrahydro - 4 - pyridyl}benzimidazolin - 2 - one

Mechanism of action: It produces sedation by blocking postsynaptic dopamine receptors in limbic system. By blocking dopamine receptor in chemoreceptor trigger zone and γ amino butyric acid receptor it acts as an antiemetic.

Use: It is used as antipsychotic and sedative. It is used as an adjunct to anesthesia to produce sedation and reduces incidence of nausea and vomiting. It is also used for psychomotor excitation and hallucination. It is used as antiemetic.

2.1.4. Dibenzoxazepines

A. Loxapine succinate (Ioxapac)

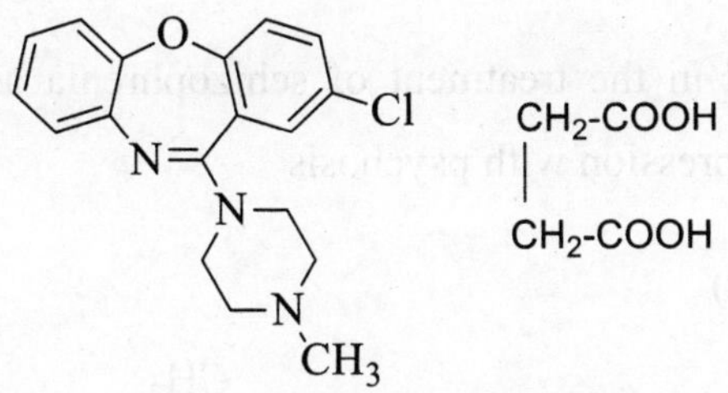

2 - Chloro - 11 - (4 - methyl - 1 - piperazinyl) dibenz - [b,f] - [1,4] - oxazepin succinate

It is a dibenzoxazepine derivative. It is an effective antipsychotic and has side effects similar to Phenothiazines.

Mechanism of action: It acts by blocking dopamine at postsynaptic receptors in the brain.

Use: It is used for symptomatic control of schizophrenia.

2.2 Atypial Antipsychotics

A. Risperidone (Zisper)

Risperidone has structural features of a hybrid molecule between a Butyrophenone and Trazodone. It is a benzisoxazole derivative.

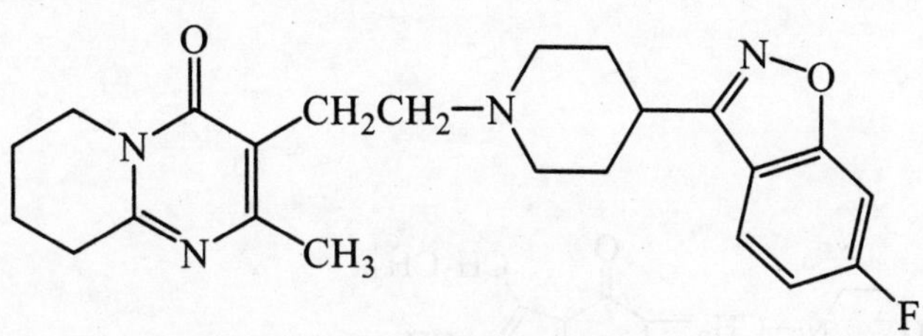

3 - {2 - [4 - (6 - Fluoro - 1, 2 - benzisoxazol - 3 - yl) - 1 - piperidinyl] ethyl} - 6, 7, 8, 9 - tetrahydro - 2 - methyl - 4H - pyrido - [1,2 - a] - pyrimidin - 4 - one

Mechanism of action: It inhibits D2 dopaminergic receptors and reduces dopaminergic neurotransmission, thereby decreases positive symptoms of schizophrenia, such as delusions and hallucinations.

Use: It is widely used in the treatment of schizophrenia and mood disorders, including bipolar disorder and depression with psychosis

B. Clozapine (Clozaril)

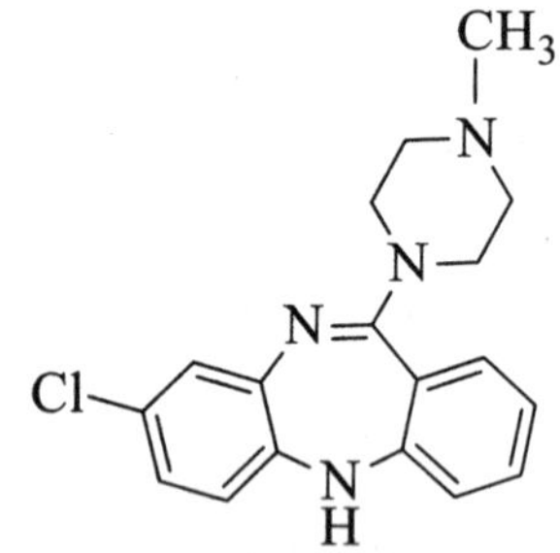

3 - Chloro - 6 - (4 - methylpiperazin-1-yl) - 11H - benzo[b] benzodiazepine

Clozapine is atypical antipsychotic drug of Dibenzo diazepine class.

Mechanism of action: It is a selective monoaminergic antagonist with high affinity for the serotonin Type 2 ($5HT_2$), dopamine Type 2 (D2), 1 and 2 adrenergic and H1 histaminergic receptors.

Use: It is mainly used for schizophrenia that does not improve following the use of other antipsychotic medications.

C. Molindone (Moban)

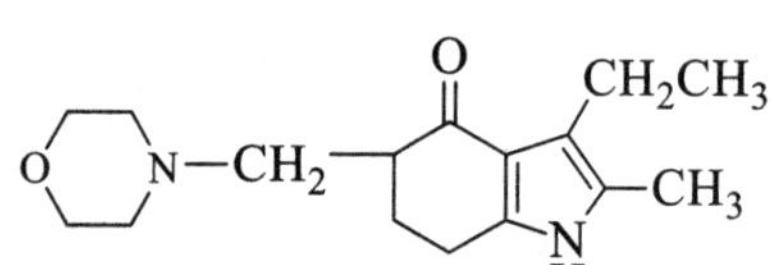

3 - Ethyl - 2 - methyl - 5 - (morpholin - 4 - ylmethyl) - 4,5,6,7 - tetrahydro - 1H - indol - 4 - one

Molindone is a dihydroindolone compound sometimes described as a typical antipsychotic class of drug.

Mechanism of action: It acts by blocking the effects of dopamine in the brain, leading to diminished symptoms of psychosis.

Uses: It is used in the treatment of schizophrenia.

D. Sulpiride (Dogmatil)

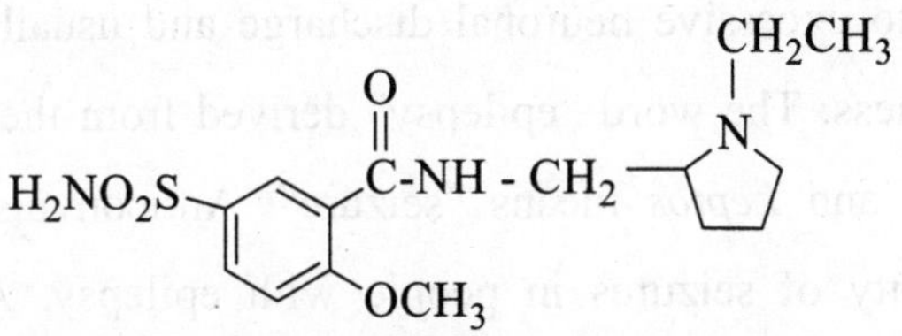

N - [(1 - Ethyl pyrrolidin - 2 - yl) methyl] - 2 - methoxy - 5 - sulfamoyl benzamide

Sulpiride is an atypical antipsychotic drug of the benzamide class

Mechanism of action: It block both dopamine D1 and D2 receptors and more selective and acts primarily as a dopamine D2 antagonist.

Uses: It is used mainly used in the treatment of psychosis associated with schizophrenia and major depressive disorder and sometimes used in low dosage to treat anxiety and mild depression.

ANTICONVULSANTS

Chapter

9

1. INTRODUCTION

Anticonvulsants are drugs used for the treatment of epileptic seizures, hence, the synonym "antiepileptic." Epilepsy is a chronic disorder characterized by paroxysmal brain dysfunction due to excessive neuronal discharge and usually associated with some alteration of consciousness. The word "epilepsy" derived from the Greek word *epi* means "upon, at, close upon" and *Leptos* means "seizure". Anticonvulsant drugs decrease the frequency and/or severity of seizures in people with epilepsy. A seizure is a physical findings or changes in behavior that occur after an episode of abnormal electrical activity in the brain. Seizures can be classified into Partial seizure (Simplex and Complex) and Generalized seizure- (Absence/petit mal, Tonic-clonic / grand mal).

The various anticonvulsant drugs have the ureide moiety as common structure (Fig. 9.1). Small changes in 'X' cause significant change in their activity towards epileptic control. Due to rapid development of molecular biological techniques newer antiepileptics like Gabapentin, Felbamate, Lamotrigine and Topiramate have emerged with limited drug-drug interaction and side effects.

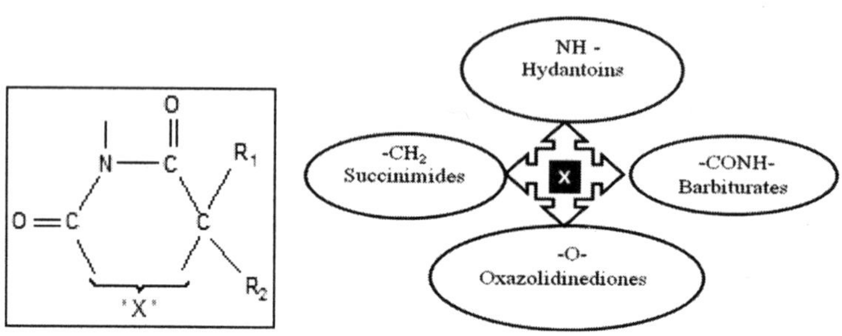

Fig. 9.1 Structure Common to Anticonvulsant Drugs

The narrow spectrum antiepileptic agents mostly work for specific types of seizures (such as partial, focal or absence, myoclonic seizures). Broad spectrum antiepileptics additionally have some effectiveness for a wide variety of seizures (partial plus absence of myoclonic seizures).

i. Narrow-spectrum antiepileptics: eg. Phenytoin, Phenobarbital, Carbamazepine, Oxcarbazepine, Gabapentin, Pregabalin, Lacosamide, Vigabatrin.

ii. Broad-spectrum antiepileptics: eg. Valproic acid, Lamotrigine, Topiramate, Zonisamide, Levetiracetam, Clonazepam, Rufinamide.

2. Mechanism of Action

The mechanism of antiepileptic drugs is not clear since the etiology of epilepsy is not yet completely understood.

- **Some drugs block sodium channel**: It has been observed that, both Na^+ and Cl^- ions are invariably present at much higher concentration outside the cell, whereas K^+ charged proteins and organic cations are more abundantly available inside the cell. Epileptic seizure causes Na^+ ion accumulation within the central neuron, which initiates enhanced synaptic nerve transmissions following presynaptic stimulation. These drugs decrease Na^+ intracellular ion by activating biochemical process that normally extrudes Na^+ ion from neurons. Prolongation of this inactive state with prolongation of the refractory period is the principle of mechanism.

- **Some drugs block calcium channel**: A low threshold calcium current govern oscillatory response in thalamic neuron.
- **Some drugs affect synaptic transmission**: Enhances GABA mediated inhibition.
- **Some drugs act on GABA:** They act by decreasing reuptake or decreasing metabolism of GABA.
- **Some drugs act on excitatory glutamatergic neurotransmission**: They block glutamatergic receptor.

3. CLASSIFICATION

I. Based on their chemical structure antiepileptics are classified as

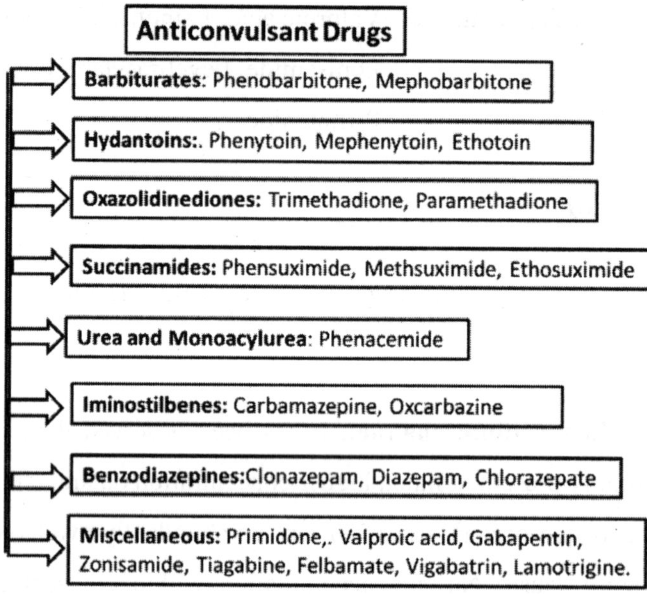

II. Based on mechanism of action antiepileptics are classified as:

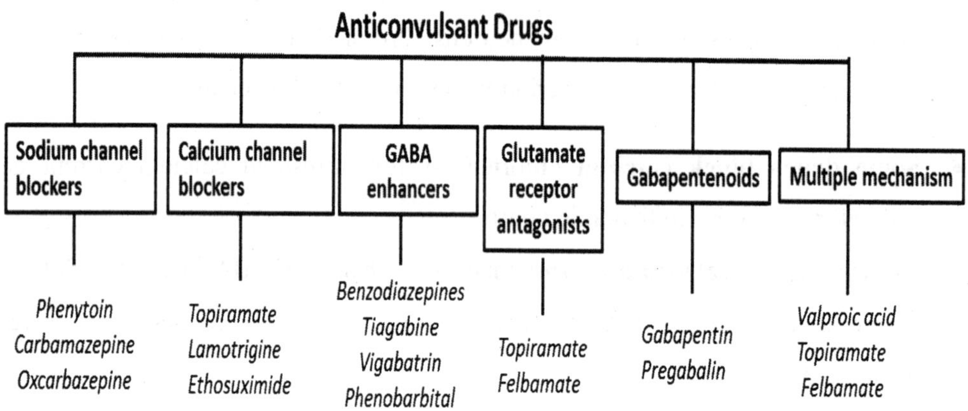

3.1 Barbiturates (For more details Refer to Chapter 7)

Most of the barbiturates are sedative and hypnotics; only few of them show anticonvulsant characters. Three important barbiturates, which exhibit anticonvulsant properties are:

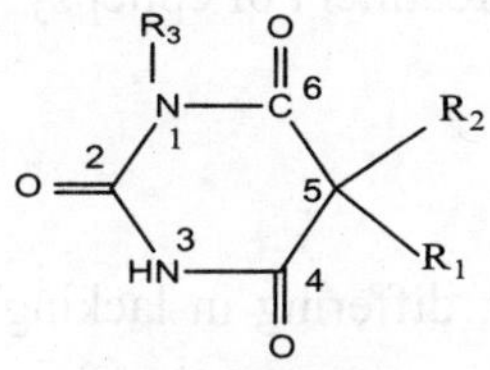

General Structure

Name	R_1	R_2	R_3
Phenobarbitone	$- C_2H_5$	$- C_6H_5$	- H
Mephobarbitone	$- C_2H_5$	$- C_6H_5$	$- CH_3$
Metharbital	$- C_2H_5$	$- C_2H_5$	$- CH_3$

A. Phenobarbital (Mudrane)

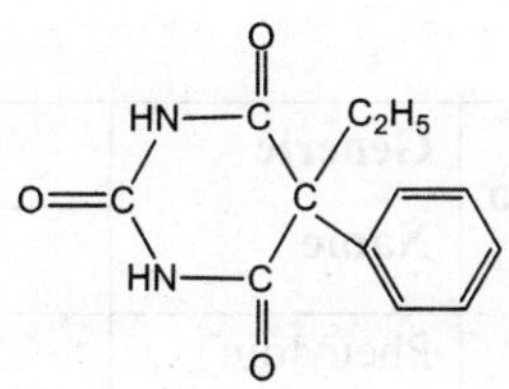

5 - Ethyl - 5 - phenyl barbituric acid

Mechanism of action: It acts as a nonselective central nervous system depressant. It promotes binding to inhibitory gamma-aminobutyric acid subtype receptors and modulates chloride currents through receptor channels. It also inhibits glutamate induced depolarizations.

Use: It is used as sedative and hypnotic. It is a drug of choice for the treatment of grand mal and petit mal epilepsy.

B. Metharbital (Gemonil)

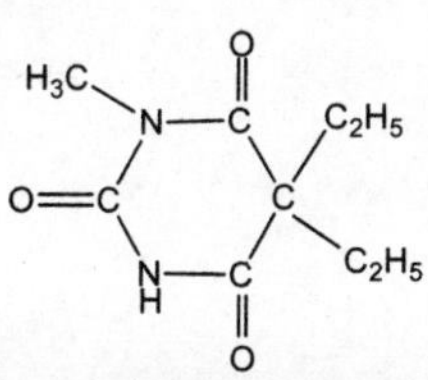

1 - Methyl - 5,5' - Diethyl barbituric acid

Mechanism of action: It binds at a distinct binding site associated with a Cl^- ionophore at the $GABA_A$ receptor, increasing the duration of time for which the Cl^- ionophore is open. The post-synaptic inhibitory effect of GABA in the thalamus is, therefore, prolonged.

Use: It is used for the treatment of short-term insomnia. It is also CNS depressants that induce drowsiness and relieve tension or nervousness. It is used in the treatment of epilepsy.

3.2 Hydantoins

The hydantoins are close structural relatives of barbituric acid, differing in lacking of 6-oxo groups. The lack of this carbonyl group decreases the acidity, so it is a weaker acid than that of barbiturates.

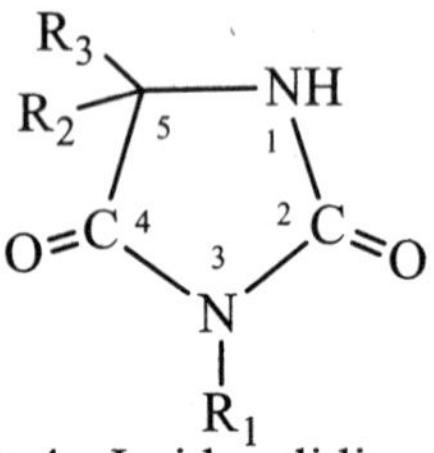

2, 4 - Imidazolidinedione

S. No	Generic Name	Substituents		
		R_1	R_2	R_3
1.	Phenytoin	- H	- C_6H_5	- C_6H_5
2.	Mephenytoin	- CH_3	- C_2H_5	- C_6H_5
3.	Ethotoin	- C_2H_5	- H	- C_6H_5

A. Phenytoin (Dilantin)

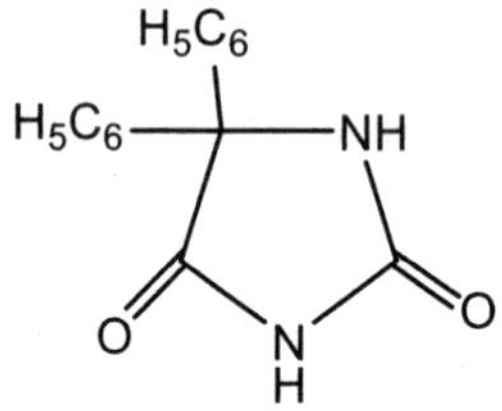

5, 5 - Diphenyl hydantoin

Synthesis

Method - I

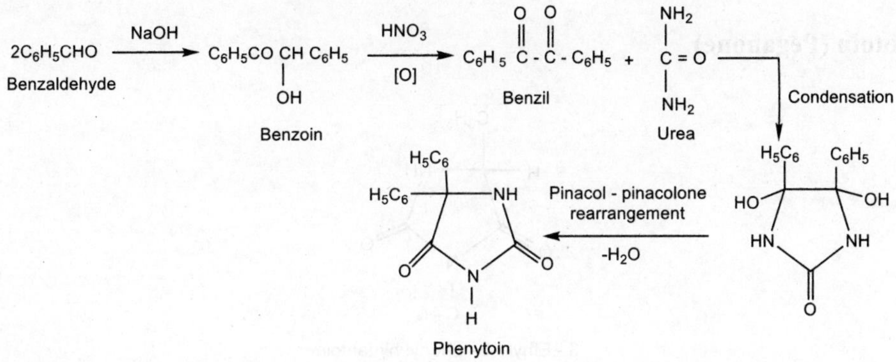

Method – II

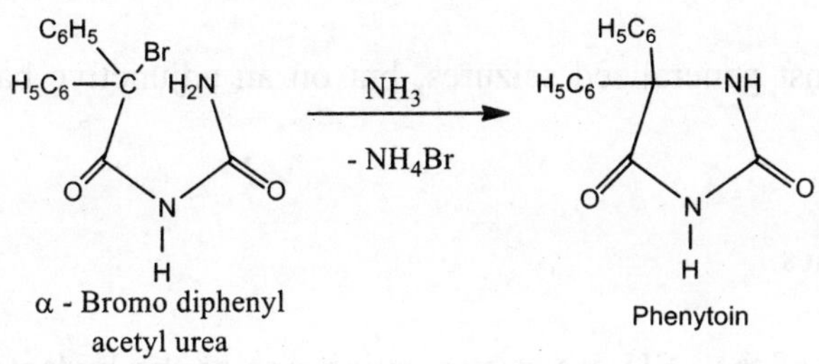

Mechanism of action: Phenytoin limit the seizure and start of new seizures activity, by regulating Na+ and Ca+ channels in neuron, enhancing the sodium-potassium activity and inhibiting the calcium movement across the neuronal membrane/neuron.

Use: It is useful against all types of seizures.

B. Mephenytoin or Methoin (Mesantoin)

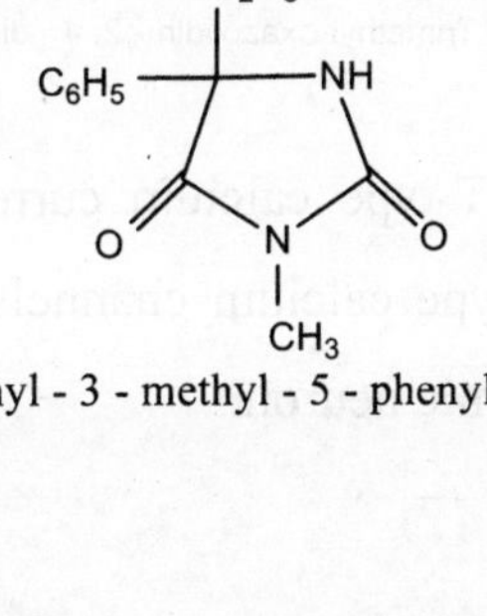

5 - Ethyl - 3 - methyl - 5 - phenyl hydantoin

Mechanism of action: Same as Phenytoin.

Use: It is used to control seizures in combination with Phenytoin.

C. Ethotoin (Peganone)

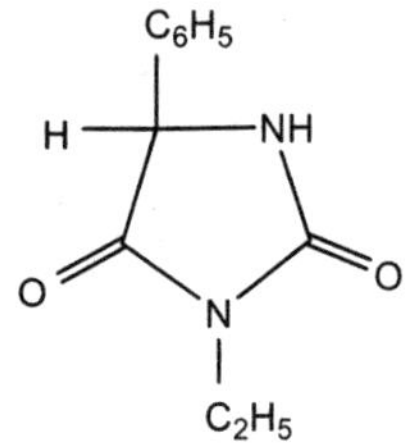

3 - Ethyl - 5 - phenyl hydantoin

Mechanism of action: Same as Phenytoin.

Use: It is used against generalized seizures, but on an adjunctive basis owing to its low potency.

3.3 Oxazolidinediones

Replacement of the -NH group at position one of the hydantoin ring with oxygen atom yields Oxazolidine - 2, 4 - dione system. Trimethadione is only clinically used.

A. Trimethadione (Trioxidone)

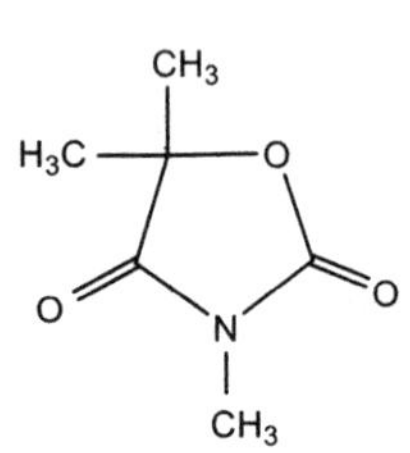

3, 5, 5 - Trimethyl oxazolidin - 2, 4 - dione

Mechanism of action: It reduces T-type calcium currents in thalamic neurons via the inhibition of voltage dependent T-type calcium channels. Low threshold calcium current governs oscillatory response in thalamic neuron.

Use: It is used in the treatment of petit mal epilepsy. Dermatological and hematological toxicities limit its clinical use.

B. Paramethadione (Paradione)

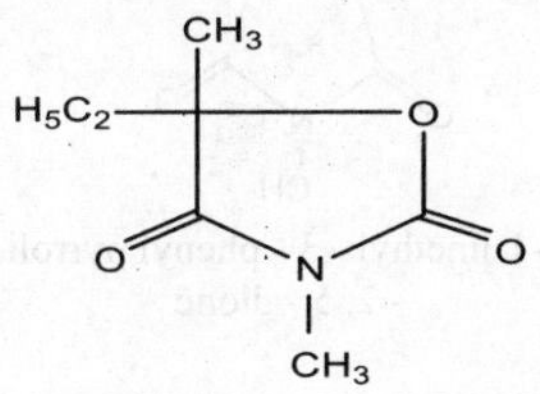

5 - Ethyl - 3, 5 - dimethyl oxazolidin - 2, 4 - dione

Mechanism of action: Same as Trimethadione.

Use: It is used in the treatment of petit mal epilepsy.

3.4 Succinimides

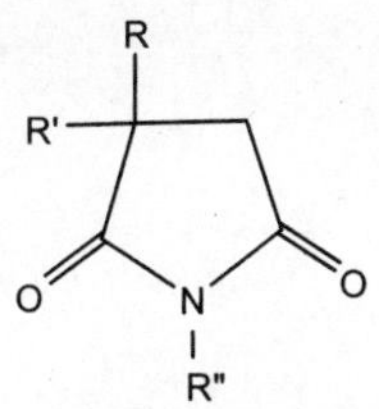

S. No	Generic name	R	R'	R"
1.	Phensuximide	$-C_6H_5$	-H	$-CH_3$
2.	Methsuximide	$-C_6H_5$	$-CH_3$	$-CH_3$
3.	Ethosuximide	$-C_2H_5$	$-CH_3$	-H

A. Phensuximide (Milontin)

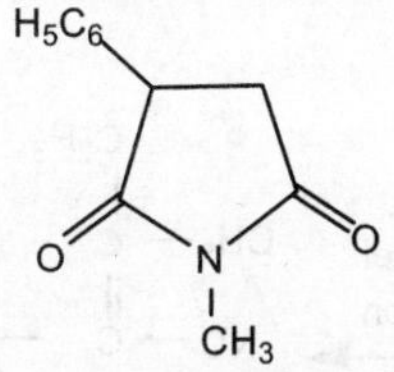

1 - Methyl - 3 - phenyl pyrrolidin - 2, 5 - dione

Mechanism of action: Its exact mechanism of action is not known but may act in inhibitory neuronal systems that are important in the generation of the three per second rhythm. Its effects may be related to its ability to inhibit depolarization-induced accumulation of cyclic AMP and cyclic GMP in brain tissue.

Use: It is used in the treatment of petit mal epilepsy.

B. Methsuximide (Petinutin)

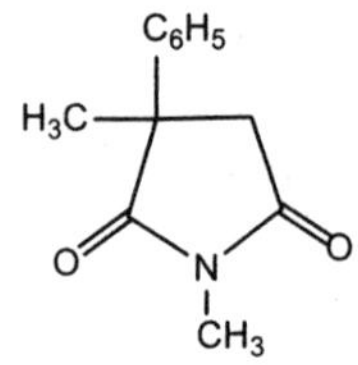

1, 3 - Dimethyl - 3 - phenyl pyrrolidin - 2, 5 - dione

Mechanism of action: It elevates the seizure threshold and reduces the frequency of attacks through depression of nerve transmission in the cortex.

Use: It is used in the treatment of petit mal epilepsy.

C. Ethosuximide (Zarontin)

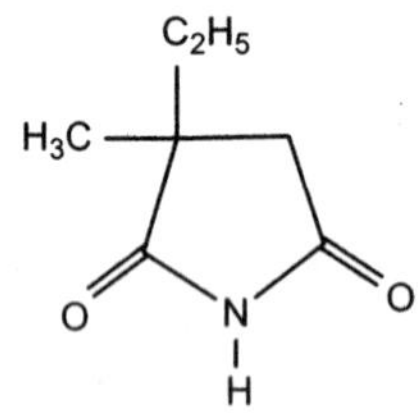

3 - Ethyl - 3 - methyl pyrrolidin - 2, 5 - dione

Synthesis

Method – I

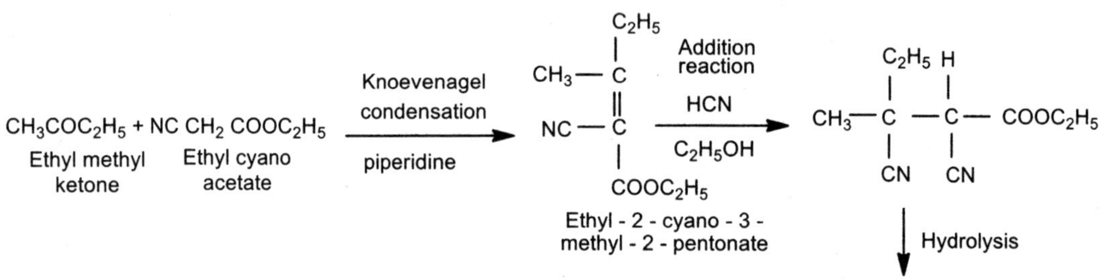

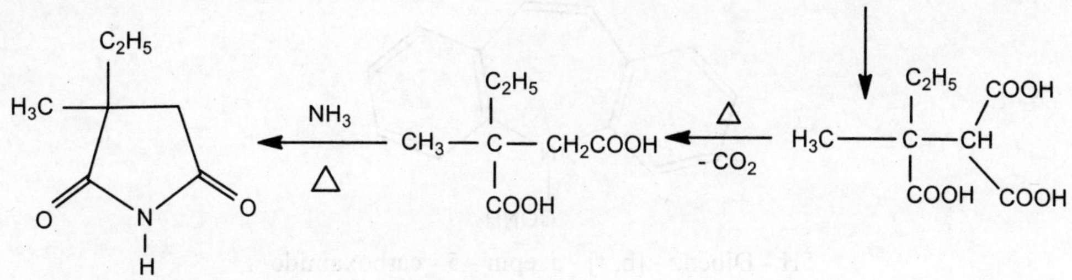

Ethosuxumide

Mechanism of action: It elevates the seizure threshold and reduces the frequency of attacks by depressing the motor cortex and elevating the threshold of CNS response to convulsive stimuli.

Use: It is effective in the cure of petit mal epilepsy.

3.5 Urea and Monoacylurea

A. Phenacemide (Phenurone)

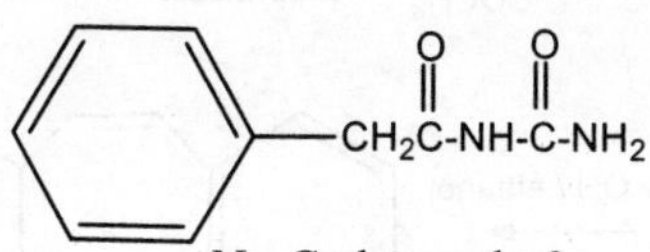

N - Carbomoyl - 2 - phenyl acetamide

Mechanism of action: It blocks neuronal sodium channels or voltage sensitive calcium channels. This suppresses neuronal depolarization and hyper synchronization causes seizures.

Use: It is used in the treatment of psychomotor epilepsy.

3.6 Imino stilbenes

A. Carbamazepine (Tegretol)

Carbamazepine contains a dibenzazepine ring system with a carbamoyl moiety hooked on to the nitrogen atom.

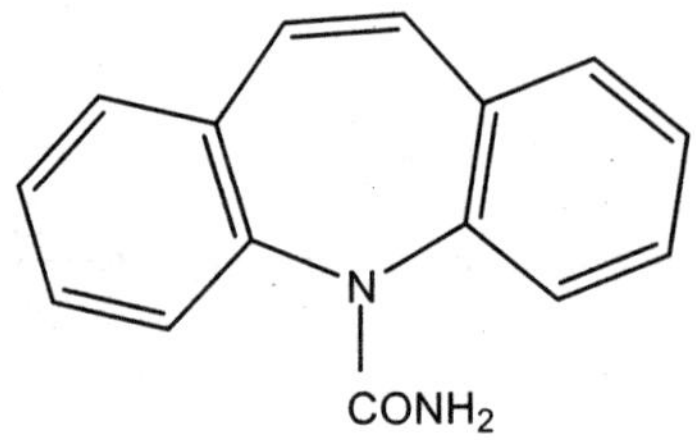

5H - Dibenz - [b, f] - azepin - 5 - carboxamide

Synthesis

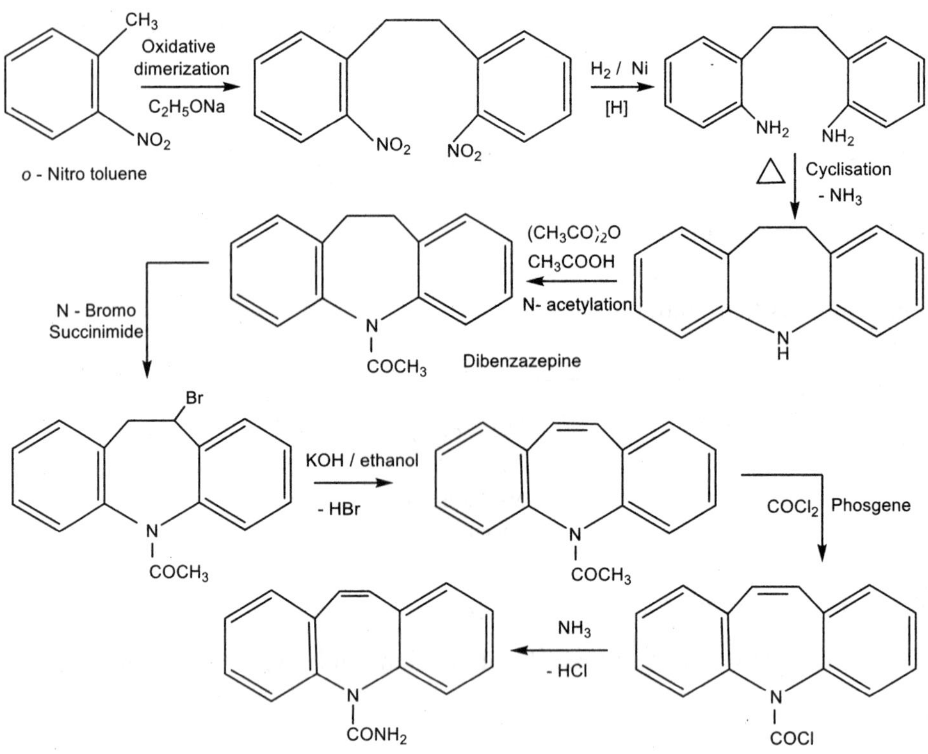

Mechanism of action: It decreases Na^+ intracellular ion by activating biochemical process that normally extrudes Na^+ ion from neurons. Prolongation of this inactive state with prolongation of the refractory period is the principle of mechanism.

Use: It is used to control grand mal and focal seizures. It is also used in the treatment of trigeminal neuralgia and treatment of manic depression.

3.7 Benzodiazepines

A. Clonazepam (Klonopin)

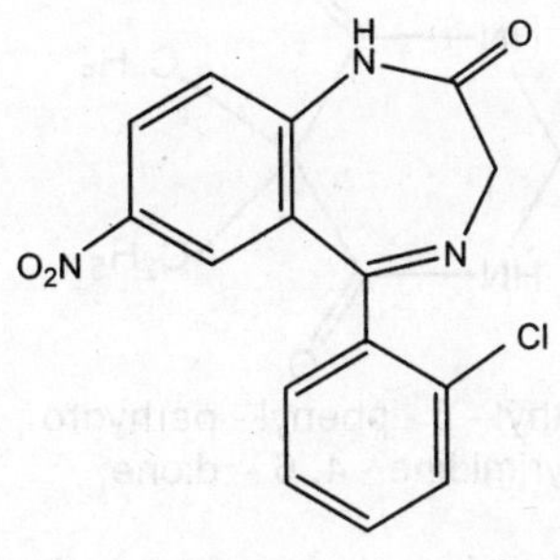

5 - (o - Chlorophenyl) - 1, 3 - dihydro - 7 - nitro - 2H - 1, 4 - benzodiazepin - 2 - one

Mechanism of action: It prevents seizures by potentiating the effects of gamma-aminobutyric acid (GABA), which is an inhibitory neurotransmitter.

Use: It is used to prevent and treat seizures and panic disorders.

3.8 Miscellaneous

A. Valproic acid (Epilim)

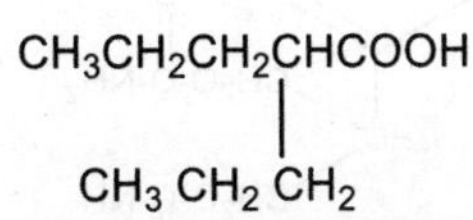

2 - Propyl pentanoic acid

Mechanism of action: It decreases seizure activity by blocking reuptake of gamma-aminobutyric acid (GABA), the common inhibitory neurotransmitter in the brain. GABA suppresses the rapid firing of neurons by inhibiting voltage-sensitive sodium channels.

Use: It is used in the treatment of grand mal, petit mal, mixed and temporal lobe epilepsy and also used in children.

B. Primidone (Mysoline)

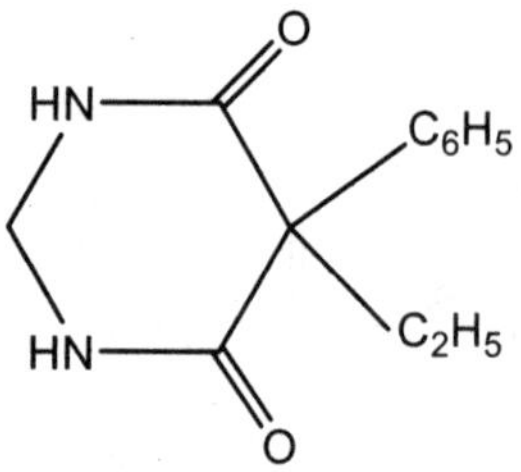

5 - Ethyl - 5 - phenyl - perhydro pyrimidine - 4, 6 - dione

Mechanism of action: It prevents seizures by decreasing excitability of neurons and increasing motor cortex's threshold of electrical stimulation.

Use: It is used as an anticonvulsant to treat partıal seizures, amyotrophic lateral sclerosis (ALS) and painful neuropathies. It is also used to treat essential tremor and other neurological conditions.

C. Felbamate (Felbatol)

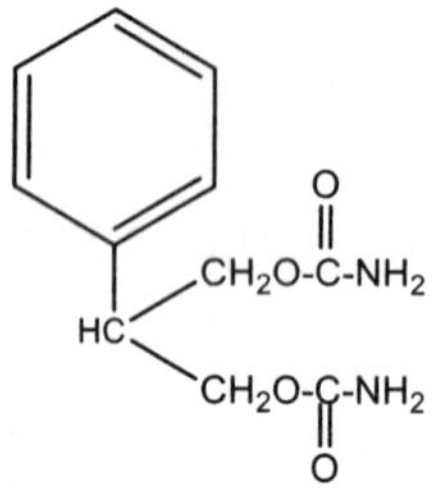

(3 - Carbamoyl oxy - 2 - phenyl propyl) carbamate

Mechanism of action: It exerts anticonvulsant action by antagonizing the amino acid glycine. When glycine binds to N-methyl-D-aspartate (NMDA) receptors in the CNS, the frequency at which receptor-gated calcium ion channels open is increased. It may raise the seizure threshold by blocking NMDA receptors so glycine can't bind to them.

Use: It is used to treat partial seizures in adults and partial and generalized seizures associated with Lennox-Gastaut syndrome in children.

D. Gabapentin (Neurontin)

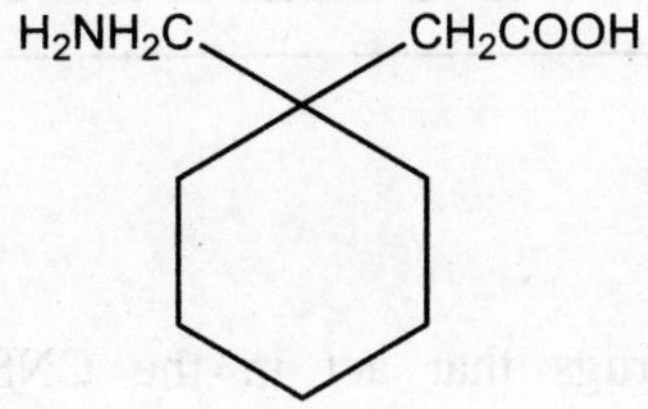

1- (Amino methyl) cyclohexaneacetic acid

Mechanism of action: It is a GABA analogue. It is s gabapentinoids, a class of drug inhibits the neurotransmitter γ-aminobutyric acid (GABA), its mechanism of action as antiepileptic involves the inhibition of alpha-2-delta subunit of voltage-gated calcium channel.

Use: It is a potent anticonvulsant, used in conjugation with other antiepileptic for the treatment and arrest of psychomotor. It is also used for neuropathic pain.

Chapter 10

GENERAL ANAESTHETICS

1. INTRODUCTION

General anesthetics are drugs that act in the CNS, causing reversible loss of consciousness, thereby causing a generalized loss of sensation. Anesthesia means, lack of feeling (derived from a Greek word). General anesthetic was introduced in clinical practice from 19th century with the use of nitrous oxide, diethyl ether and chloroform (of these, only Nitrous oxide is still used).

The general anesthetic causes the following effects for patients undergoing surgical procedures:

- Unconsciousness
- Sedation and reduce anxiety
- Analgesia
- Immobility
- Amnesia
- Skeletal muscle relaxation and
- Decrease of autonomic responses

No single drug provides all these desirable properties several categories of drugs are combined to produce optimal anesthetic activity. General anesthetics bring about descending depression of the central nervous system, starting with cerebral cortex, the basal ganglia, the cerebellum and finally the spinal cord. They are used to block the pain signals travelling through the nervous system.

2. MECHANISM OF ACTION

The anesthetic drug is thought to act by interrupting the function of central nervous system. Although all parts of the nervous system are affected by anesthetic agents, the main targets appear to be the cortex, thalamus, hippocampus, midbrain reticular formation and spinal cord. Mechanisms underlying the anesthetic effect are not known. It appears that a variety of molecular mechanism may contribute to general anesthetic activity.

Earlier theories of anesthesia postulated interaction with the lipid membrane bilayer.

- Meyer and Overton's "lipid theory" - a direct relationship exists between lipid solubility of agent and its anesthetic potency. According to this theory, anesthesia occurs when sufficient concentration of anesthetic is achieved in lipid bilayer. When general anesthetic is dissolved in lipid bilayer and membranes, they cause disordering or increased fluidity of the membrane. This may inactivate the protein essential functioning of CNS or ion channel, which would remain open resulting in chloride ion influx leading to synaptic hyper polarization, which inhibits neuronal function.

According to the new polysynaptolytic theory general anesthetics inhibit reversible neurotransmission in many synapses of CNS

- **Ligand-gated ion channels:** Many intravenous anesthetic agents mediate their effects by potentiating the activity of GABA (γ-aminobutyric acid) at inhibitory $GABA_A$ receptor. General anesthetics bind to $GABA_A$ receptors in a hydrophobic pocket located in the transmembrane domain and stabilize the open form of the Cl- channel causes neuronal hyperpolarization and ultimately inhibition of neuronal activity.

- **Two-pore domain K+ channels**: Volatile and gaseous anaesthetics activate K+ channel, causing K+ efflux thus reducing membrane excitability. This may contribute to the analgesic, hypnotic and immobilizing effects of these agents.

- **NMDA receptors:** Unlike other anesthetics, Nitrous oxide and Ketamine do not have actions on $GABA_A$ receptors. Glutamate, the major excitatory neurotransmitter in the CNS, activates an important site of action for these anesthetics. Ketamine inhibits the excitatory neurotransmitter glutamate at NMDA receptors. It functions at the thalamus (which relays sensory impulses from reticular activating system to the cerebral cortex) and the limbic cortex (which is involved with the awareness of sensation.

3. CLASSIFICATION

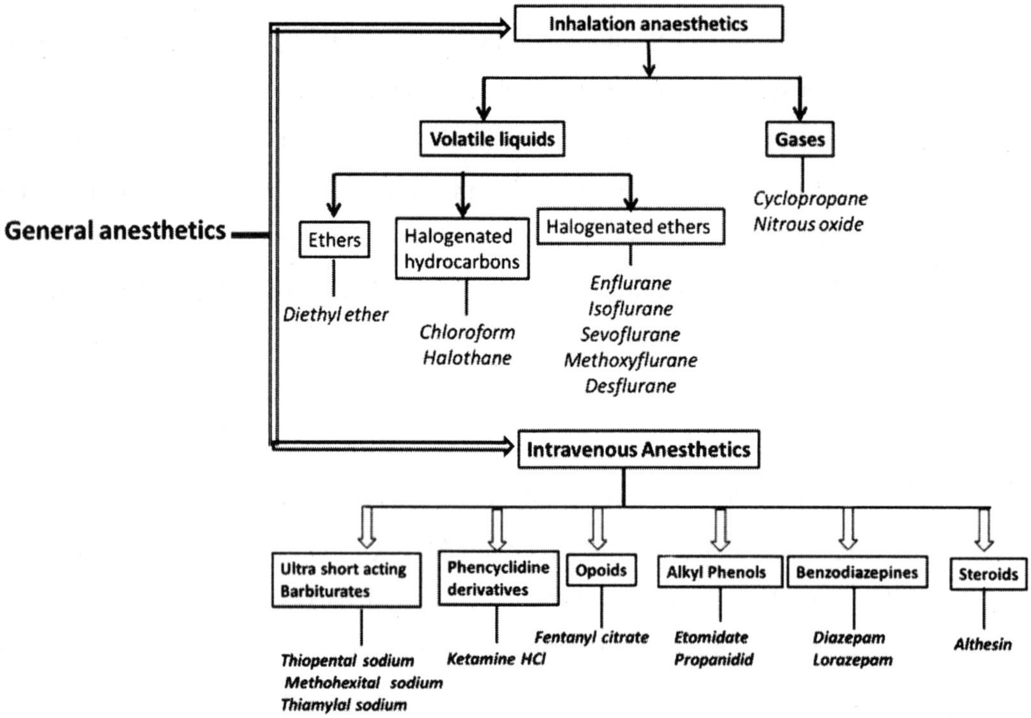

3.1 Inhalation Anaesthetics

Inhalation anesthetics are used for induction and maintenance of general anesthesia as well as sedation. Ether, Chloroform, Trichloroethylene, Cyclopropane, Methoxyflurane and Enflurane, inhalation anesthetics were once widely used have now been replaced by Sevoflurane, Isoflurane and Desflurane which have improved pharmacokinetic properties, fewer side effects and are non-flammable. The older agent, Nitrous oxide is still used widely (especially in obstetric practice). Diethyl ether is not used now-a-days mainly because of the flammability and explosiveness of its vapor. Queen Victoria delivered her 8th child in Chloroform anesthesia. Chloroform is sweetish odour volatile liquid but it is no longer used because of its hepato and cardio toxicity. Its hepatotoxic metabolite is phosgene, once a suffocating chemical warfare agent.

The replacement of hydrogen from low molecular weight ether and hydrocarbon by halogen results halogenated hydrocarbons with increased anaesthetic potency and proportional decrease in its flammability. But this halogen substitution is also accompanied by an increase in toxicity, which has limited the use as anesthetics. Among, the halogens fluorinated hydrocarbons have decreased toxicity, flammability and boiling point with increased anesthetics potency. Halogenated anesthetic agents are likely to cause cardiac dysrhythmias.

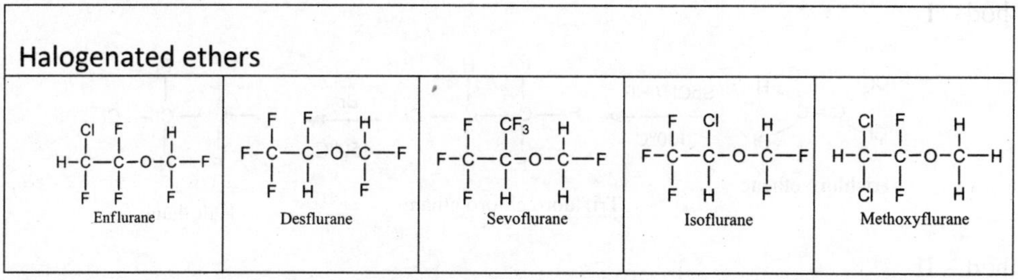

Inhalation anesthetics could be either volatile liquids or gases and they are administered through inhalation process. Mostly, they are administered via endotracheal tube that goes down to the throat and deliver the drugs directly to the lungs; this is done because most of the inhaled anaesthetics are irritating to the airway. Volatile anaesthetics (e.g. Isoflurane, Sevoflurane) are delivered in air, oxygen or oxygen–nitrous oxide mixtures as the carrier gas. Movement of these agents from lungs to various body compartments depent upon their solubility in blood and tissues as well as on blood flow, which play a major role in induction.

A. Halothane (Fluothane)

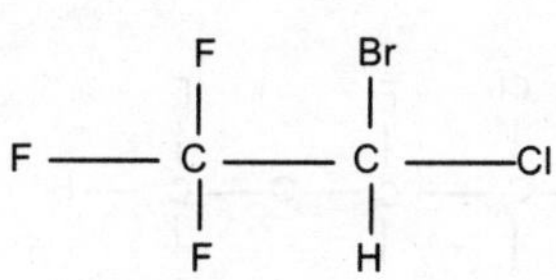

2 - Bromo - 2 - chloro - 1, 1, 1-
trifluro ethane

Halothane is a volatile, non-flammable fluorinated hydrocarbon. It is the only inhalational anaesthetic agent containing a bromine atom. It does not produce potent analgesia. It is non-explosive, rapid acting; pleasant smelling muscle relaxant and compatible with other drugs and it is more popular than other agents. It is twice as potent as chloroform and four times as that of ether. Its use has been limited due to its idiosyncratic hepatotoxicity.

Synthesis

Method – I

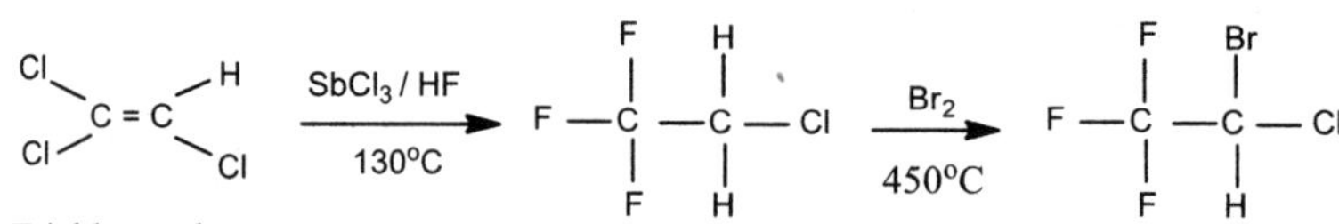

Trichloro ethene Trifluoro chloro ethane Halothane

Method – II

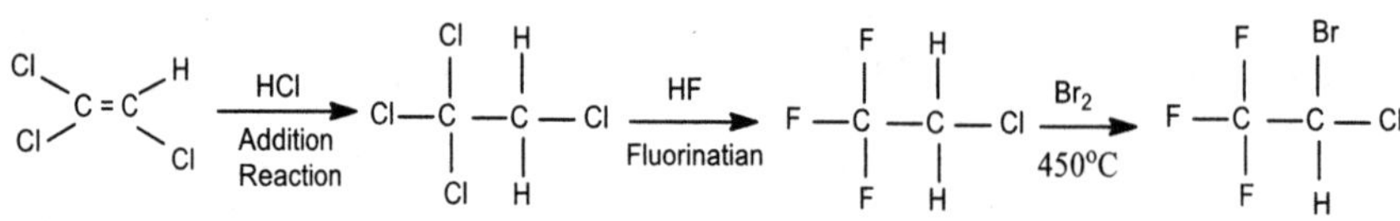

Trichloro ethene Tetrachloro ethane Trifluoro chloro ethane Halothane

Mechanism of action: It act on multiple ion channels, which ultimately depresses nerve conduction, breathing, cardiac contractility. It also binds to potassium channels in cholinergic neurons and also to NMDA.

Use: It is a potent, safe and frequently employed general inhalation anaesthetic.

B. Enflurane (Erthrane)

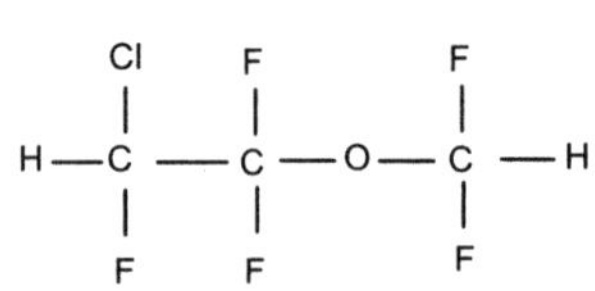

1- Difluro methoxy - 2 - chloro 1, 1, 2 - triifluoro ethane

It is a halogenated ether. It is a structural isomer of Isoflurane. It vaporizes readily but it is liquid at room temperature.

Mechanism of action: It activates calcium dependent *ATPase* in the sarcoplasmic reticulum by increasing the fluidity of the lipid membrane. It also binds to the GABA receptor potassium channel, the glycine receptor and antagonizes the glutamate receptor.

Use: It is used for induction and maintenance of general anesthesia. It is also used to analgesia for vaginal delivery.

C. Isoflurane (Isorane)

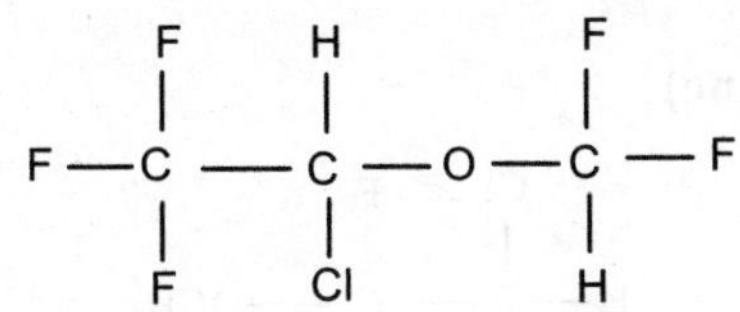

1- Difluoro methoxy - 1- chloro - 2, 2, 2 - trifluoroethane

Isoflurane is closely related to Enflurane. It is an isomer of Enflurane, non-inflammable liquid vaporizes readily. It is a racemic mixture of R- and S- optical isomer. Isoflurane does not induce cardiac arrhythmias or sensitize the heart to catecholamines. However, like other halogenated gases, it produces dose-dependent hypotension. It has a pungent odor and stimulates respiratory and is therefore not used for inhalation induction.

Mechanism of action: Same as Enflurane.

Use: It is used as inhalation anaesthetics for maintenance of general anesthesia induced by another drug. It is frequently used in veterinary practice.

D. Sevoflurane (Sevorane)

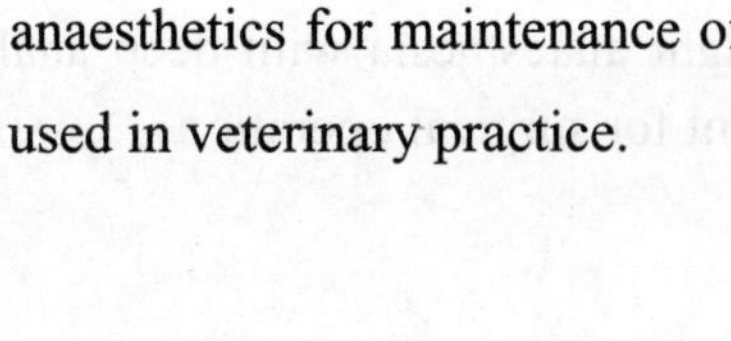

2 - Fluoro methoxy - 1, 1, 1, 3, 3, 3 - hexafluoropropane

Sevoflurane is a sweet smelling, non-flammable highly fluorinated ether, often used inhalation anesthetics nowadays. It can be given by mask because it does not cause irritation. This makes it suitable for inhalation induction in pediatric patients. It has a rapid onset and recovery due to low blood solubility. It should not be used in patients with aortic stenosis.

Mechanism of action: Same as Enflurane.

Use: It is used as an inhalation anaesthetic.

E. Methoxyflurane (Penthrane)

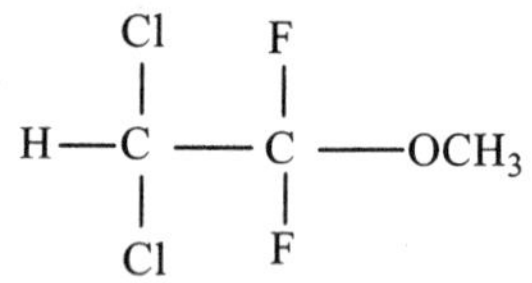

1- Methoxy - 2, 2 - dichloro - 1, 1 - difluoroethane

Methoxyflurane is freely soluble in lipid, so the partition co-efficient (blood / gas) is large, consequently recovery is slow. It produces an excellent anaesthesia and good muscle relaxation. It is a volatile liquid with boiling point about 105°C. It does not have a high vapor pressure at room temperature, so the concentration in the inspired air is low.

Mechanism of action: Same as Enflurane.

Use: It is employed to cause light anaesthesia with deep analgesic and muscle relaxation feature, which make it convenient for surgical operation.

F. Desflurane (Suprane)

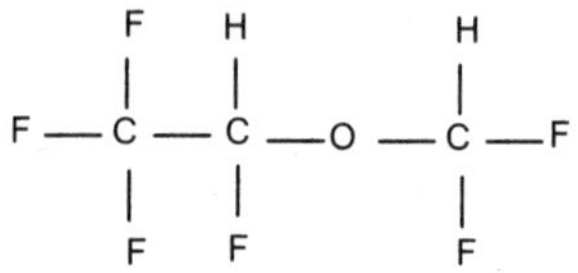

2 - (Difluoro methoxy) - 1, 1, 1, 2 - tetrafluoro ethane

Desflurane is a pungent, volatile fluorinated methyl ethyl ether which is non-flammable. It is liquid at room temperature. Since its boiling point is close to room temperature a specially designed heated vaporizer is used to deliver the drug either with oxygen or nitrous oxide.

Mechanism of action: Same as Enflurane.

Use: It is used as an inhalation agent for induction or maintenance of anaesthesia for adult and not recommended for pediatric use.

3.2 Intravenous Anesthetics

Intravenous anesthetic causes unconsciousness when administered parenterally. They are also classified as

- Inducing agents :
    - ✓ Ultra Short acting: Barbiturates, Propofol and Etomidate
- Slow acting drugs:
    - ✓ Benzodiazepines: Diazepam, Lorazepam and Midazolam
    - ✓ Dissociative anesthetics: Ketamine
    - ✓ Opioid analgesic: Fentanyl

Intravenous anesthetics act more rapidly, producing unconsciousness in about 20 seconds, as soon as the drug reaches the brain from its site of injection and then maintained by inhalation anesthetic.

3.2.1 Ultra Short Acting Barbiturates

A. Thiopental sodium (Thiopen)

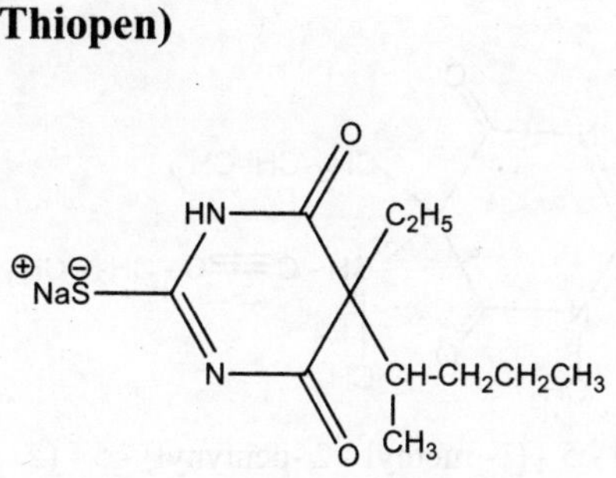

5 - Ethyl - 5 - (1- methyl butyl) - 2 - thio barbituric acid

Thiopental is an ultra-short acting barbiturate. It is used to produce quick anaesthesia and initiate anaesthesia.

Mechanism of action: It depresses the CNS and inhibits ascending transmission of impulses in the reticular formation. Thiopental may enhance or mimic inhibitory action of δ-aminobutyric acid, thereby causing anticonvulsant effect and producing sedation and hypnosis.

Use: It belongs to the category of ultra-short acting barbiturates, usually administered intravenously for the production of complete anaesthesia for short duration. It is also used as a basal anaesthesia.

B.Thiamylal sodium (Citosol)

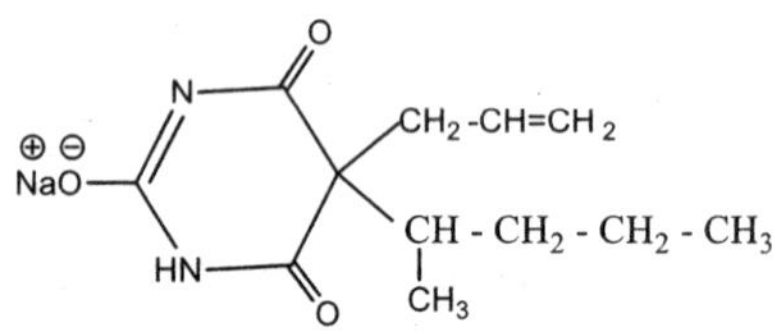

Sodium - 5 - allyl - 5 - (1 - methyl butyl) - 2 -thiobarbiturate

Mechanism of action: It binds at a distinct binding site associated with a Cl^- ionophore at the $GABA_A$ receptor, increasing the duration of time for which the Cl^- ionophore is open. The post-synaptic inhibitory effect of GABA in the thalamus is, therefore, prolonged.

Use: It is an ultra-short acting barbiturate used as intravenous anaesthetic.

C. Methohexital sodium (Brevital)

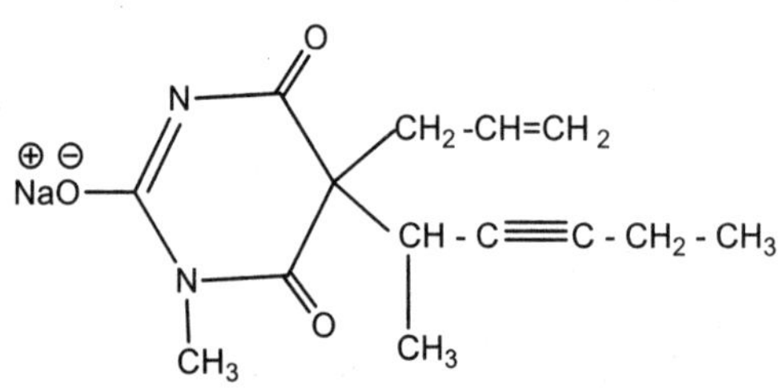

1- Methyl - 5 - (1- methyl - 2 -pentynyl) - 5 - (2 - propenyl) barbituric acid

Synthesis

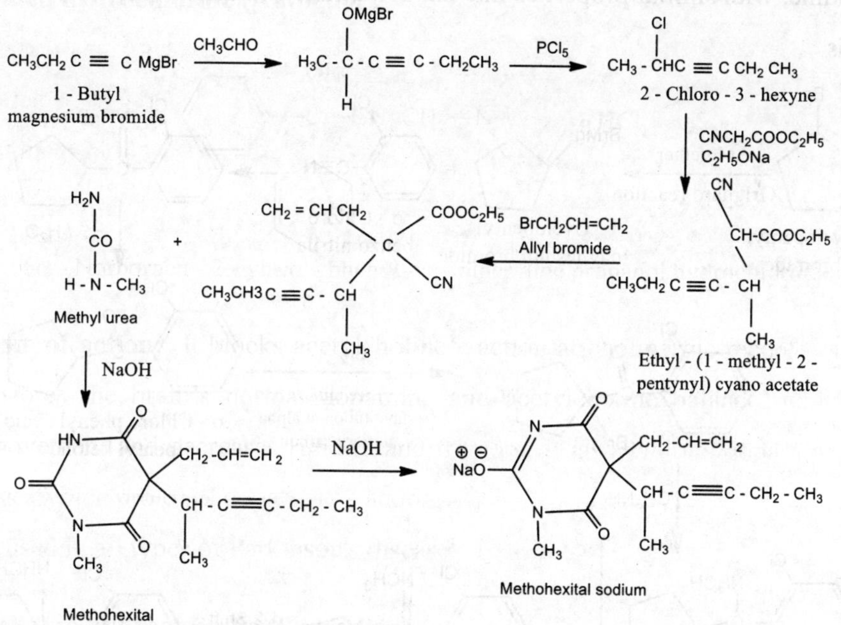

Mechanism of action: Same as Thiamylal sodium.

Use: It is useful for short surgical operation such as oral surgery, gynecological investigation and electroconvulsive therapy.

3.2.2.2 Phencyclidine Derivative

A. Ketamine hydrochloride (Aneket)

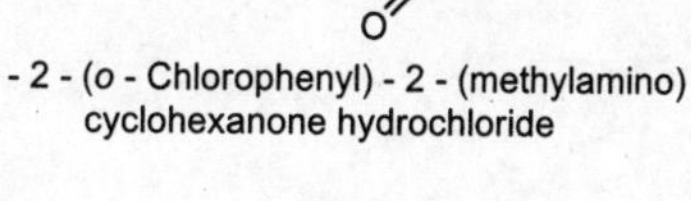

(±) - 2 - (*o* - Chlorophenyl) - 2 - (methylamino) cyclohexanone hydrochloride

It is a dissociative anesthetic. It is a short-acting, non-barbiturate anesthetic, induces a dissociated state in which the patient is unconscious (but may appear to be awake) and does not feel pain. Ketamine is described as unique drug as provides sedation, amnesia and analgesic and no other drug in clinical practice possess all three features. It is an analogue of phencyclidine, with similar properties like hallucinations and dream-like state.

Synthesis

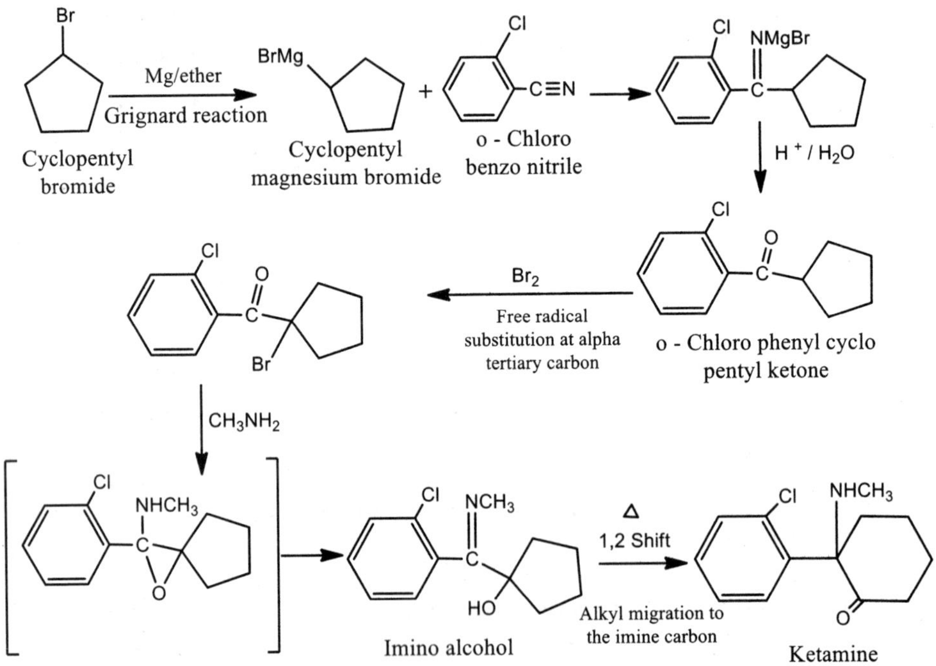

Mechanism of action: it inhibits the excitatory neurotransmitter glutamate at NMDA receptors. It functions at the thalamus (which relays sensory impulses from reticular activating system to the cerebral cortex) and the limbic cortex (which is involved with the awareness of sensation).

Use: It is an intravenous anaesthetic agent and drug of choice for short surgical operation and mainly used as induction anesthesia in children and elderly people.

Chapter 11

NARCOTIC ANALGESICS

1. INTRODUCTION

Analgesics are agents which relieve pain by acting centrally to elevate pain threshold without disturbing consciousness or altering other sensory modalities. The term opiate is used to describe alkaloid molecule derived from opium, which in turn derived from the juice of opium poppy, *Papaver somniferum* eg., Morphine and Codeine. Opioid refers to all the compounds either natural or synthetic which have the functional properties of opiate.

Narcotics are drugs derived from opium or opium like copounds with analgesic effect associated with significant alteration of mood and behavior by producing depression of the central nervous system. These analgesics tend to produce euphoria, which is an important factor in their addictive property, which limits their use. Other limitations include respiratory depression, decreased gastrointestinal motility leading to constipation, increased biliary tract pressure and pruritis due to histamine release. Drugs of this group are used as analgesic but also possess numerous other useful properties. For example Morphine is used to induce sleep in the presence of pain, suppress cough and facilitate anaesthesia.

2. CLASSIFICATION

Narcotic analgesics are classified on the basis of chemical structure as follows:

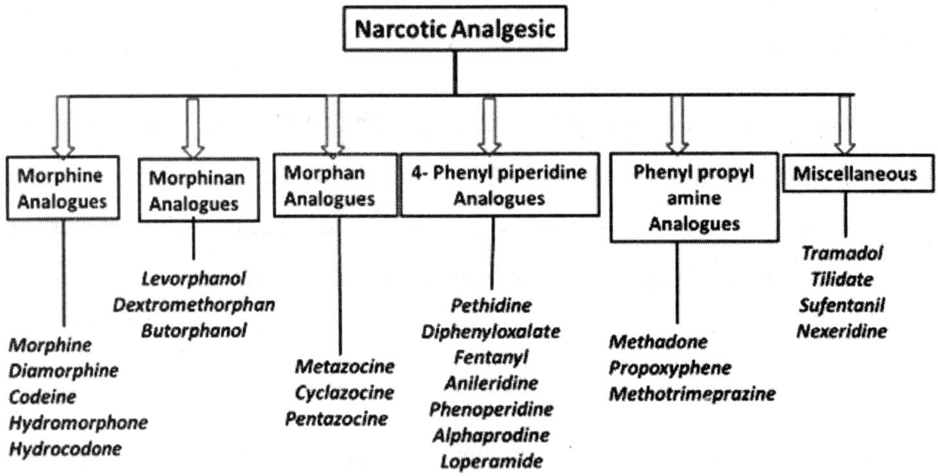

2.1 Morphine and its Related Compounds

Morphine is one of the most abundant opioid found in opium. It is regarded as the gold standard or benchmark of analgesic used to relieve intense pain. Morphine is named after the Roman god of sleep Morpheus. It is an alkaloid isolated from the juice of unriped seed capsule of the poppy plant *Papaver somniferum*. Opium contains numerous alkaloids and they are divided into two main types:

(i) Phenanthrene type: Morphine, Codeine, Thebaine.

(ii) Benzylisoquinoline type. eg. Papaverine, Noscapine.

The Morphine group act on CNS as depressant and stimulant. Papaverine group has antispasmodic action on the smooth muscles. Though Morphine is a potent analgesic, the side effects like, repiratory depression, addiction and sedation associated with Morphine, initiated the attempts for modification of this structure.

2.1.1 Chemistry of Morphine

- The structure of Morphine is composed of five fused rings - pentacyclic structure consisting of a benzene ring (A), two partially unsaturated cyclohexane rings (B and C), a piperidine ring (D) and a dihydrofuran ring (E). Rings A, B and C are the phenanthrene ring system.

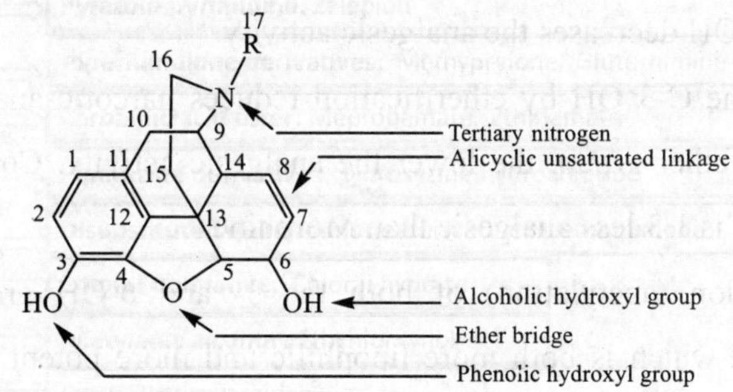

- Two hydroxyl functional groups, a C_3-phenolic OH and a C_6-allylic OH
- An ether linkage between C_4 and C_5,
- Double bond between C_7 and C_8,
- Tertiary amine function at position 17,
- It has five chiral centers with absolute stereochemistry 5(R), 6(S), 9(R), 13(S) and 14(R). The naturally occurring isomer is levo (-) rotatory.

2.1.2 Structure Activity Relationships

The prototypic narcotic analgesic is (-)-Morphine is a complex pentacyclic skeleton. This complex structure is responsible for number of adverse effect associated with Morphine. By applying molecular dissection concept the pharmacodynamically essential part is identified. In this, various skeletons are gradually removed one by one.

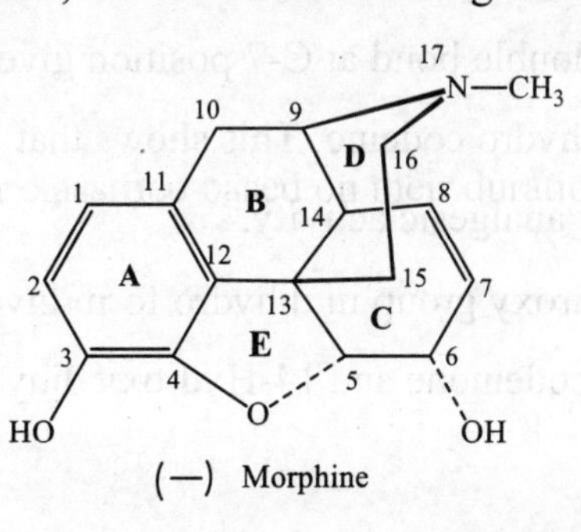

(—) Morphine

The various series obtained through the application of this concept are:

(i) Modification of Ring A

- The ring A and 3- OH group is crucial for analgesic activity. Any substitution on phenyl ring diminishes activity.
- Phenolic OH is essential for binding with μ and κ receptors. Modification of phenolic -OH decreases the analgesic activity.
- Altering the C-3 OH by etherification reduces narcotic analgesic activity and the larger the ether group, the lower the analgesic activity. Codeine (Methyl ether of morphine) is 1/3 less analgesic than Morphine.
- Esterification (acetylation) of both the 3- and 6-OH groups yields Heroin, a compound which is both more lipophilic and more potent. But they have greater side effects and have severe tolerance and dependence characteristics.

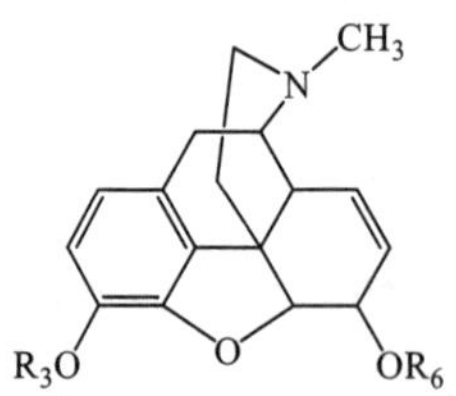

Compound Name	**R3**	**R6**
Codeine	CH_3 -	H-
Heroin	CH_3CO-	CH_3CO-

(ii) Modification of Ring C (alicyclic ring)

- The alcoholic hydroxyl group at C-6 when methylated, esterified, oxidized, removed or replaced by halogen, analgesic activity as well as toxicity of the compound increases. In other word 6-OH of Morphine are not required for analgesic activity.
- The saturation of the double bond at C-7 position gives more potent compound. eg: Dihydro morphine, Dihydro codeine. This shows that 7,8-double bond of Morphine also is not required for analgesic activity.
- Introduction of 14-hydroxy group in dihydro form gives more potent compound. eg 14- Hydroxy dihydro codeinone and 14-Hydroxy dihydromorphinone.

- Annelation – Bridging of C_6 and C_{14} through ethylene linkage yields Thebaine compounds such as Etorphine which are 200 times more potent than Morphine potent analgesics. These compounds typically used to immobilize large animals (elephants).
- Replacement of the N-methyl group of the Thebaine with a methylcyclopropyl group yields compounds with mixed agonist/antagonist or partial agonist activity. For example, Buprenorphine HC1 (Buprenex) is a mixed agonist /antagonist.

(iii) Modification of Ring D

- Tertiary nitrogen is necessary for good opioid activity.
- Replacement of Morphine's N-methyl group by a hydrogen atom as in Nor-morphine reduces analgesic activity to 1/8th that of morphine.
- Replacement of Morphine's N-methyl group with larger alkyl groups reduces activity. However, substitution with aralkyl group significantly increases analgesic activity eg N-Phenethylnormorphine.
- Replacement of Morphine's N-methyl group with an allyl group (-CH_2-CH=CH_2), a methylcyclopropyl group or a methylcyclobutyl group results in the emergence of opiate receptor antagonist activity.
- Three of these compounds - Naloxone, Naltrexone and Nalmefene - are pure opiate antagonists (at μ, k and δ receptors).

(iv) Morphinan Analogues

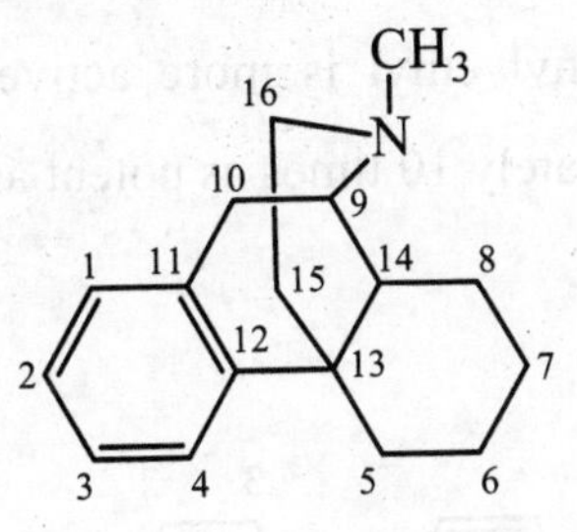

- The ethereal linkage is not required for analgesic activity.

- Removal of ether (ring E) bridge between the C_4 and C_5 atom named as Morphinans has increased analgesic activity. The *levo* form of morphinan possess analgesic activity, while the *dextro* form is cough suppressant.
- Levorphanol and Butorphanol are examples of morphinan series. Levorphanol is eight times more active than Morphine. Butorphanol is a mixed agonist and antagonist.

(v) Benzomorphans or Morphans

- Lack of ring C and E of morphine retains the activity and these compounds are named as 6,7- Benzomorphans.

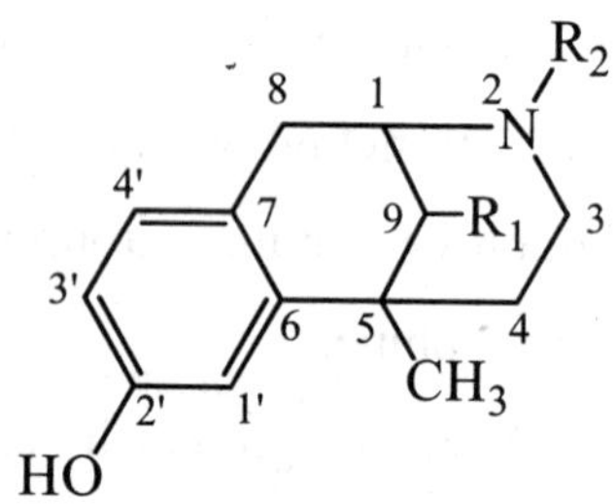

- Pentazocine is a classical example from benzomorphan series. It is the mixed agonist-antagonist analgesic to be marketed. It is an agonist at the kappa and sigma opioid receptors and has a weak antagonist action at the mu receptor.
- The trimethyl compound ($R_1 = R_2$: CH_3) is more active than dimethyl (R_1= H, R_2 = CH_3) compound. N-phenyl ethyl is more active than trimethyl compounds. eg. Phenazocine is approximately 10 times as potent as morphine

(vi) 4-Phenyl piperidine

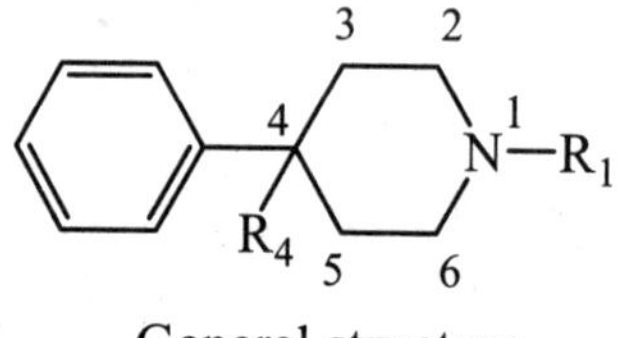

General structure

- Removal of ring B, C and E (with only A and D) known as 4-Phenyl piperidine class possess analgesic activity, which opened new search of simpler, relatively small and structurally uncomplicated analgesics.

- Mepheridine is a major drug from this series with 1/4th of potency of Morphine. The reversed ester of Meperidine, the propionoxy compound was most active, being 5 times more active than Meperidine. eg. Prodines.

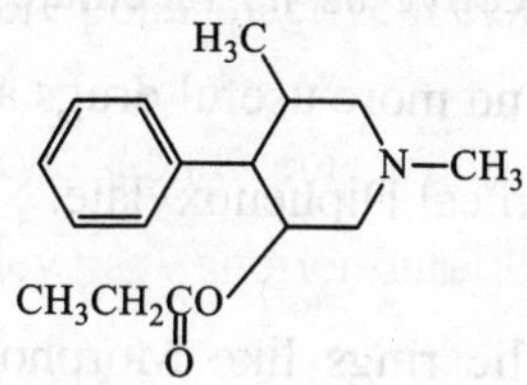

- Introduction of *m*-hydroxy group in phenyl ring increases the activity since it is similar to C_3-OH of Morphine eg. Bemidone. Replacement of ester moiety by a ketone function in a Bemidone results in Ketobemidone is equivalent to Morphine in activity.

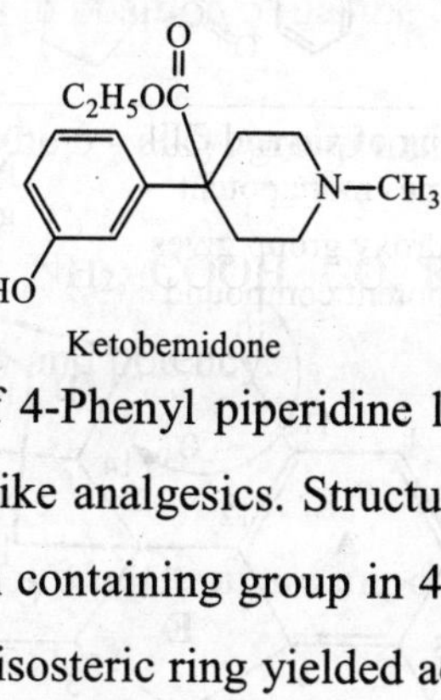

Ketobemidone

- Structural modifications of 4-Phenyl piperidine lead to the discovery of Fentanyl group which is Morphine like analgesics. Structural modification of Fentanyl, like introducing a small oxygen containing group in 4th position of piperidine ring and replacing phenyl ring with isosteric ring yielded active compounds with lower side effects. Example Alfentanil and Sufentanil.

(vii) **Methadone Series**

The further simplification of Morphine nucleus by opening the nitrogen ring resulted into Methadone series of compound.

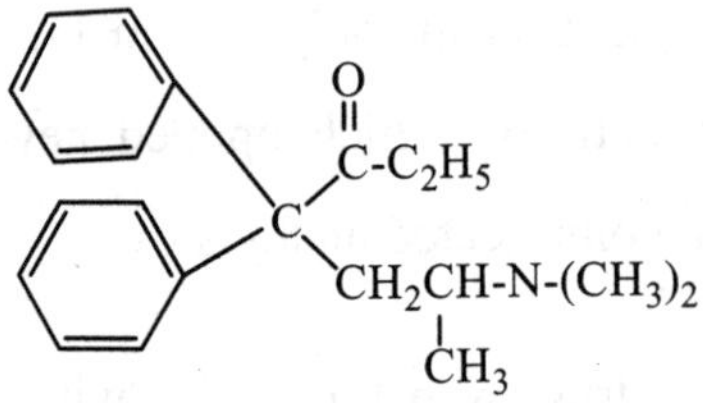

Methadone

- Methadone is orally active and has longer duration of action. The *levo* isomer of Methadone is twice as effective as its racemates. Many variations in Methadone structure have been made and more useful drugs are analgesic Acetylmethadols and Propoxyphene and antidiarrheal Diphenoxylate.

- Replacement of heterocyclic rings like Morpholine and Piperidine for dimethyl amino group gives a compound as potent as Methadone with Morphine like properties. eg. Racemoramide.

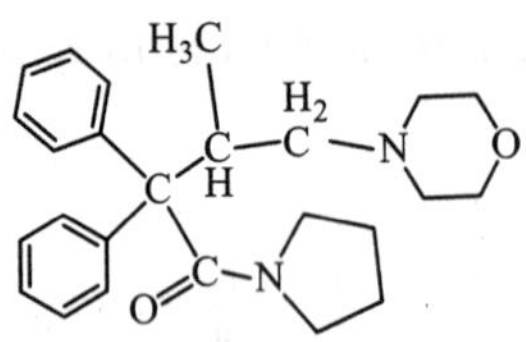

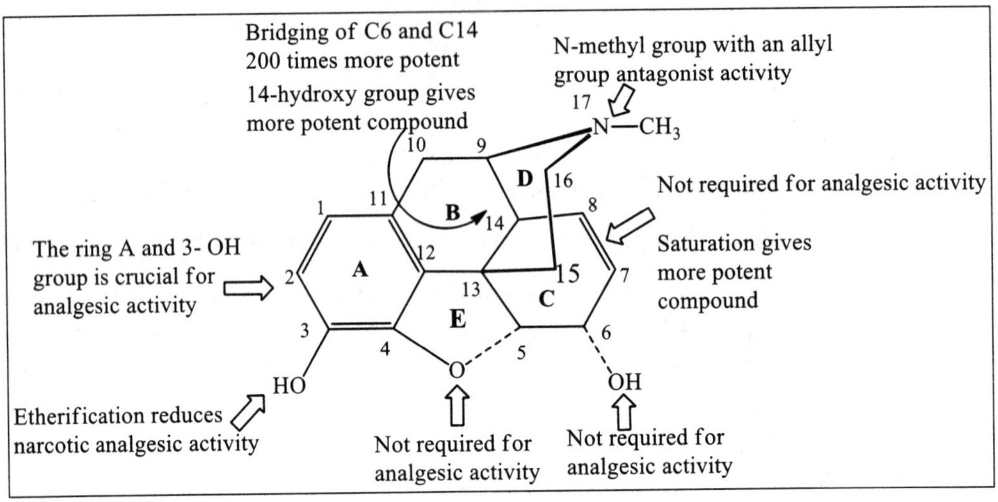

Fig.11.1 Summary of SAR

A.Morphine sulphate (Roxanol)

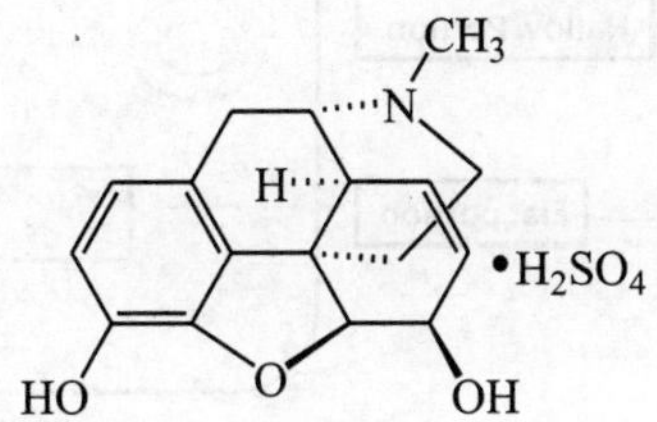

Mechanism of action: Morphine causes analgesia by selectively acting on receptor situated both in the higher centre and spinal cord. It activates specific opiate receptors (δ, μ and k) each of which are involved in controlling different brain functions. Binding of Morphine to the μ opioid receptor results in hyperpolarization of the neuron leading to the inhibition of release of nociceptive neurotransmitters causing an analgesic effect and increased pain tolerance due to reduced neuronal excitability. In the central nervous and gastrointestinal systems, Morphine exhibits effects including analgesia, sedation, anxiolysis, euphoria, respiratory depression and gastrointestinal system smooth muscle contraction. The structure features, which are recognized to be essential for the perfect fit of a narcotic analgesic on receptors, are represented below:

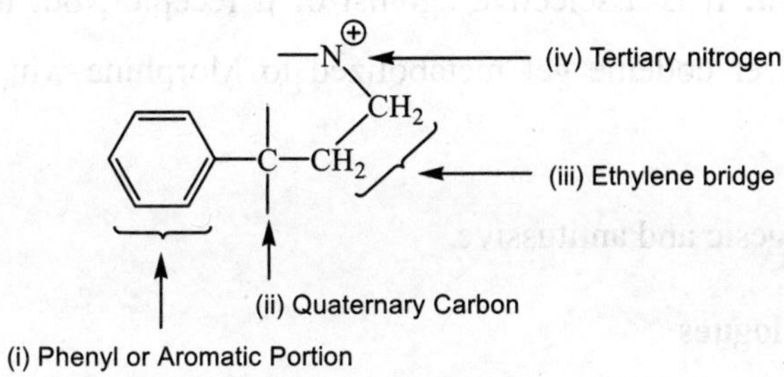

Opioid receptor composed of three prominent parts:

- A flat portion which holds aromatic part by Vander-Waal's force.
- A cavity or a hallow portion which entraps ethylene bridge
- An anionic site which holds the 3° Nitrogen, which get ionized at physiological pH.

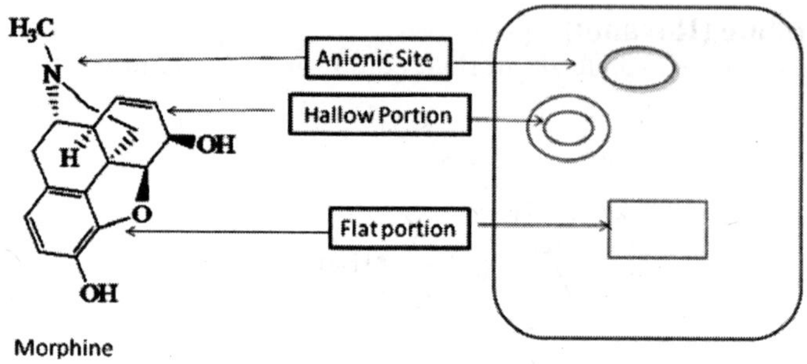

Fig. 11.2 Diagram of the surface of Analgesic receptor site with the corresponding lower surface of the drug molecule

Use: It is used to relieve moderate to severe pain.

B. Codeine (Nurofen Plus)

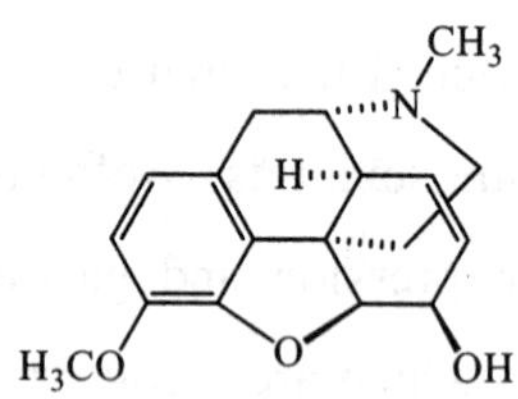

Codeine

Mechanism of action: It is a selective agonist of μ receptor, but its affinity is weak to opoid receptor. In liver codeine get metabolized to Morphine which is ten times more potent agonist.

Use: It is a mild analgesic and antitussive.

2.2 Morphinan Analogues

A.Levorphanol tartrate (Levo-Dromoran)

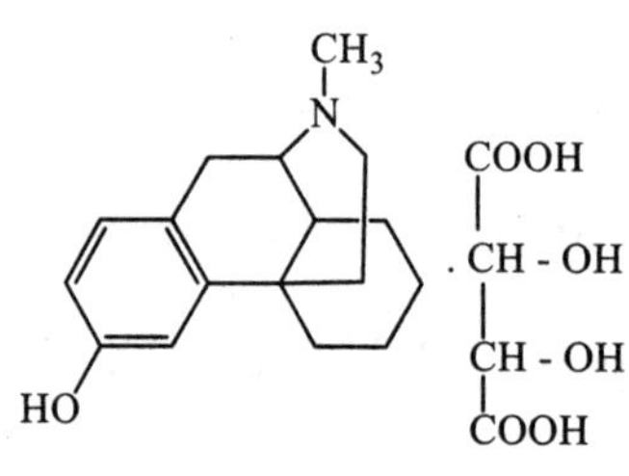

17 - Methyl morphinan - 3 - ol

Levorphanol is 8 times more potent than Morphine. The removal of 4, 5 - epoxide and saturation of double bond at C_7 and C_8, increases flexibility and affinity to all subtype of opioid receptors.

Mechanism of action: It mimics the actions of endogenous peptides at μ opioid receptor in both brain and the spinal cord to alter the transmission and perception of pain.

Use: It is used to releive moderate to high pain in biliary and renal colic, myocardial infarction in serious trauma and cancer pain.

2.3 Morphan Analogues

A. Pentazocine (Talwin)

Pentazocine is a mixed agonist / antagonist.

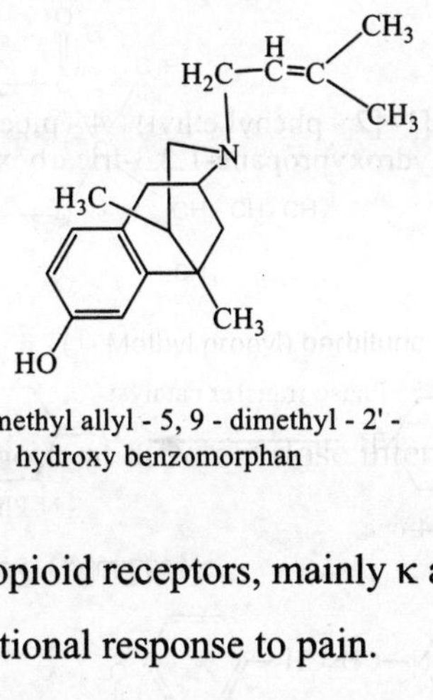

2 - Dimethyl allyl - 5, 9 - dimethyl - 2' - hydroxy benzomorphan

Mechanism of action: It binds to opioid receptors, mainly κ and σ receptors, at many CNS sites to alter perception of and emotional response to pain.

Use: It is a synthetic analgesic agent, used to control moderate to acute pain.

2.4 4 - Phenyl Piperidine Analogues

A. Meperidine hydrochloride (Pethidine)

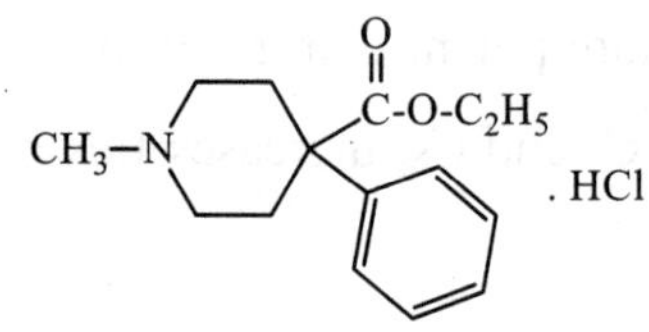

4 - Ethoxy carbonyl - 1 - methyl -
4 - phenyl piperidine

Mechanism of action: It stimulates μ and κ receptors, which alters the perception of and emotional response to pain.

Use: It is a synthetic narcotic analgesic possesses the action and uses similar to Morphine.

B. Fentanyl citrate (Sublimaze)

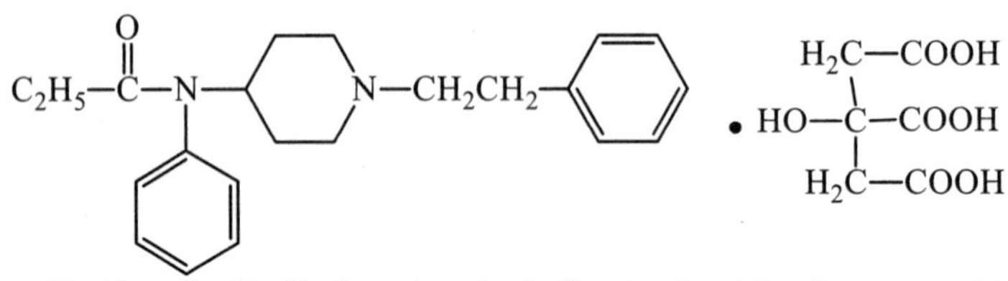

N - Phenyl - *N* - [1- [2 - phenyl ethyl) - 4 - piperidinyl]propanamide - 2-hydroxypropane-1,2,3-tricarboxylic acid

Synthesis

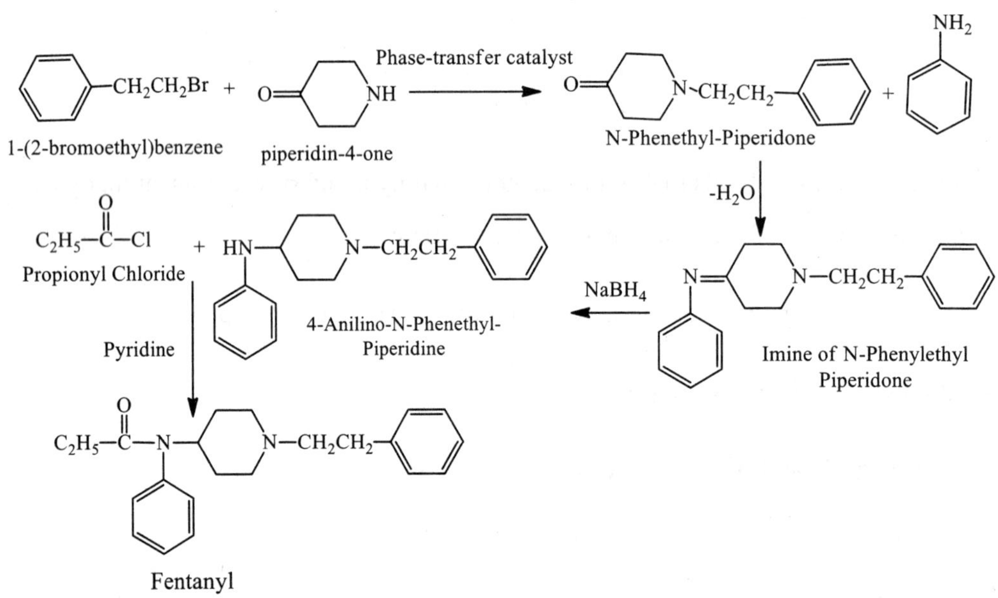

Mechanism of action: It binds to μ-receptor in the central nervous system (CNS) thereby mimicking the effects of endogenous opiates, altering perception of and emotional response to pain by inhibiting ascending pain pathways. Fentanyl may alter neuro-transmitter release from afferent nerves responsive to painful stimuli and it causes respiratory depression by acting directly on respiratory centers in the brain stem.

Use: It is a potent narcotic analgesics with anesthetic properties.

C. Diphenoxylate hydrochloride (Lamotil)

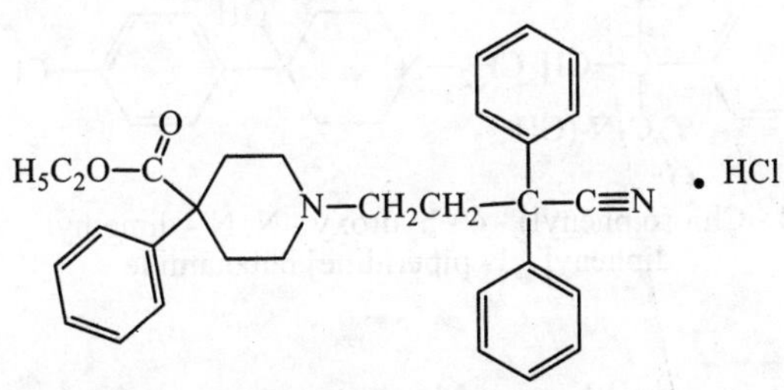

Ethyl - 1 - (3 - Cyano - 3, 3 - diphenyl propyl) - 4 - phenyl - 4 - piperidine carboxylate

Mechanism of action: It is an opiate receptor agonists that stimulate μ receptors in GI to decrease the peristalsis and constrict the sphincters. It has a direct effect on circular smooth muscle of the bowel, that conceivably results in segmentation and prolongation of gastrointestinal transit time.

Use: It is used to treat diarrhea.

D. Anileridine hydrochloride (Leritine)

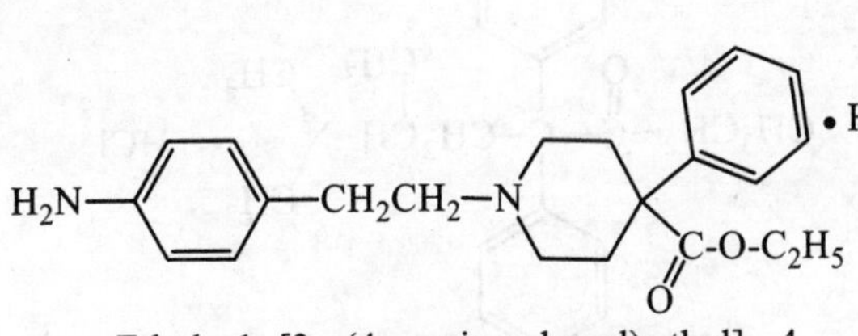

Ethyl - 1- [2 - (4 - amino phenyl) ethyl] - 4 - phenyl - 4 - piperidine carboxylate

Mechanism of action: It binds to opioid receptors in the central nervous sytem (CNS) and mimics the endogenous opioids resulting in a decrease of nociceptive neurotransmitters and eventually an analgesic effect.

Use: It is a narcotic pain reliever used to treat moderate to severe pain.

E. Loperamide hydrochloride (Imodium)

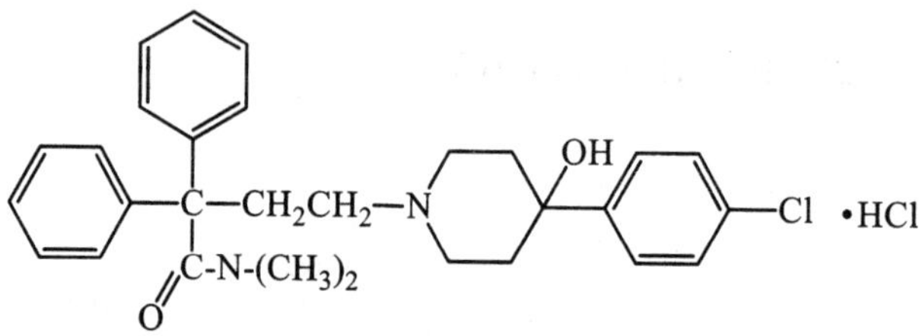

4 - [(4 - Chloro phenyl) - 4 - hydroxy - N, N - dimethyl - α, α - diphenyl - 1- piperidine] butanamide

Mechanism of action: It is a mild opioid μ-receptor agonist but is used largely for the treatment of diarrhea rather than pain. Loperamide acts as a potent opiate agonist in the intestine and reduces intestinal motility, causing a slowing of intestinal transport and increased resorption of water and electrolytes, actions that are helpful in treating diarrhea.

Use: It is a safe and effective opioid derived anti-diarrheal agent

2.5 Phenylpropylamine Analogues

A. Methadone hydrochloride (Dolophine)

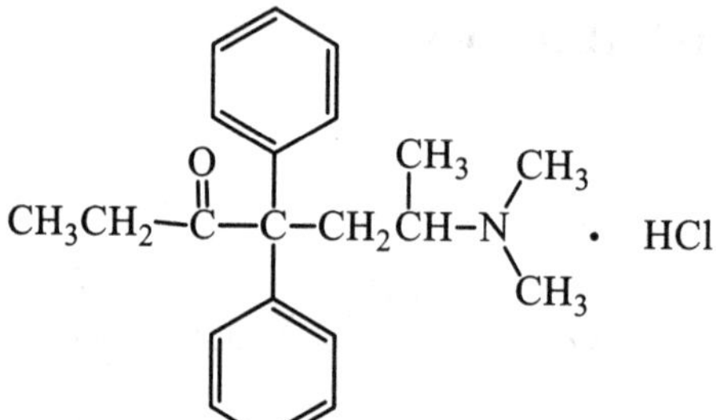

6 - Dimethyl amino - 4, 4 - diphenyl heptan - 3 - one

Synthesis

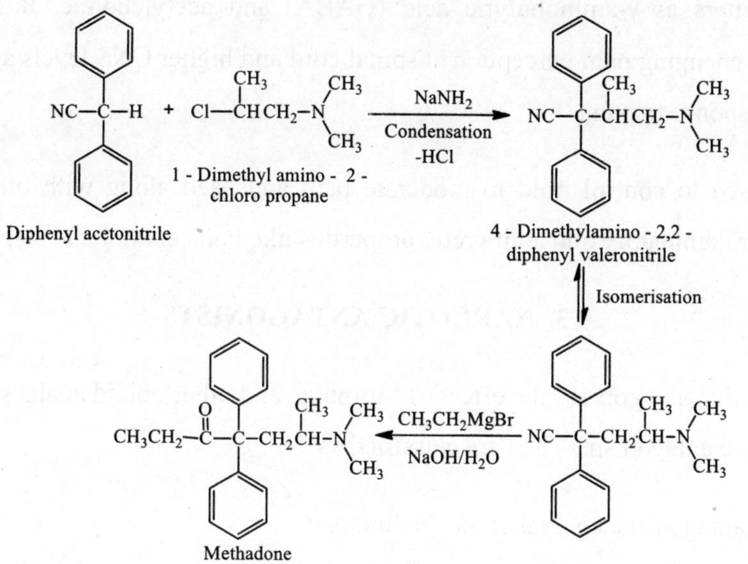

Levomethadone is the biologically active enantiomere (10-15 times more pain relieving) because it has a higher affinity to opioid receptors than its *dextro* enantiomer.

Mechanism of action: It binds to opioid receptors in spinal cord and higher levels of CNS to produce analgesia and euphoric effects.

Use: It is a potent narcotic analgesic. It also exerts sedation and antitussive properties.

B. Propoxyphene hydrochloride or Dextropropoxyphene (Darvocet – N)

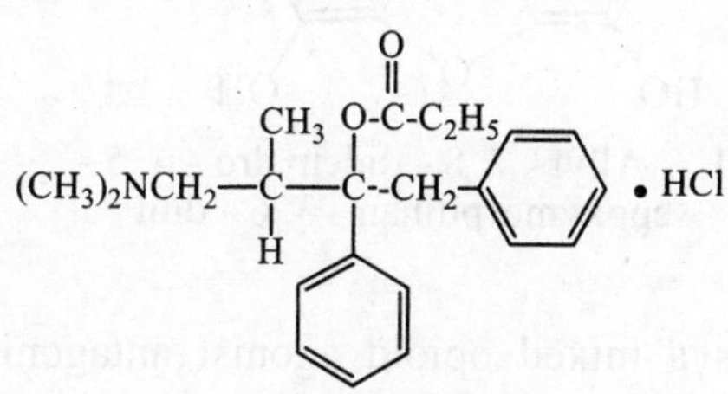

(2S, 3R) - (±) - 4 - (Dimethylamino) - 3 - methyl - 1, 2 - diphenyl - 2 - butanyl propionate

Only the *dextro* isomer has an analgesic effect; the *levo* isomer appears to exert an antitussive effect.

Mechanism of action: It strongly agonizes μ-receptors, blocking release of such inhibitory neurotransmitters as γ-aminobutyric acid (GABA) and acetylcholine. It also mediates analgesia by changing pain perception at spinal cord and higher CNS levels and by altering emotional response to pain.

Use: It is used to control mild to moderate pain and used along with other analgesics having anti inflammatory and antipyretic properties like Paracetamol and Aspirin.

3. NARCOTIC ANTAGONISTS

Drug that antagonizes the effect of Morphine and other opioid analgesics act mainly by competitive antagonism. They are classified as

i) Pure antagonists. eg. Naloxone, Naltrexone

ii) Partial agonists of Nalorphine type. eg. Nalorphine, Levallorphan, Cyclazocine.

iii) Partial agonists of Morphine type. eg. Propiram, Profadol.

A. Nalorphine hydrochloride (Nalline)

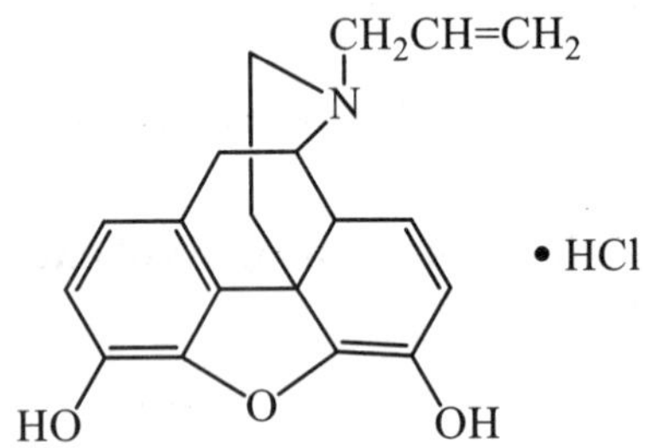

17 - Allyl - 7, 8 - didehydro - 4, 5 - epoxymorphinan - 3, 6 - diol

Mechanism of action: It is a mixed opioid agonist–antagonist. It acts at two opioid receptors at the μ-receptor it has antagonistic effects and at the κ-receptors it exerts high-efficacy agonistic characteristics.

Use: It is a narcotic antagonist effectively employed antidote to reverse narcotic over dose and in challenge test to determine opoid depression.

B. Naloxone hydrochloride (Narcan)

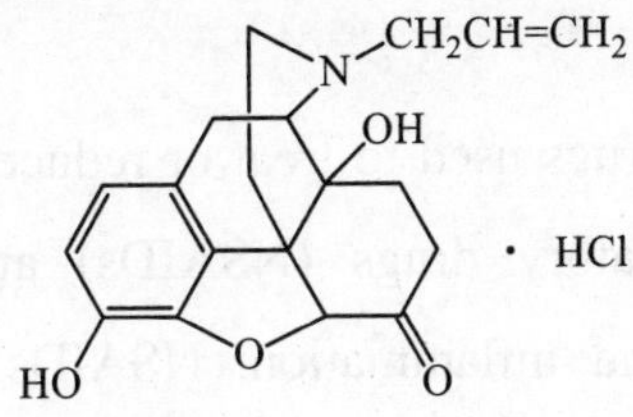

17 - Allyl - 5 - epoxy - 3, 14 - dihydroxy morphinan - 6 - one

Mechanism of action: It antagonizes the opioid effects by competing at μ-opioid receptor.

Use: It is a specific narcotic antagonist possess no morphine-like properties. It has been found to reverse narcotic analgesic. It is used in combination with opoid to reduce the risk of opoid misuse.

C. Levallorphan tartrate (Naloxifan)

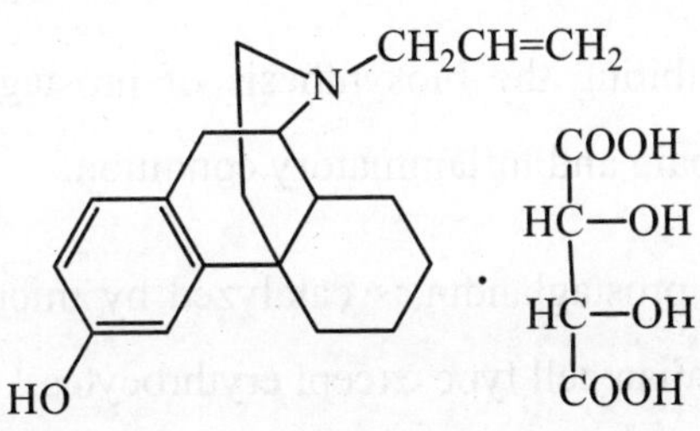

17 - Allyl morphinan - 3 - ol

Mechanism of action: It is a mixed agonist and antagonist. It antagonizes opioid effects by competing μ-receptor and as agonist wth κ receptor.

Use: It is a potent synthetic analgesic very much chemically and pharmacologically related to Morphine.

ANTI-INFLAMMATORY DRUGS

Chapter 12

1. INTRODUCTION

Anti-inflammatory are drugs used to treat or reduces inflammation or swelling. Non-steroidal anti-inflammatory drugs (NSAIDs) are one of the most commonly prescribed drugs for pain and inflammation. NSAIDs are drugs with analgesic (pain reducing) antipyretic (fever reducing) and anti-inflammatory properties. NSAIDs are non-narcotic (they do not induce stupor) which distinguishes it from steroidal anti-inflammatory drugs (Corticosteroids). Specific uses include the treatment of headaches, arthritis, sports injuries and menstrual cramps, acute pain and inflammation, osteoarthritis, rheumatoid arthritis, spondylitis, painful shoulder, acute gouty arthritis and postoperative pain.

2. MECHANISM OF ACTION

- NSAIDs act by inhibiting the biosynthesis of prostaglandin, which is the basic cause behind fever, pain and inflammatory condition.
- The biosynthesis of prostaglandin is catalyzed by microsomal enzyme present in almost every mammalian cell type except erythrocytes.
- Prostaglandin is a naturally occurring 20 carbon cyclo pentane fatty acid derivatives derived from arachidonic acid.

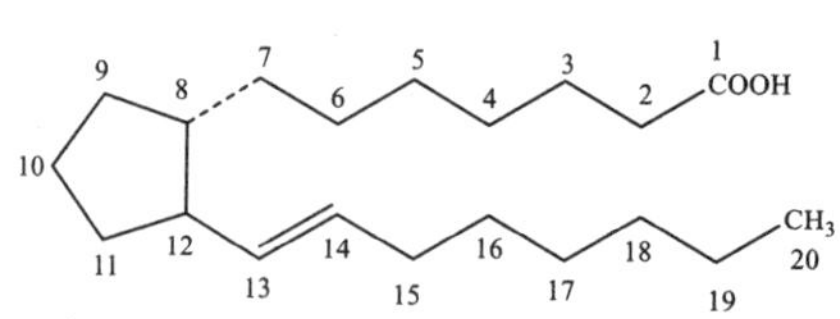

Fig. 12.1 General Structure of Prostaglandin

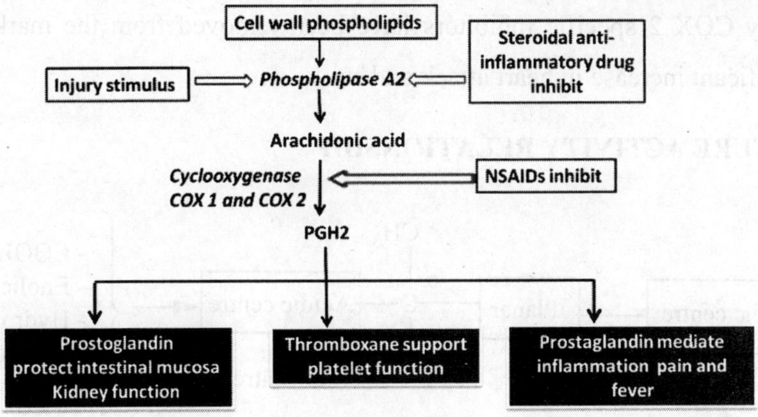

Fig 12.2 Mechanism of NSAIDs

- Arachidonic acid is released from membrane phospholipids as a response to inflammation stimuli by the enzyme *phospholipase* A_2.
- Prostaglandin (PGH_2), prostacyclin (PGI_2) and thromboxane A_2 (TxA_2) are produced by arachidonic acid by *cyclooxygenase* (also known as *prostaglandin synthase*)
- *Cyclooxygenase* exist two isoforms COX 1 and COX 2.
- *Cyclooxygenase 3* (COX 3) has been recently identified.
- COX 1 perform in physiological condition such as homeostasis of the entire organism, protect stomach from limiting acid secretion, renal function and platelet aggregation (promote blood clotting)
- COX 2 is generated during inflammation by pathological stimulus.
- Both COX enzymes produces prostaglandin that promote fever and pain.
- NSAID's block COX enzyme and reduces the production of prostaglandin and also reduces inflammatory symptoms. Since prostaglandin that protect stomach and produce blood clotting is also reduced that block both COX 1 and COX 2 enzymes causes ulcers in stomach and increased risk of bleeding.
- Selective COX 2 inhibitors may eliminate side effects associated with NSAID'S due to COX 1 inhibition such as gastric and renal effect.

- Many COX 2 specific inhibitors have been removed from the market due to its significant increase in heart attack and stroke.

3. STRUCTURE ACTIVITY RELATIONSHIP

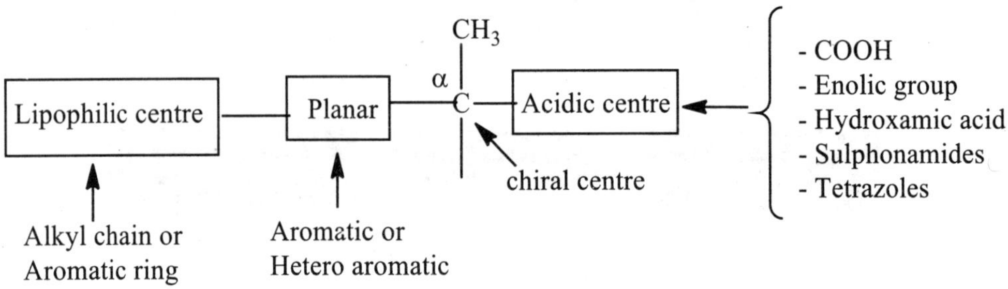

Fig. 12.3 Schematic Representation of SAR of NSAIDs

- In general, NSAIDs structurally (Fig. 12.3) consists of acidic moiety which can be represented by carboxylic acid group, an enolic group, a hydroxamic acid group, a sulfonamide or a tetrazole ring.
- The centre of acidity is attached to a planar aromatic or hetero aromatic ring.
- The centre of acidity is generally located one carbon adjacent to the planar surface. This distance plays a critical role, because as the distance increases the activity of the drug diminishes.
- Aryl and hetero-aryl derivatives are common, since they correlate with the double bond at 5 - and 8 - position of the arachidonic acid.
- Amide or ester derivatives of carboxylic acids are usually attributed to the metabolic hydrolysis products.
- Substitution of a methyl group on the α-carbon increases the anti-inflammatory activity. Groups larger than methyl show a decline in activity.
- The resulting α-methyl acetic or 2 - substituted propionic acid has been given a class name profen.
- The introduction of methyl group in α-position creates a chiral center; the anti-inflammatory activity is associated with S (+) enantiomer.

- The activity is further enhanced by an addition of lipophilic group alkyl or additional aromatic ring, which is non-coplanar with the original aromatic or hetero-aromatic ring. This lipophilic area corresponds to the double bond region at the position 11- of arachidonic acid.

4. CLASSIFICATION

Anti-inflammatory Drugs

- **Heteroaryl acetic acid analogues :** Indomethacin, Tolmetin, Zomepirac
- **Aryl acetic acid analogues :** Sulindac, Ibufenac, Diclofenac sodium
- **Aryl propionic acid analogues:** Ibuprofen, Flubiprofen, Ketoprofen, Naproxen
- **Oxicams :** Piroxicam, Meloxicam,Tenoxicam
- **Salicylic acid analogues:** Aspirin, Salol, Salsalate, Salicylic acid
- ***P*- Amino phenol derivatives:** Acetaminophen, Phenacetin
- **Pyrozolone and Pyrazolidones :** Antipyrine, Dipyrone, Phenylbutazone, Oxyphenbutazone
- **N- Arylanthranilic acid derivatives :** Mefenamic acid, Meclofenamate, Ketorolac
- **Selective Cox-2 inhibitiors:** Celecoxib, Rofecoxib, Valdecoxib
- **Miscellaneous :** Gold compounds, Allopurinol

4.1 Heteroaryl Acetic acid Analogues

A. Indomethacin (Microcid)

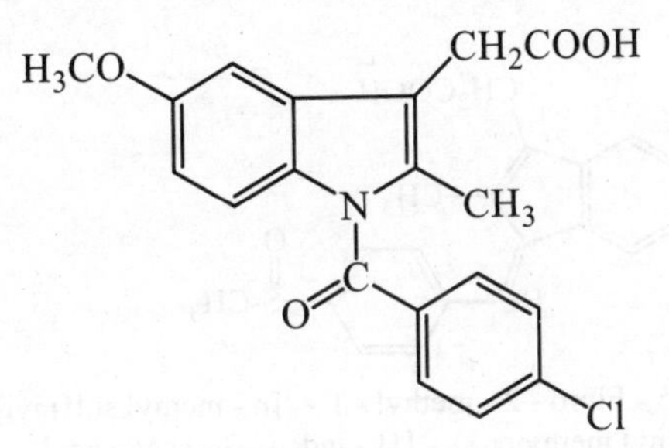

1 - (p - Chloro benzoyl) - 5 - methoxy - 2 - methyl indole - 3 - acetic acid

Use: It is used as anti-inflammatory, analgesic in rheumatic arthritis, spondylitis and to lesser extent in gout.

B. Tolmetin (Tolectin)

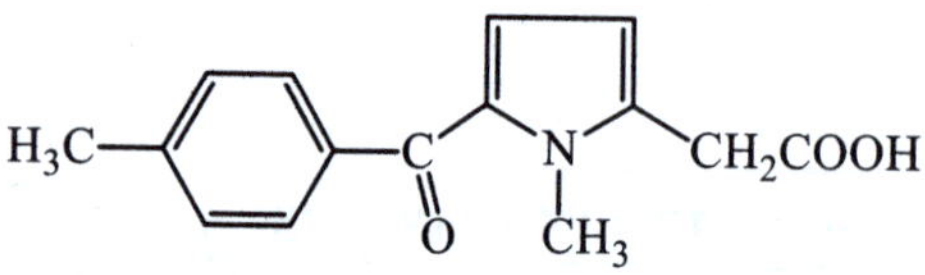

1- Methyl - 5 - (4 - methyl benzoyl) pyrrole - 2 - acetic acid

Use: It is used in acute and chronic rheumatic arthritis.

C. Zomepirac (Zomax)

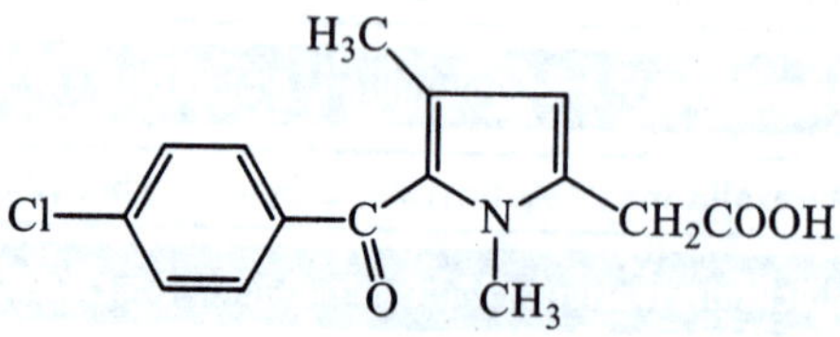

2 - [5 - (4 - chloro benzoyl) - 1, 4 - Dimethyl -pyrrole - 2 -yl] acetic acid

Use: It is used as analgesic and anti-inflammatory drug.

4.2 Aryl Aceticacid Analogues

A. Sulindac (Clinoril)

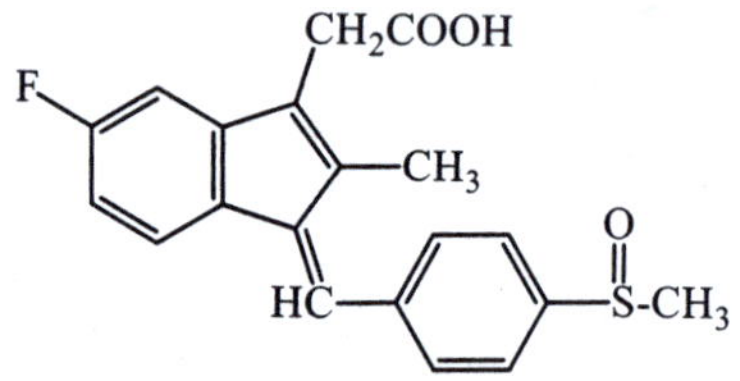

(1Z) - 5 - Fluro - 2 - methyl - 1 - {[p - methyl sulfinyl] phenyl methylene} - 1H - inden - 3 - acetic acid

Sulindac is a prodrug, the sulfoxide functional group is reduced to active sulfide metabolite. The Z-isomer is more potent anti-inflammatory than the E-isomer.

Use: It has analgesic, antipyretic and anti - inflammatory properties. It is usually employed in the treatment of rheumatic and muscular skeletal disorders, acute gouty arthritis and osteoarthritis.

B. Diclofenac (Voltaren)

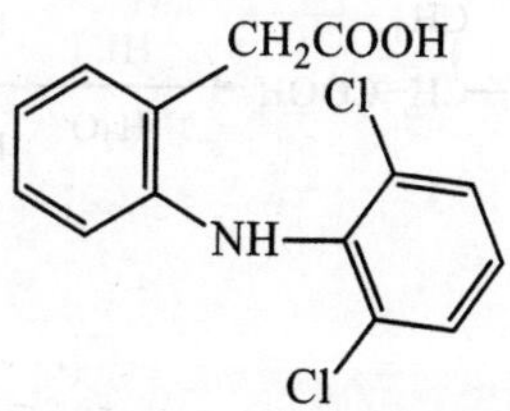

o - (2, 6, - Dichloro anilino) phenyl acetic acid

Use: It is used in the treatment of rheumatic arthritis.

4.3 Aryl Propionic acid Analogues

These compounds are also known as propionic acid derivatives. In this series of compound, potency of it increases by the introduction of α - methyl group on acetic acid moiety.

A. Ibuprofen (Advil)

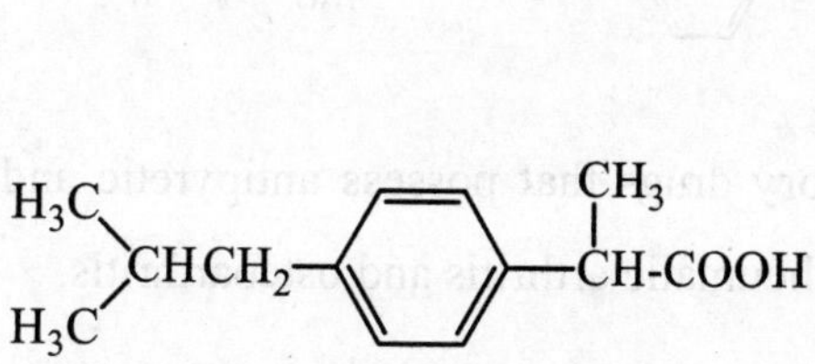

2 - (4- Isobutyl phenyl) - propionic acid

Ibuprofen is administered as a racemic mixture. The R-enantiomer undergoes extensive interconversion to the S-enantiomer *in vivo*. The S-enantiomer is believed to be the more pharmacologically active enantiomer. Ibuprofen is produced industrially as racemates.

Synthesis

Method - 1

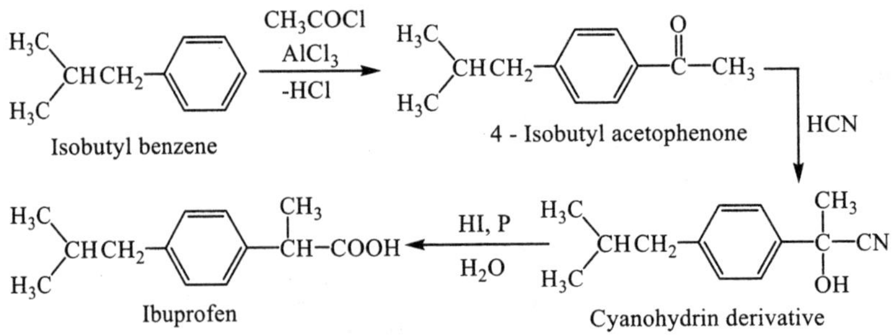

Method - II

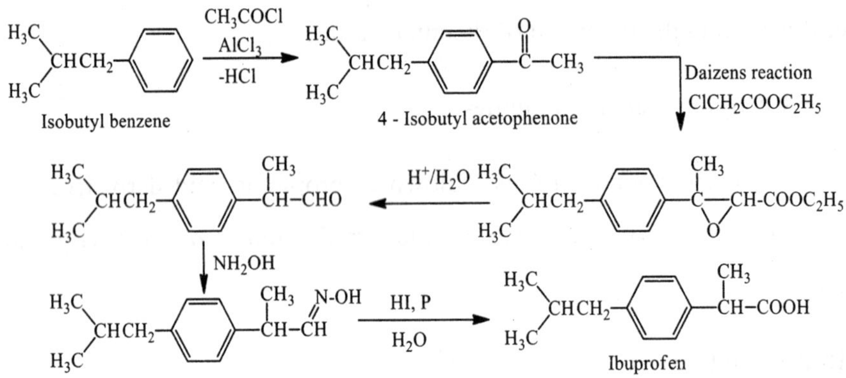

Use: It is anti-inflammatory drugs that possess antipyretic and analgesic properties. It is used for the treatment of rheumatic arthritis and osteoarthritis.

C. Naproxen (Naprosyn)

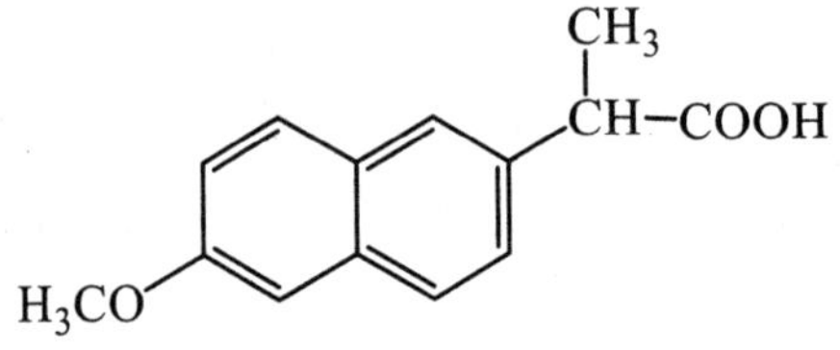

(±) - 2 - (6 - Methoxy - 2 - naphthyl) - propionic acid

Use: It has analgesic, anti-inflammatory and antipyretic activities. It is used in the treatment of rheumatic arthritis, dysmenorrhea and acute gout.

4.4 Oxicams

A. Piroxicam(Dolonex)

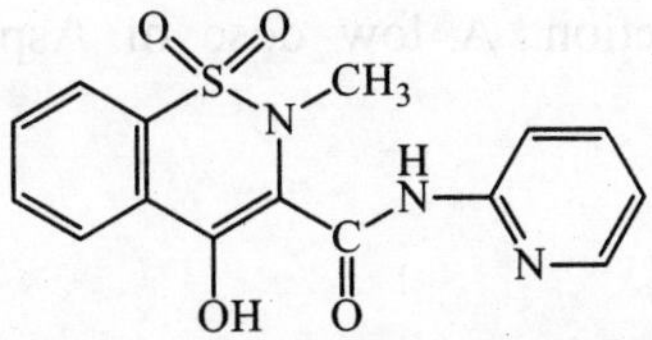

4 - Hydroxy - 2 - methyl - N - 2 - pyridyl - 2H - 1, 2 - benzothiazine - 3 - carboxamide - 1,1 - dioxide

Use: It is used in the treatment of rheumatic arthritis and osteoarthritis.

4.5 Salicylic Acid Analogues

A. Sodium salicylate (Cleanoderm)

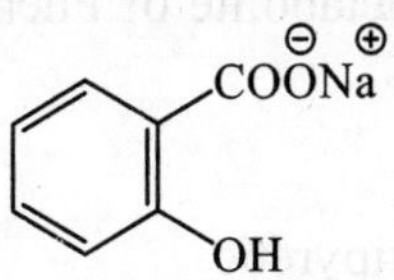

2 - Hydroxy sodium benzoate

Use: It is generally used for the treatment of fever and the relief of pain. It also possesses anti-inflammatory actions similar to Aspirin. It is recommended in acute rheumatic fever and in the symptomatic therapy of gout. It also possesses antifungal activity.

B. Aspirin (or) Acetyl salicylic acid (Ecosprin)

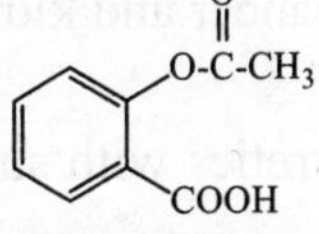

Acetyl salicylic acid

Aspirin is chemically named as acetyl salicylic acid, which is a Prodrug of Salicylic acid. Salts of Aspirin have fewer undesirable side effects than Aspirin. It is usually recommended for bed time dosage.

Use: It is used as an antipyretic, anti-inflammatory and analgesic in a variety of conditions. It also inhibits platelet function; it has been employed prophylactically to minimize the incidence of myocardial infarction. A low dose of Aspirin reduces heart attack and thrombotic stroke.

4.6 p-Aminophenol Analogues

A. Acetaminophen (or) Paracetamol (Crocin/Calpol)

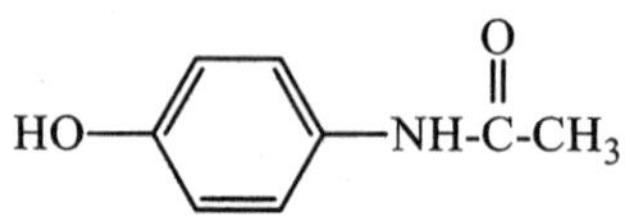

4 - Hydroxy acetanilide

Paracetamol is an active metabolite of Phenacetin, but it is not toxic at therapeutic dose like Phenacetin.

Use: It is used as analgesic and antipyretic.

B. Phenacetin (Condradol)

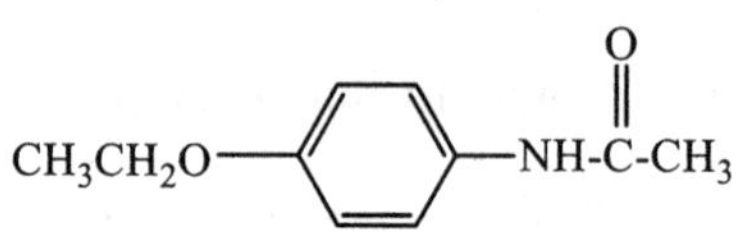

p - Ethoxy acetanilide

Phenacetin was the first analgesic in 1887 to come to the market. Its analgesic effect is due to its action on sensory tract of the spinal card. Its use is declined due to its adverse effect which includes certain cancer and kidney damage.

Use: It is used as analgesic and antipyretics with similar effect as Aspirin. It is more toxic than Paracetamol.

4.7 Pyrazolones and Pyrazolidinones

A. Antipyrine (or) Phenazone (Auralgan)

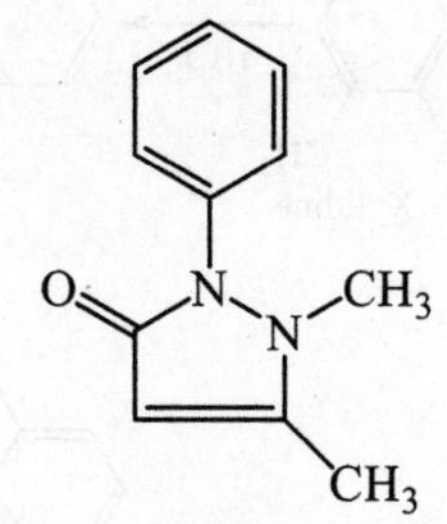

2, 3 - Dimethyl - 1 - phenyl - 3 - pyrazolin - 5 - one

Use: It is used as antipyretics and also possess local anaesthetic activity.

B. Phenylbutazone (Flanil)

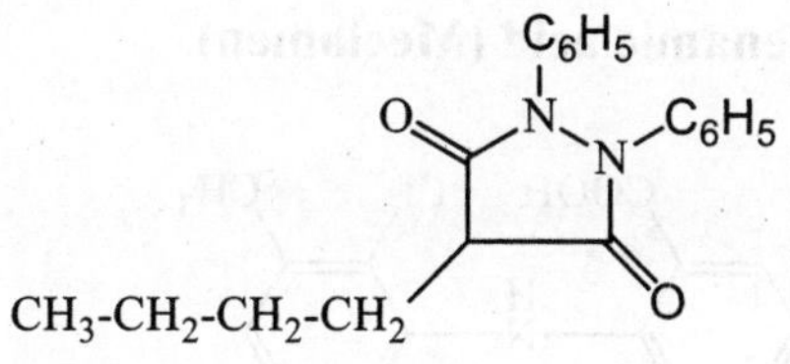

4 - Butyl - 1, 2 - diphenyl pyrazolidin - 3, 5 - dione

Use: It is used in osteoarthritis, rheumatic arthritis, spondylitis and Reiter's disease.

4.8 N- Arylanthranilic Acid Derivatives

A. Mefenamic acid (Mefegesic)

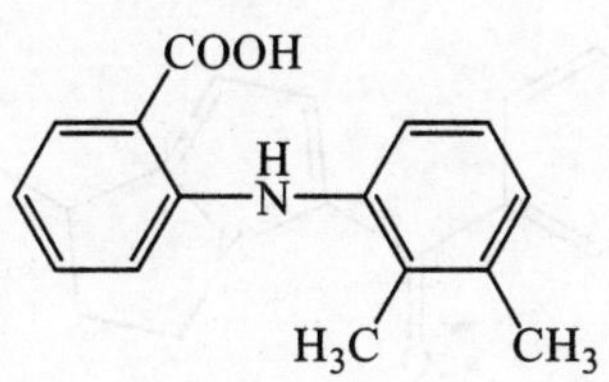

N - (2, 3 - Xylyl) anthranilic acid

Synthesis

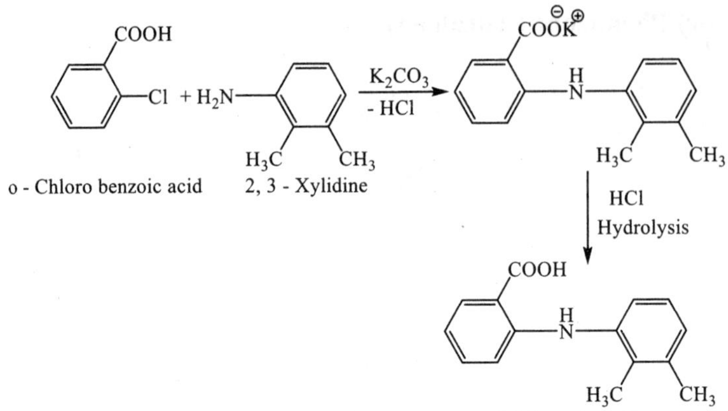

Mefenamic acid

Use: It is used as analgesic drug usually used in the treatment of dysmenorrhea and mild pain.

B. Meclofenamate (or) Meclofenamic acid (Meclomen)

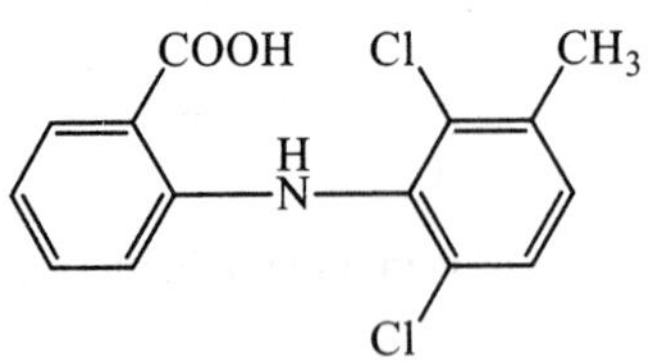

N - (2, 6 - dichloro - m - tolyl) anthranilic acid

Use: It has analgesic, anti-inflammatory and antipyretic properties. It is used in the treatment of acute and chronic rheumatic arthritis and osteoarthritis.

C. Ketorolac (Toradol)

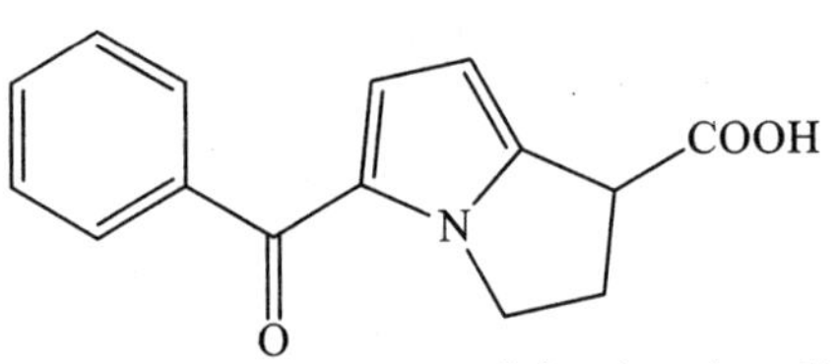

5-Benzoyl-2,3-dihydro-1*H*-pyrrolizine-1-carboxylic acid

Ketorolac is a synthetic pyrrolizine carboxylic acid derivative

Use: It is used to treat moderate to severe pain.

Index